Genetic, Epigenetic, Environmental, and Pharmacological Models for Neuroscience, Neurologic Diseases, and Psychiatric Disorders: Advancement in Bench-to-Bedside Translational Research

Genetic, Epigenetic, Environmental, and Pharmacological Models for Neuroscience, Neurologic Diseases, and Psychiatric Disorders: Advancement in Bench-to-Bedside Translational Research

Editor

Masaru Tanaka

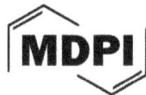

Basel • Beijing • Wuhan • Barcelona • Belgrade • Novi Sad • Cluj • Manchester

Editor
Masaru Tanaka
University of Szeged (HUN-REN-SZTE)
Szeged
Hungary

Editorial Office
MDPI
St. Alban-Anlage 66
4052 Basel, Switzerland

This is a reprint of articles from the Special Issue published online in the open access journal *Biomedicines* (ISSN 2227-9059) (available at: https://www.mdpi.com/journal/biomedicines/special_issues/psychiatric_disorders_biom).

For citation purposes, cite each article independently as indicated on the article page online and as indicated below:

Lastname, A.A.; Lastname, B.B. Article Title. *Journal Name* **Year**, *Volume Number*, Page Range.

ISBN 978-3-7258-0821-2 (Hbk)
ISBN 978-3-7258-0822-9 (PDF)
doi.org/10.3390/books978-3-7258-0822-9

© 2024 by the authors. Articles in this book are Open Access and distributed under the Creative Commons Attribution (CC BY) license. The book as a whole is distributed by MDPI under the terms and conditions of the Creative Commons Attribution-NonCommercial-NoDerivs (CC BY-NC-ND) license.

Contents

About the Editor vii

Preface ix

Masaru Tanaka and László Vécsei
From Lab to Life: Exploring Cutting-Edge Models for Neurological and Psychiatric Disorders
Reprinted from: *Biomedicines* **2024**, *12*, 613, doi:10.3390/biomedicines12030613 1

Beate Rassler, Katarzyna Blinowska, Maciej Kaminski and Gert Pfurtscheller
Analysis of Respiratory Sinus Arrhythmia and Directed Information Flow between Brain and Body Indicate Different Management Strategies of fMRI-Related Anxiety
Reprinted from: *Biomedicines* **2023**, *11*, 1028, doi:10.3390/biomedicines11041028 10

Georgios Papageorgiou, Dimitrios Kasselimis, Nikolaos Laskaris and Constantin Potagas
Unraveling the Thread of Aphasia Rehabilitation: A Translational Cognitive Perspective
Reprinted from: *Biomedicines* **2023**, *11*, 2856, doi:10.3390/biomedicines11102856 35

Katalin Borbély, Miklós Emri, István Kenessey, Márton Tóth, Júlia Singer, Péter Barsi, et al.
PET/MRI in the Presurgical Evaluation of Patients with Epilepsy: A Concordance Analysis
Reprinted from: *Biomedicines* **2022**, *10*, 949, doi:10.3390/biomedicines10050949 49

Lidio Lima de Albuquerque, Milan Pantovic, Mitchell Clingo, Katherine Fischer, Sharon Jalene, Merrill Landers, et al.
A Single Application of Cerebellar Transcranial Direct Current Stimulation Fails to Enhance Motor Skill Acquisition in Parkinson's Disease: A Pilot Study
Reprinted from: *Biomedicines* **2023**, *11*, 2219, doi:10.3390/biomedicines11082219 63

Gen Inoue, Yuhei Ohtaki, Kazue Satoh, Yuki Odanaka, Akihito Katoh, Keisuke Suzuki, et al.
Sedation Therapy in Intensive Care Units: Harnessing the Power of Antioxidants to Combat Oxidative Stress
Reprinted from: *Biomedicines* **2023**, *11*, 2129, doi:10.3390/biomedicines11082129 78

Bo Chen, Shunhui Wei, See Wee Low, Charlene Priscilla Poore, Andy Thiam-Huat Lee, Bernd Nilius and Ping Liao
TRPM4 Blocking Antibody Protects Cerebral Vasculature in Delayed Stroke Reperfusion
Reprinted from: *Biomedicines* **2023**, *11*, 1480, doi:10.3390/biomedicines11051480 93

Eleonóra Spekker, Zsuzsanna Bohár, Annamária Fejes-Szabó, Mónika Szűcs, László Vécsei and Árpád Párdutz
Estradiol Treatment Enhances Behavioral and Molecular Changes Induced by Repetitive Trigeminal Activation in a Rat Model of Migraine
Reprinted from: *Biomedicines* **2022**, *10*, 3175, doi:10.3390/biomedicines10123175 107

Ilnur I. Salafutdinov, Dilara Z. Gatina, Maria I. Markelova, Ekaterina E. Garanina, Sergey Yu. Malanin, Ilnaz M. Gazizov, et al.
A Biosafety Study of Human Umbilical Cord Blood Mononuclear Cells Transduced with Adenoviral Vector Carrying Human Vascular Endothelial Growth Factor cDNA In Vitro
Reprinted from: *Biomedicines* **2023**, *11*, 2020, doi:10.3390/biomedicines11072020 125

Anna Ikonnikova, Anastasia Anisimova, Sergey Galkin, Anastasia Gunchenko, Zhabikai Abdukhalikova, Marina Filippova, et al.
Genetic Association Study and Machine Learning to Investigate Differences in Platelet Reactivity in Patients with Acute Ischemic Stroke Treated with Aspirin
Reprinted from: *Biomedicines* **2022**, *10*, 2564, doi:10.3390/biomedicines10102564 . . . . **143**

Justyna Sobolewska-Nowak, Katarzyna Wachowska, Artur Nowak, Agata Orzechowska, Agata Szulc, Olga Płaza and Piotr Gałecki
Exploring the Heart–Mind Connection: Unraveling the Shared Pathways between Depression and Cardiovascular Diseases
Reprinted from: *Biomedicines* **2023**, *11*, 1903, doi:10.3390/biomedicines11071903 . . . . **159**

Felice Festa, Silvia Medori and Monica Macrì
Move Your Body, Boost Your Brain: The Positive Impact of Physical Activity on Cognition across All Age Groups
Reprinted from: *Biomedicines* **2023**, *11*, 1765, doi:10.3390/biomedicines11061765 . . . . **190**

Andrea De Micheli, Umberto Provenzani, Kamil Krakowski, Dominic Oliver, Stefano Damiani, Natascia Brondino, et al.
Physical Health and Transition to Psychosis in People at Clinical High Risk
Reprinted from: *Biomedicines* **2024**, *12*, 523, doi:10.3390/biomedicines12030523 . . . . **217**

About the Editor

Masaru Tanaka

Masaru Tanaka, M.D., Ph.D. is a Senior Research Fellow in the Danube Neuroscience Research Laboratory, HUN-REN-SZTE Neuroscience Research Group, Hungarian Research Network, University of Szeged (HUN-REN-SZTE). His scientific interest includes depression anxiety, dementia pain, their comorbid nature, and translational research in neurological diseases and psychiatric disorders. His current research focuses on the antidepressant, anxiolytic, and nootropic effects of neuropeptide, neurohormones and tryptophan metabolites, and their analogues in preclinical of neuropsychiatric diseases. He is an editorial board member of Frontiers in Neuroscience, Frontiers in Psychiatry, Anesthesia Research, the Journal of Integrative Neuroscience, Advances in Clinical Experimental Medicine, Biology and Life Sciences, and Biomedicines, among others. He obtained a PhD in Medicine and an MD in general Medicine from the University of Szeged, and a bachelors' degree in Biophysics from the university of Illinois, Urbana-Champaign.

Preface

Neuroscience, neurology, and psychiatry are all dynamic fields that seek to understand the complex mechanisms that govern brain function and dysfunction. They also intend to develop effective treatments for a wide range of neurological and psychiatric disorders. Recent advances in molecular biology, genetics, epigenetics, pharmacology, and neuroimaging have shed new light on the causes, pathophysiology, diagnosis, and treatment of these disorders. However, translating these basic research findings into clinical applications and improving patients' quality of life is still a challenge.

Neuroplasticity, the brain's extraordinary ability to reorganize and adapt throughout life, is a major focus of these disciplines. Neuroplasticity encompasses a variety of mechanisms such as synaptic plasticity, neurogenesis, and changes in neuronal connectivity that are required for learning, memory, and recovery from injury or disease. In addition to understanding neuroplasticity, non-invasive brain stimulation techniques such as transcranial magnetic stimulation and transcranial direct current stimulation have emerged as potential therapeutic tools. These techniques can modulate neuroplasticity by inducing changes in cortical excitability and connectivity, potentially providing relief for symptoms associated with depression, schizophrenia, and chronic pain.

This Special Issue invited original research articles and reviews on genetic, epigenetic, environmental, and pharmacological models of neuroscience, neurologic diseases, and psychiatric disorders. The goal was to highlight the latest developments and innovations in bench-to-bedside translational research, as well as the opportunities and limitations of various models and methods. The Special Issue received 12 high-quality submissions from authors worldwide, covering a wide range of topics and disorders. The articles presented novel findings and perspectives on the molecular and cellular mechanisms, genetic and epigenetic factors, environmental influences, pharmacological interventions, and biomarkers of these disorders. The articles also discussed the challenges and future directions of translational research in neuroscience, neurology, and psychiatry.

Masaru Tanaka
Editor

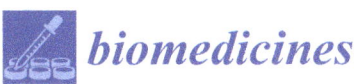

Editorial

From Lab to Life: Exploring Cutting-Edge Models for Neurological and Psychiatric Disorders

Masaru Tanaka [1,*,†] and László Vécsei [1,2,†]

1. HUN-REN-SZTE Neuroscience Research Group, Hungarian Research Network, University of Szeged (HUN-REN-SZTE), Danube Neuroscience Research Laboratory, Tisza Lajos krt. 113, H-6725 Szeged, Hungary; vecsei.laszlo@med.u-szeged.hu
2. Department of Neurology, Albert Szent-Györgyi Medical School, University of Szeged, Semmelweis u. 6, H-6725 Szeged, Hungary
* Correspondence: tanaka.masaru.1@med.u-szeged.hu; Tel.: +36-62-342-847
† These authors contributed equally to this work.

1. Introduction

Neuroscience, neurology, and psychiatry are rapidly evolving fields that aim to understand the complex mechanisms underlying brain function and dysfunction, as well as to develop effective interventions for various neurological and psychiatric disorders [1–3]. Recent advances in molecular biology, genetics, epigenetics, pharmacology, and neuroimaging have provided new insights into the etiology, pathophysiology, diagnosis, and treatment of these disorders [4–8]. However, there are still many challenges and gaps in translating basic research findings into clinical applications and improving the quality of life of patients and their families [9–11]. One pivotal area of interest within these disciplines is neuroplasticity, the brain's remarkable ability to reorganize and adapt throughout life [12–16]. Neuroplasticity encompasses various mechanisms, including synaptic plasticity, neurogenesis, and alterations in neuronal connectivity, which underpin crucial processes such as learning, memory, and recovery from injury or disease [17–20]. In tandem with understanding neuroplasticity, non-invasive brain stimulation (NIBS) techniques such as transcranial magnetic stimulation (TMS) and transcranial direct current stimulation (tDCS) have emerged as promising therapeutic modalities [21–23]. These techniques can modulate neuroplasticity by inducing changes in cortical excitability and connectivity, offering potential avenues for ameliorating symptoms associated with conditions such as depression, schizophrenia (SCZ), and chronic pain [24–26]. Research indicates that NIBS holds promise for enhancing cognitive function, alleviating mood disturbances, and reducing pain perception by targeting specific brain regions implicated in these processes [27–29]. Moreover, combining NIBS with cognitive training, psychotherapy, or pharmacotherapy may enhance treatment outcomes synergistically [30–33].

To address these challenges and gaps, this Special Issue invited original research articles and reviews focusing on genetic, epigenetic, environmental, and pharmacological models for neuroscience, neurologic diseases, and psychiatric disorders. We aimed to showcase the latest developments and innovations in bench-to-bedside translational research, as well as highlight the opportunities and limitations of various models and methods [34–36]. We also aimed to foster interdisciplinary collaboration and communication among researchers and clinicians working in different fields and domains. The Special Issue received 12 high-quality submissions from authors across the world, covering a wide range of topics and disorders, such as Alzheimer's disease, Parkinson's disease (PD), Huntington's disease, SCZ, bipolar disorder, depression, anxiety, autism, addiction, and pain. The articles presented novel findings and perspectives on the molecular and cellular mechanisms, genetic and epigenetic factors, environmental influences, pharmacological interventions, and biomarkers of these disorders, complementing previous research [37–39].

Citation: Tanaka, M.; Vécsei, L. From Lab to Life: Exploring Cutting-Edge Models for Neurological and Psychiatric Disorders. *Biomedicines* **2024**, *12*, 613. https://doi.org/10.3390/biomedicines12030613

Received: 4 March 2024
Accepted: 6 March 2024
Published: 8 March 2024

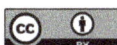

Copyright: © 2024 by the authors. Licensee MDPI, Basel, Switzerland. This article is an open access article distributed under the terms and conditions of the Creative Commons Attribution (CC BY) license (https:// creativecommons.org/licenses/by/ 4.0/).

The articles also discussed the challenges and future directions of translational research in neuroscience, neurology, and psychiatry. Below, we briefly summarize the main contributions and implications of each article.

2. Special Issue Articles

2.1. Neurostimulation and Neuroimaging Techniques for Neurological and Psychiatric Disorders

Neuroimaging techniques and brain stimulation such as functional magnetic resonance imaging (fMRI), positron emission tomography/magnetic resonance imaging (MRI) (PET/MRI), electroencephalography, and TMS are powerful tools for exploring the brain mechanisms underlying language processing and recovery in various neurological and psychiatric disorders [40–44]. These techniques can measure hemodynamic, metabolic, and electrophysiological changes in the brain regions involved in language function, as well as modulate their activity and connectivity [42,45,46]. By applying these techniques to different populations, such as patients with fMRI-related anxiety, epilepsy, or aphasia, researchers can gain insights into the factors that affect language performance and plasticity and develop novel interventions to enhance language rehabilitation [47–49].

Rassler et al. investigate how healthy subjects cope with anxiety during fMRI scans by analyzing their heart rate, respiration, and brain activity [50]. The authors found that different subjects use different strategies, such as activating a neural pacemaker or entraining brain oscillations with respiration, to modulate their anxiety level. The article also discusses the implications of these findings for understanding the neural mechanisms of anxiety and its treatment. Papageorgiou et al. reviewed the current state and challenges of aphasia rehabilitation, a field that aims to restore language functions after stroke [51]. This article discusses how translational neuroscience, which bridges basic science and clinical practice, can provide insights into the neural mechanisms of neuroplasticity and language recovery. Additionally, it suggests that domain-general cognitive processes support language, which implies that non-linguistic factors may affect aphasia treatment outcomes. The article concludes that a multidisciplinary and translational approach is needed to advance the knowledge and practice of aphasia rehabilitation.

Borbély et al. evaluated the concordance between PET/MRI and electroclinical data in the presurgical evaluation of patients with epilepsy [52]. Their study found that PET/MRI had a high concordance rate with electroclinical data, suggesting that PET/MRI could be a valuable tool in the presurgical evaluation of patients with epilepsy. The study highlights the potential of PET/MRI in improving the accuracy of presurgical evaluation and reducing the risk of complications associated with epilepsy surgery. The findings of this study could have significant implications for the management of patients with epilepsy, particularly those who are candidates for surgery. de Albuquerque et al. investigated the effect of a single application of cerebellar transcranial direct current stimulation (c-tDCS) on motor skill acquisition in PD [53]. The pilot study found that a single application of c-tDCS failed to enhance motor skill acquisition in the condition. The study highlights the need for further research to determine the optimal parameters and duration of c-tDCS to improve motor skill acquisition in the disease. The findings of this study could have significant implications for the development of new therapeutic strategies for PD.

2.2. Antioxidant and Anti-Inflammatory Therapies for Neurologic Diseases and Stroke

Neurological disorders, such as stroke, migraine, and epilepsy, are characterized by impairments in brain function and structure, which can have an impact on patients' quality of life and survival [54–57]. Finding effective therapeutic interventions to prevent or treat these disorders presents a significant challenge for biomedical research. In this regard, three articles published in this Special Issue investigate the effects of various pharmacological or hormonal treatments on brain function and structure in animal models or human patients suffering from various neurological disorders [58–60]. They use a variety of methods to assess the outcomes of the interventions, including biochemical assays, behavioral tests, and neuroimaging techniques [61–63]. Their findings shed new light on the mechanisms and potential benefits of these interventions for the prevention and treatment of neurological disorders.

Inoue et al. investigated the potential of sedation therapy in intensive care units (ICUs) to combat oxidative stress by harnessing the power of antioxidants [58]. The research aimed to determine whether common sedatives, such as propofol, thiopental, and dexmedetomidine, have direct free radical scavenging activity. The study identified the direct radical-scavenging activity of various sedatives used in clinical settings and reported a representative case of traumatic brain injury wherein thiopental administration demonstrated antioxidant effects. The findings suggest the potential for the redevelopment of sedatives containing thiopental as an antioxidant therapy, highlighting the importance of further research in this area. The study provides valuable insights into the potential dual benefits of sedatives in ICUs, serving as both sedative agents and antioxidants, which could have significant implications for the management of critically ill patients requiring sedation in ICUs.

Chen et al. used a rat model to investigate the ability of M4P, a TRPM4-blocking antibody, to protect the cerebral vasculature during delayed stroke reperfusion [59]. The study found that M4P reduced mortality rates and infarct volume, improved vascular integrity, and improved cerebral blood flow and functional recovery after delayed stroke reperfusion. These findings suggest that TRPM4-blocking antibodies have therapeutic potential in reducing vascular injury associated with delayed stroke reperfusion, opening up a promising avenue for the development of stroke therapies. Spekker et al. investigated the effect of estradiol treatment on the behavioral and molecular changes induced by repetitive trigeminal activation in a migraine rat model [60]. These changes were found to be enhanced by estradiol treatment, suggesting that estradiol may have a modulatory effect on the pathophysiology of migraine. The study sheds light on the potential role of estradiol in migraine-related mechanisms, emphasizing its significance in migraine research. These studies provide valuable insights into novel treatment approaches for neurological disorders, emphasizing the need for further research in these areas [64].

2.3. Genetic and Epigenetic Factors in Neurologic Diseases and Stroke

Stroke is a neurological condition that arises when the flow of blood to a specific area of the brain is disrupted, resulting in brain injury and the impairment of multiple functions [65–67]. Stroke is a significant contributor to mortality and impairment on a global scale, necessitating urgent biomedical research to identify effective interventions and preventive measures [68–70]. In this context, two articles explore the role of human umbilical cord blood cells, which are a rich source of stem cells and growth factors, in the context of stroke [71,72]. Salafutdinov et al. evaluated the biosafety of human umbilical cord blood mononuclear cells transduced with an adenoviral vector containing human vascular endothelial growth factor cDNA in vitro [71]. The study assessed the transduction efficacy, transgene expression, transcriptome analysis, and secretome profiling of genetically modified cells, yielding valuable insights into their safety and potential applications. The findings add to our understanding of the biosafety aspects of this cellular modification, which is important for the development of new therapeutic strategies. Ikonnikova et al. used a genetic association study and machine learning to investigate platelet reactivity differences in aspirin-treated patients with acute ischemic stroke [72]. The study sought to understand the contribution of genetic features to laboratory aspirin resistance as measured by platelet aggregation, thereby providing insights into the genetic variations that influence platelet reactivity in the context of ischemic stroke and aspirin treatment. The study's findings add to ongoing efforts to understand the genetic determinants of aspirin resistance, a major concern in ischemic stroke care. These studies offer valuable knowledge about the safety and potential uses of genetically modified cells and the genetic factors that affect platelet reactivity in the context of ischemic stroke and aspirin treatment. They emphasize the need for additional research in these fields.

2.4. Physical and Mental Health Interactions in Psychiatric Disorders

Physical health and mental health are closely intertwined and affect each other in various ways [73–75]. For example, physical illnesses can increase the risk of developing mental disorders, and vice versa [76–78]. To better understand and intervene in these complex and bidirectional relationships, a translational and multidisciplinary approach is needed that bridges the gap between basic and clinical research and incorporates different perspectives and methods from various disciplines [79–81]. In this context, the three articles published in this Special Issue of *Biomedicines* adopt such an approach and use various methods and data sources, such as epidemiological studies, randomized controlled trials, meta-analyses, systematic reviews, and clinical guidelines, to provide evidence-based and comprehensive insights into the interactions between physical health and mental health in different populations and contexts [82–84]. Their results have important implications for the prevention and treatment of various neurological and psychiatric disorders.

Sobolewska-Nowak et al. investigated the relationship between depression and cardiovascular disease, focusing on common risk factors such as obesity, diabetes, and physical inactivity. The study emphasizes the importance of interdisciplinary collaboration and the incorporation of depression screening into the treatment of cardiac conditions, highlighting the bidirectional relationship between these health issues and the need to address mental health in cardiovascular care [82]. The study by Festa et al. highlights the positive impact of physical activity on cognition across all age groups, emphasizing the benefits of exercise on attention, memory, and executive functions. The study emphasizes the importance of better understanding the mechanisms underlying these effects, as well as the development of appropriate intervention programs based on age and comorbidity, in order to maximize the cognitive benefits of physical activity [83].

The study by De Micheli et al. investigated the relationship between physical health and the transition to psychosis in people at clinically high risk [84]. The research highlights the importance of monitoring physical health outcomes in individuals at clinically high risk for psychosis, emphasizing the need for public health strategies to promote physical health in this population. The study underscores the bidirectional relationship between physical and mental health, highlighting the need for integrated care to improve outcomes in individuals at clinically high risk for psychosis. These studies advocate for integrated care and the promotion of healthy behaviors to improve overall health outcomes, recognizing the interconnectedness of physical and mental health.

3. Conclusions

Neurological and psychiatric disorders are among the most prevalent and debilitating conditions that affect millions of people worldwide [85–87]. Despite the advances in neuroscience and neurology, the etiology and pathogenesis of these disorders remain largely unknown, and contemporary treatments are often inadequate or associated with adverse effects [88–91]. Therefore, there is an urgent need to develop new and effective strategies to prevent, diagnose, and treat these disorders [92–94]. To achieve this goal, it is essential to establish reliable and relevant models that can recapitulate the complex interactions between the genetic, epigenetic, environmental, and pharmacological factors that contribute to the onset and progression of these disorders [95–97]. Moreover, it is important to identify novel targets and mechanisms that can modulate the molecular and functional changes that occur in the brain and peripheral tissues of patients with these disorders [98–102].

This Special Issue on Genetic, Epigenetic, Environmental, and Pharmacological Models for Neuroscience, Neurologic Diseases, and Psychiatric Disorders: Advancement in Bench-to-Bedside Translational Research has presented a collection of 12 articles that cover a wide range of topics and methods in the field of neuroscience and neurology. The articles have demonstrated the importance and challenges of developing and validating animal and cellular models that can mimic the complex pathophysiology and phenotypes of human neurological and psychiatric disorders. The articles have also highlighted the potential of novel pharmacological and non-pharmacological interventions that can modulate the molecular and functional alterations underlying these disorders. The Special Issue has provided valuable insights and perspectives for advancing translational research from basic science to clinical applications. We hope that this Special Issue will stimulate further research and collaboration among researchers and clinicians who share the common goal of improving the diagnosis, prevention, and treatment of neurological and psychiatric disorders. We also hope that this Special Issue will inspire new ideas and innovations that can bridge the gap between bench and bedside and ultimately benefit patients and society. We thank all the authors and reviewers for their contributions to this Special Issue, and we invite the readers to explore the diverse and exciting topics that are presented in this collection.

Author Contributions: Conceptualization, M.T.; writing—original draft preparation, M.T.; writing—review and editing, M.T. and L.V. visualization, M.T.; supervision, M.T. and L.V.; project administration, M.T.; funding acquisition, M.T. and L.V. All authors have read and agreed to the published version of the manuscript.

Funding: This work was supported by the National Research, Development, and Innovation Office—NKFIH K138125, SZTE SZAOK-KKA No: 2022/5S729, and the HUN-REN Hungarian Research Network.

Institutional Review Board Statement: Not applicable.

Informed Consent Statement: Not applicable.

Data Availability Statement: Data sharing is not applicable to this article.

Conflicts of Interest: The authors declare no conflicts of interest.

Abbreviations

c-tDCS	Cerebellar transcranial direct current stimulation.
fMRI	Functional magnetic resonance imaging.
ICUs	Intensive care units.
MRI	Magnetic resonance imaging.
PD	Parkinson's disease.
PET	Positron emission tomography.
SCZ	Schizophrenia.
tDCS	Transcranial direct current stimulation.
TMS	Transcranial magnetic stimulation.

References

1. Bassett, D.S.; Sporns, O. Network neuroscience. *Nat. Neurosci.* **2017**, *20*, 353–364. [CrossRef]
2. Huys, Q.J.; Maia, T.V.; Frank, M.J. Computational psychiatry as a bridge from neuroscience to clinical applications. *Nat. Neurosci.* **2016**, *19*, 404–413. [CrossRef]
3. Insel, T.R.; Quirion, R. Psychiatry as a clinical neuroscience discipline. *JAMA* **2005**, *294*, 2221–2224. [CrossRef]
4. Sullivan, P.F.; Posthuma, D. Biological pathways and networks implicated in psychiatric disorders. *Curr. Opin. Behav. Sci.* **2015**, *2*, 58–68. [CrossRef]
5. Geschwind, D.H.; Flint, J. Genetics and genomics of psychiatric disease. *Science* **2015**, *349*, 1489–1494. [CrossRef]
6. Grezenko, H.; Ekhator, C.; Nwabugwu, N.U.; Ganga, H.; Affaf, M.; Abdelaziz, A.M.; Rehman, A.; Shehryar, A.; Abbasi, F.A.; Bellegarde, S.B. Epigenetics in neurological and psychiatric disorders: A comprehensive review of current understanding and future perspectives. *Cureus* **2023**, *15*, e43960. [CrossRef]
7. Nathan, P.J.; Phan, K.L.; Harmer, C.J.; Mehta, M.A.; Bullmore, E.T. Increasing pharmacological knowledge about human neurological and psychiatric disorders through functional neuroimaging and its application in drug discovery. *Curr. Opin. Pharmacol.* **2014**, *14*, 54–61. [CrossRef]
8. Iorio-Morin, C.; Sarica, C.; Elias, G.J.; Harmsen, I.; Hodaie, M. Neuroimaging of psychiatric disorders. *Prog. Brain Res.* **2022**, *270*, 149–169.
9. Insel, T.R. Translating scientific opportunity into public health impact: A strategic plan for research on mental illness. *Arch. Gen. Psychiatry* **2009**, *66*, 128–133. [CrossRef]
10. Schumann, G.; Binder, E.B.; Holte, A.; de Kloet, E.R.; Oedegaard, K.J.; Robbins, T.W.; Walker-Tilley, T.R.; Bitter, I.; Brown, V.J.; Buitelaar, J. Stratified medicine for mental disorders. *Eur. Neuropsychopharmacol.* **2014**, *24*, 5–50. [CrossRef]

11. Di Luca, M.; Destrebecq, F.; Kramer, S. Future of the aging brain: Bridging the gap between research and policy. *Aging Brain* **2021**, *1*, 100002. [CrossRef]
12. Tanaka, M.; Schmidt, A.; Hassel, S. Case Reports in Neuroimaging and Stimulation. *Front. Psychiatry* **2023**, *14*, 1264669.
13. Tanaka, M.; Diano, M.; Battaglia, S. Insights into structural and functional organization of the brain: Evidence from neuroimaging and non-invasive brain stimulation techniques. *Front. Psychiatry* **2023**, *14*, 1225755. [CrossRef]
14. Tortora, F.; Hadipour, A.L.; Battaglia, S.; Falzone, A.; Avenanti, A.; Vicario, C.M. The role of Serotonin in fear learning and memory: A systematic review of human studies. *Brain Sci.* **2023**, *13*, 1197. [CrossRef] [PubMed]
15. Gandhi, A.B.; Kaleem, I.; Alexander, J.; Hisbulla, M.; Kannichamy, V.; Antony, I.; Mishra, V.; Banerjee, A.; Khan, S. Neuroplasticity Improves Bipolar Disorder: A Review. *Cureus* **2020**, *12*, e11241. [CrossRef]
16. Rădulescu, I.; Drăgoi, A.M.; Trifu, S.C.; Cristea, M.B. Neuroplasticity and depression: Rewiring the brain's networks through pharmacological therapy (Review). *Exp. Ther. Med.* **2021**, *22*, 1131. [CrossRef]
17. Battaglia, S.; Nazzi, C.; Thayer, J.F. Genetic differences associated with dopamine and serotonin release mediate fear-induced bradycardia in the human brain. *Transl. Psychiatry* **2024**, *14*, 24. [CrossRef]
18. Battaglia, S.; Nazzi, C.; Thayer, J. Heart's tale of trauma: Fear-conditioned heart rate changes in post-traumatic stress disorder. *Acta Psychiatr. Scand.* **2023**. [CrossRef]
19. Battaglia, S.; Nazzi, C.; Thayer, J. Fear-induced bradycardia in mental disorders: Foundations, current advances, future perspectives. *Neurosci. Biobehav. Rev.* **2023**, *149*, 105163. [CrossRef]
20. Jászberényi, M.; Thurzó, B.; Bagosi, Z.; Vécsei, L.; Tanaka, M. The Orexin/Hypocretin System, the Peptidergic Regulator of Vigilance, Orchestrates Adaptation to Stress. *Biomedicines* **2024**, *12*, 448. [CrossRef]
21. Terranova, C.; Rizzo, V.; Cacciola, A.; Chillemi, G.; Calamuneri, A.; Milardi, D.; Quartarone, A. Is there a future for non-invasive brain stimulation as a therapeutic tool? *Front. Neurol.* **2019**, *9*, 1146. [CrossRef]
22. Bandeira, I.D.; Lins-Silva, D.H.; Barouh, J.L.; Faria-Guimarães, D.; Dorea-Bandeira, I.; Souza, L.S.; Alves, G.S.; Brunoni, A.R.; Nitsche, M.; Fregni, F. Neuroplasticity and non-invasive brain stimulation in the developing brain. *Prog. Brain Res.* **2021**, *264*, 57–89.
23. Hanoglu, L.; Velioglu, H.A.; Hanoglu, T.; Yulug, B. Neuroimaging-guided transcranial magnetic and direct current stimulation in MCI: Toward an individual, effective and disease-modifying treatment. *Clin. EEG Neurosci.* **2023**, *54*, 82–90. [CrossRef]
24. Battaglia, S.; Di Fazio, C.; Mazzà, M.; Tamietto, M.; Avenanti, A. Targeting Human Glucocorticoid Receptors in Fear Learning: A Multiscale Integrated Approach to Study Functional Connectivity. *Int. J. Mol. Sci.* **2024**, *25*, 864. [CrossRef]
25. Battaglia, M.R.; Di Fazio, C.; Battaglia, S. Activated tryptophan-kynurenine metabolic system in the human brain is associated with learned fear. *Front. Mol. Neurosci.* **2023**, *16*, 1217090. [CrossRef]
26. Battaglia, S.; Di Fazio, C.; Vicario, C.M.; Avenanti, A. Neuropharmacological modulation of N-methyl-D-aspartate, noradrenaline and endocannabinoid receptors in fear extinction learning: Synaptic transmission and plasticity. *Int. J. Mol. Sci.* **2023**, *24*, 5926. [CrossRef]
27. Xu, Y.; Qiu, Z.; Zhu, J.; Liu, J.; Wu, J.; Tao, J.; Chen, L. The modulation effect of non-invasive brain stimulation on cognitive function in patients with mild cognitive impairment: A systematic review and meta-analysis of randomized controlled trials. *BMC Neurosci.* **2019**, *20*, 2. [CrossRef] [PubMed]
28. Brunoni, A.R.; Palm, U. Transcranial direct current stimulation in psychiatry: Mood disorders, schizophrenia and other psychiatric diseases. In *Practical Guide to Transcranial Direct Current Stimulation: Principles, Procedures and Applications*; Springer: Cham, Switzerland, 2019; pp. 431–471.
29. Kong, Q.; Li, T.; Reddy, S.; Hodges, S.; Kong, J. Brain stimulation targets for chronic pain: Insights from meta-analysis, functional connectivity and literature review. *Neurotherapeutics* **2023**, *21*, e00297. [CrossRef] [PubMed]
30. Gregorio, F.; Battaglia, S. Advances in EEG-based functional connectivity approaches to the study of the central nervous system in health and disease. *Adv. Clin. Exp. Med.* **2023**, *32*, 607–612. [CrossRef]
31. Di Gregorio, F.; Steinhauser, M.; Maier, M.E.; Thayer, J.F.; Battaglia, S. Error-related cardiac deceleration: Functional interplay between error-related brain activity and autonomic nervous system in performance monitoring. *Neurosci. Biobehav. Rev.* **2024**, *157*, 105542. [CrossRef]
32. Ippolito, G.; Bertaccini, R.; Tarasi, L.; Di Gregorio, F.; Trajkovic, J.; Battaglia, S.; Romei, V. The role of alpha oscillations among the main neuropsychiatric disorders in the adult and developing human brain: Evidence from the last 10 years of research. *Biomedicines* **2022**, *10*, 3189. [CrossRef] [PubMed]
33. Balogh, L.; Tanaka, M.; Török, N.; Vécsei, L.; Taguchi, S. Crosstalk between existential phenomenological psychotherapy and neurological sciences in mood and anxiety disorders. *Biomedicines* **2021**, *9*, 340. [CrossRef] [PubMed]
34. Tanaka, M.; Szabó, Á.; Vécsei, L.; Giménez-Llort, L. Emerging translational research in neurological and psychiatric diseases: From in vitro to in vivo models. *Int. J. Mol. Sci.* **2023**, *24*, 15739. [CrossRef] [PubMed]
35. Tanaka, M.; Vécsei, L. Editorial of Special Issue "Crosstalk between Depression, Anxiety, and Dementia: Comorbidity in Behavioral Neurology and Neuropsychiatry". *Biomedicines* **2021**, *9*, 517. [CrossRef]
36. Tanaka, M.; Szabó, Á.; Vécsei, L. Integrating Armchair, Bench, and Bedside Research for Behavioral Neurology and Neuropsychiatry: Editorial. *Biomedicines* **2022**, *10*, 2999. [CrossRef]
37. Tanaka, M.; Vécsei, L. Monitoring the redox status in multiple sclerosis. *Biomedicines* **2020**, *8*, 406. [CrossRef]

38. Tanaka, M.; Bohár, Z.; Vécsei, L. Are kynurenines accomplices or principal villains in dementia? Maintenance of kynurenine metabolism. *Molecules* **2020**, *25*, 564. [CrossRef]
39. de Oliveira Zanuso, B.; Dos Santos, A.R.d.O.; Miola, V.F.B.; Campos, L.M.G.; Spilla, C.S.G.; Barbalho, S.M. Panax ginseng and aging related disorders: A systematic review. *Exp. Gerontol.* **2022**, *161*, 111731. [CrossRef] [PubMed]
40. Shah, N.J.; Oros-Peusquens, A.-M.; Arrubla, J.; Zhang, K.; Warbrick, T.; Mauler, J.; Vahedipour, K.; Romanzetti, S.; Felder, J.; Celik, A. Advances in multimodal neuroimaging: Hybrid MR–PET and MR–PET–EEG at 3 T and 9.4 T. *J. Magn. Reson.* **2013**, *229*, 101–115. [CrossRef] [PubMed]
41. Yen, C.; Lin, C.L.; Chiang, M.C. Exploring the Frontiers of Neuroimaging: A Review of Recent Advances in Understanding Brain Functioning and Disorders. *Life* **2023**, *13*, 1472. [CrossRef]
42. Jiang, S.; Carpenter, L.L.; Jiang, H. Optical neuroimaging: Advancing transcranial magnetic stimulation treatments of psychiatric disorders. *Vis. Comput. Ind. Biomed. Art* **2022**, *5*, 22. [CrossRef] [PubMed]
43. Liloia, D.; Crocetta, A.; Cauda, F.; Duca, S.; Costa, T.; Manuello, J. Seeking Overlapping Neuroanatomical Alterations between Dyslexia and Attention-Deficit/Hyperactivity Disorder: A Meta-Analytic Replication Study. *Brain Sci.* **2022**, *12*, 1367. [CrossRef] [PubMed]
44. Liloia, D.; Manuello, J.; Costa, T.; Keller, R.; Nani, A.; Cauda, F. Atypical local brain connectivity in pediatric autism spectrum disorder? A coordinate-based meta-analysis of regional homogeneity studies. *Eur. Arch. Psychiatry Clin. Neurosci.* **2024**, *274*, 3–18. [CrossRef] [PubMed]
45. Shibasaki, H. Human brain mapping: Hemodynamic response and electrophysiology. *Clin. Neurophysiol.* **2008**, *119*, 731–743. [CrossRef] [PubMed]
46. Hallett, M.; Di Iorio, R.; Rossini, P.M.; Park, J.E.; Chen, R.; Celnik, P.; Strafella, A.P.; Matsumoto, H.; Ugawa, Y. Contribution of transcranial magnetic stimulation to assessment of brain connectivity and networks. *Clin. Neurophysiol.* **2017**, *128*, 2125–2139. [CrossRef] [PubMed]
47. Gaston, T.E.; Nair, S.; Allendorfer, J.B.; Martin, R.C.; Beattie, J.F.; Szaflarski, J.P. Memory response and neuroimaging correlates of a novel cognitive rehabilitation program for memory problems in epilepsy: A pilot study. *Restor. Neurol. Neurosci.* **2019**, *37*, 457–468. [CrossRef]
48. Reid, L.B.; Boyd, R.N.; Cunnington, R.; Rose, S.E. Interpreting intervention induced neuroplasticity with fMRI: The case for multimodal imaging strategies. *Neural Plast.* **2016**, *2016*, 2643491. [CrossRef]
49. Elkana, O.; Frost, R.; Kramer, U.; Ben-Bashat, D.; Schweiger, A. Cerebral language reorganization in the chronic stage of recovery: A longitudinal fMRI study. *Cortex* **2013**, *49*, 71–81. [CrossRef]
50. Rassler, B.; Blinowska, K.; Kaminski, M.; Pfurtscheller, G. Analysis of Respiratory Sinus Arrhythmia and Directed Information Flow between Brain and Body Indicate Different Management Strategies of fMRI-Related Anxiety. *Biomedicines* **2023**, *11*, 1028. [CrossRef]
51. Papageorgiou, G.; Kasselimis, D.; Laskaris, N.; Potagas, C. Unraveling the Thread of Aphasia Rehabilitation: A Translational Cognitive Perspective. *Biomedicines* **2023**, *11*, 2856. [CrossRef]
52. Borbély, K.; Emri, M.; Kenessey, I.; Tóth, M.; Singer, J.; Barsi, P.; Vajda, Z.; Pál, E.; Tóth, Z.; Beyer, T. Pet/Mri in the presurgical evaluation of patients with epilepsy: A concordance analysis. *Biomedicines* **2022**, *10*, 949. [CrossRef]
53. de Albuquerque, L.L.; Pantovic, M.; Clingo, M.; Fischer, K.; Jalene, S.; Landers, M.; Mari, Z.; Poston, B. A Single Application of Cerebellar Transcranial Direct Current Stimulation Fails to Enhance Motor Skill Acquisition in Parkinson's Disease: A Pilot Study. *Biomedicines* **2023**, *11*, 2219. [CrossRef]
54. Ribeiro de Souza, F.; Sales, M.; Rabelo Laporte, L.; Melo, A.; Manoel da Silva Ribeiro, N. Body structure/function impairments and activity limitations of post-stroke that predict social participation: A systematic review. *Top. Stroke Rehabil.* **2023**, *30*, 589–602. [CrossRef]
55. Hubbard, C.S.; Khan, S.A.; Keaser, M.L.; Mathur, V.A.; Goyal, M.; Seminowicz, D.A. Altered brain structure and function correlate with disease severity and pain catastrophizing in migraine patients. *eneuro* **2014**, *1*, e20.14. [CrossRef]
56. Guekht, A.B.; Mitrokhina, T.V.; Lebedeva, A.V.; Dzugaeva, F.K.; Milchakova, L.E.; Lokshina, O.B.; Feygina, A.A.; Gusev, E.I. Factors influencing on quality of life in people with epilepsy. *Seizure* **2007**, *16*, 128–133. [CrossRef]
57. Nemeth, V.L.; Must, A.; Horvath, S.; Király, A.; Kincses, Z.T.; Vécsei, L. Gender-specific degeneration of dementia-related subcortical structures throughout the lifespan. *J. Alzheimer's Dis.* **2017**, *55*, 865–880. [CrossRef]
58. Inoue, G.; Ohtaki, Y.; Satoh, K.; Odanaka, Y.; Katoh, A.; Suzuki, Y.; Tomita, Y.; Eiraku, M.; Kikuchi, K.; Harano, K. Sedation Therapy in Intensive Care Units: Harnessing the Power of Antioxidants to Combat Oxidative Stress. *Biomedicines* **2023**, *11*, 2129. [CrossRef] [PubMed]
59. Chen, B.; Wei, S.; Low, S.W.; Poore, C.P.; Lee, A.T.-H.; Nilius, B.; Liao, P. TRPM4 Blocking Antibody Protects Cerebral Vasculature in Delayed Stroke Reperfusion. *Biomedicines* **2023**, *11*, 1480. [CrossRef] [PubMed]
60. Spekker, E.; Bohár, Z.; Fejes-Szabó, A.; Szűcs, M.; Vécsei, L.; Párdutz, Á. Estradiol Treatment Enhances Behavioral and Molecular Changes Induced by Repetitive Trigeminal Activation in a Rat Model of Migraine. *Biomedicines* **2022**, *10*, 3175. [CrossRef] [PubMed]
61. Cauda, F.; Nani, A.; Liloia, D.; Manuello, J.; Premi, E.; Duca, S.; Fox, P.T.; Costa, T. Finding specificity in structural brain alterations through Bayesian reverse inference. *Hum. Brain Mapp.* **2020**, *41*, 4155–4172. [CrossRef] [PubMed]

62. Manuello, J.; Costa, T.; Cauda, F.; Liloia, D. Six actions to improve detection of critical features for neuroimaging coordinate-based meta-analysis preparation. *Neurosci. Biobehav. Rev.* **2022**, *137*, 104659. [CrossRef] [PubMed]
63. Nani, A.; Manuello, J.; Mancuso, L.; Liloia, D.; Costa, T.; Vercelli, A.; Duca, S.; Cauda, F. The pathoconnectivity network analysis of the insular cortex: A morphometric fingerprinting. *NeuroImage* **2021**, *225*, 117481. [CrossRef] [PubMed]
64. Tajti, J.; Szok, D.; Csáti, A.; Szabó, Á.; Tanaka, M.; Vécsei, L. Exploring novel therapeutic targets in the common pathogenic factors in migraine and neuropathic pain. *Int. J. Mol. Sci.* **2023**, *24*, 4114. [CrossRef]
65. Jiang, X.; Andjelkovic, A.V.; Zhu, L.; Yang, T.; Bennett, M.V.; Chen, J.; Keep, R.F.; Shi, Y. Blood-brain barrier dysfunction and recovery after ischemic stroke. *Prog. Neurobiol.* **2018**, *163*, 144–171. [CrossRef] [PubMed]
66. Marshall, R.S. The functional relevance of cerebral hemodynamics: Why blood flow matters to the injured and recovering brain. *Curr. Opin. Neurol.* **2004**, *17*, 705–709. [CrossRef]
67. Lyu, J.; Xie, D.; Bhatia, T.N.; Leak, R.K.; Hu, X.; Jiang, X. Microglial/Macrophage polarization and function in brain injury and repair after stroke. *CNS Neurosci. Ther.* **2021**, *27*, 515–527. [CrossRef]
68. Thrift, A.G.; Thayabaranathan, T.; Howard, G.; Howard, V.J.; Rothwell, P.M.; Feigin, V.L.; Norrving, B.; Donnan, G.A.; Cadilhac, D.A. Global stroke statistics. *Int. J. Stroke* **2017**, *12*, 13–32. [CrossRef]
69. Lekoubou, A.; Nguyen, C.; Kwon, M.; Nyalundja, A.D.; Agrawal, A. Post-stroke Everything. *Curr. Neurol. Neurosci. Rep.* **2023**, *23*, 785–800. [CrossRef]
70. Mead, G.E.; Sposato, L.A.; Sampaio Silva, G.; Yperzeele, L.; Wu, S.; Kutlubaev, M.; Cheyne, J.; Wahab, K.; Urrutia, V.C.; Sharma, V.K. A systematic review and synthesis of global stroke guidelines on behalf of the World Stroke Organization. *Int. J. Stroke* **2023**, *18*, 499–531. [CrossRef]
71. Salafutdinov, I.I.; Gatina, D.Z.; Markelova, M.I.; Garanina, E.E.; Malanin, S.Y.; Gazizov, I.M.; Izmailov, A.A.; Rizvanov, A.A.; Islamov, R.R.; Palotás, A. A Biosafety Study of Human Umbilical Cord Blood Mononuclear Cells Transduced with Adenoviral Vector Carrying Human Vascular Endothelial Growth Factor cDNA In Vitro. *Biomedicines* **2023**, *11*, 2020. [CrossRef]
72. Ikonnikova, A.; Anisimova, A.; Galkin, S.; Gunchenko, A.; Abdukhalikova, Z.; Filippova, M.; Surzhikov, S.; Selyaeva, L.; Shershov, V.; Zasedatelev, A. Genetic Association Study and Machine Learning to Investigate Differences in Platelet Reactivity in Patients with Acute Ischemic Stroke Treated with Aspirin. *Biomedicines* **2022**, *10*, 2564. [CrossRef]
73. Koban, L.; Gianaros, P.J.; Kober, H.; Wager, T.D. The self in context: Brain systems linking mental and physical health. *Nat. Rev. Neurosci.* **2021**, *22*, 309–322. [CrossRef] [PubMed]
74. Morrey, L.B.; Roberts, W.O.; Wichser, L. Exercise-related mental health problems and solutions during the COVID-19 pandemic. *Curr. Sports Med. Rep.* **2020**, *19*, 194. [CrossRef] [PubMed]
75. Kivimäki, M.; Batty, G.D.; Pentti, J.; Shipley, M.J.; Sipilä, P.N.; Nyberg, S.T.; Suominen, S.B.; Oksanen, T.; Stenholm, S.; Virtanen, M. Association between socioeconomic status and the development of mental and physical health conditions in adulthood: A multi-cohort study. *Lancet Public Health* **2020**, *5*, e140–e149. [CrossRef] [PubMed]
76. Momen, N.C.; Plana-Ripoll, O.; Agerbo, E.; Benros, M.E.; Børglum, A.D.; Christensen, M.K.; Dalsgaard, S.; Degenhardt, L.; de Jonge, P.; Debost, J.-C.P. Association between mental disorders and subsequent medical conditions. *N. Engl. J. Med.* **2020**, *382*, 1721–1731. [CrossRef] [PubMed]
77. Nielsen, R.E.; Banner, J.; Jensen, S.E. Cardiovascular disease in patients with severe mental illness. *Nat. Rev. Cardiol.* **2021**, *18*, 136–145. [CrossRef] [PubMed]
78. De Hert, M.; Correll, C.U.; Bobes, J.; Cetkovich-Bakmas, M.; Cohen, D.; Asai, I.; Detraux, J.; Gautam, S.; Möller, H.-J.; Ndetei, D.M. Physical illness in patients with severe mental disorders. I. Prevalence, impact of medications and disparities in health care. *World Psychiatry* **2011**, *10*, 52. [CrossRef] [PubMed]
79. Edmondson, D.; Conroy, D.; Romero-Canyas, R.; Tanenbaum, M.; Czajkowski, S. Climate change, behavior change and health: A multidisciplinary, translational and multilevel perspective. *Transl. Behav. Med.* **2022**, *12*, 503–515. [CrossRef] [PubMed]
80. Erdemir, A.; Mulugeta, L.; Ku, J.P.; Drach, A.; Horner, M.; Morrison, T.M.; Peng, G.C.; Vadigepalli, R.; Lytton, W.W.; Myers, J.G., Jr. Credible practice of modeling and simulation in healthcare: Ten rules from a multidisciplinary perspective. *J. Transl. Med.* **2020**, *18*, 369. [CrossRef]
81. Craske, M.G.; Herzallah, M.M.; Nusslock, R.; Patel, V. From neural circuits to communities: An integrative multidisciplinary roadmap for global mental health. *Nat. Ment. Health* **2023**, *1*, 12–24. [CrossRef]
82. Sobolewska-Nowak, J.; Wachowska, K.; Nowak, A.; Orzechowska, A.; Szulc, A.; Płaza, O.; Gałecki, P. Exploring the heart–mind connection: Unraveling the shared pathways between depression and cardiovascular diseases. *Biomedicines* **2023**, *11*, 1903. [CrossRef]
83. Festa, F.; Medori, S.; Macrì, M. Move Your Body, Boost Your Brain: The Positive Impact of Physical Activity on Cognition across All Age Groups. *Biomedicines* **2023**, *11*, 1765. [CrossRef]
84. De Micheli, A.; Provenzani, U.; Krakowski, K.; Oliver, D.; Damiani, S.; Brondino, N.; McGuire, P.; Fusar-Poli, P. Physical Health and Transition to Psychosis in People at Clinical High Risk. *Biomedicines* **2024**, *2024*, 523. [CrossRef]
85. Feigin, V.L.; Vos, T.; Nichols, E.; Owolabi, M.O.; Carroll, W.M.; Dichgans, M.; Deuschl, G.; Parmar, P.; Brainin, M.; Murray, C. The global burden of neurological disorders: Translating evidence into policy. *Lancet Neurol.* **2020**, *19*, 255–265. [CrossRef]
86. Hyman, S.E. Psychiatric Disorders: Grounded in Human Biology but Not Natural Kinds. *Perspect. Biol. Med.* **2021**, *64*, 6–28. [CrossRef]

87. Vigo, D.; Thornicroft, G.; Atun, R. Estimating the true global burden of mental illness. *Lancet Psychiatry* **2016**, *3*, 171–178. [CrossRef] [PubMed]
88. Sheppard, O.; Coleman, M. Alzheimer's Disease: Etiology, Neuropathology and Pathogenesis. In *Alzheimer's Disease: Drug Discovery*; Huang, X., Ed.; Exon Publications Copyright: Brisbane, AU, USA, 2020.
89. Blokhin, I.O.; Khorkova, O.; Saveanu, R.V.; Wahlestedt, C. Molecular mechanisms of psychiatric diseases. *Neurobiol. Dis.* **2020**, *146*, 105136. [CrossRef]
90. Akhtar, A.; Andleeb, A.; Waris, T.S.; Bazzar, M.; Moradi, A.R.; Awan, N.R.; Yar, M. Neurodegenerative diseases and effective drug delivery: A review of challenges and novel therapeutics. *J. Control. Release* **2021**, *330*, 1152–1167. [CrossRef]
91. Semahegn, A.; Torpey, K.; Manu, A.; Assefa, N.; Tesfaye, G.; Ankomah, A. Psychotropic medication non-adherence and its associated factors among patients with major psychiatric disorders: A systematic review and meta-analysis. *Syst. Rev.* **2020**, *9*, 17. [CrossRef]
92. Tanaka, M.; Chen, C. Towards a mechanistic understanding of depression, anxiety, and their comorbidity: Perspectives from cognitive neuroscience. *Front. Behav. Neurosci.* **2023**, *17*, 1268156. [CrossRef]
93. Matias, J.N.; Achete, G.; Campanari, G.S.d.S.; Guiguer, E.L.; Araújo, A.C.; Buglio, D.S.; Barbalho, S.M. A systematic review of the antidepressant effects of curcumin: Beyond monoamines theory. *Aust. N. Z. J. Psychiatry* **2021**, *55*, 451–462. [CrossRef]
94. Buglio, D.S.; Marton, L.T.; Laurindo, L.F.; Guiguer, E.L.; Araújo, A.C.; Buchaim, R.L.; Goulart, R.d.A.; Rubira, C.J.; Barbalho, S.M. The role of resveratrol in mild cognitive impairment and Alzheimer's disease: A systematic review. *J. Med. Food* **2022**, *25*, 797–806. [CrossRef]
95. Polyák, H.; Galla, Z.; Nánási, N.; Cseh, E.K.; Rajda, C.; Veres, G.; Spekker, E.; Szabó, Á.; Klivényi, P.; Tanaka, M. The tryptophan-kynurenine metabolic system is suppressed in cuprizone-induced model of demyelination simulating progressive multiple sclerosis. *Biomedicines* **2023**, *11*, 945. [CrossRef]
96. Barbalho, S.M.; Bueno Ottoboni, A.M.M.; Fiorini, A.M.R.; Guiguer, E.L.; Nicolau, C.C.T.; Goulart, R.d.A.; Flato, U.A.P. Grape juice or wine: Which is the best option? *Crit. Rev. Food Sci. Nutr.* **2020**, *60*, 3876–3889. [CrossRef]
97. Barbalho, S.M.; Direito, R.; Laurindo, L.F.; Marton, L.T.; Guiguer, E.L.; Goulart, R.d.A.; Tofano, R.J.; Carvalho, A.C.; Flato, U.A.P.; Capelluppi Tofano, V.A. Ginkgo biloba in the aging process: A narrative review. *Antioxidants* **2022**, *11*, 525. [CrossRef]
98. Tanaka, M.; Szabó, Á.; Körtési, T.; Szok, D.; Tajti, J.; Vécsei, L. From CGRP to PACAP, VIP, and Beyond: Unraveling the Next Chapters in Migraine Treatment. *Cells* **2023**, *12*, 2649. [CrossRef]
99. Gruchot, J.; Herrero, F.; Weber-Stadlbauer, U.; Meyer, U.; Küry, P. Interplay between activation of endogenous retroviruses and inflammation as common pathogenic mechanism in neurological and psychiatric disorders. *Brain Behav. Immun.* **2023**, *107*, 242–252. [CrossRef]
100. Northoff, G.; Hirjak, D.; Wolf, R.C.; Magioncalda, P.; Martino, M. All roads lead to the motor cortex: Psychomotor mechanisms and their biochemical modulation in psychiatric disorders. *Mol. Psychiatry* **2021**, *26*, 92–102. [CrossRef]
101. Küpeli Akkol, E.; Tatlı Çankaya, I.; Şeker Karatoprak, G.; Carpar, E.; Sobarzo-Sánchez, E.; Capasso, R. Natural Compounds as Medical Strategies in the Prevention and Treatment of Psychiatric Disorders Seen in Neurological Diseases. *Front. Pharmacol.* **2021**, *12*, 669638. [CrossRef]
102. Yohn, S.E.; Weiden, P.J.; Felder, C.C.; Stahl, S.M. Muscarinic acetylcholine receptors for psychotic disorders: Bench-side to clinic. *Trends Pharmacol. Sci.* **2022**, *43*, 1098–1112. [CrossRef]

Disclaimer/Publisher's Note: The statements, opinions and data contained in all publications are solely those of the individual author(s) and contributor(s) and not of MDPI and/or the editor(s). MDPI and/or the editor(s) disclaim responsibility for any injury to people or property resulting from any ideas, methods, instructions or products referred to in the content.

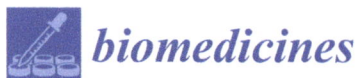

Article

Analysis of Respiratory Sinus Arrhythmia and Directed Information Flow between Brain and Body Indicate Different Management Strategies of fMRI-Related Anxiety

Beate Rassler [1,*], Katarzyna Blinowska [2,3], Maciej Kaminski [3] and Gert Pfurtscheller [4]

1. Carl-Ludwig-Institute of Physiology, University of Leipzig, 04103 Leipzig, Germany
2. Nalecz Institute of Biocybernetics and Biomedical Engineering, Polish Academy of Sciences, 02-109 Warsaw, Poland; katarzyna.blinowska@fuw.edu.pl
3. Faculty of Physics, University of Warsaw, 02-093 Warsaw, Poland; maciek.kaminski@fuw.edu.pl
4. Institute of Neural Engineering, Graz University of Technology, 8010 Graz, Austria; pfurtscheller@tugraz.at
* Correspondence: beate.rassler@medizin.uni-leipzig.de; Tel.: +49-341-9715565

Abstract: Background: Respiratory sinus arrhythmia (RSA) denotes decrease of cardiac beat-to-beat intervals (RRI) during inspiration and RRI increase during expiration, but an inverse pattern (termed negative RSA) was also found in healthy humans with elevated anxiety. It was detected using wave-by-wave analysis of cardiorespiratory rhythms and was considered to reflect a strategy of anxiety management involving the activation of a neural pacemaker. Results were consistent with slow breathing, but contained uncertainty at normal breathing rates (0.2–0.4 Hz). Objectives and methods: We combined wave-by-wave analysis and directed information flow analysis to obtain information on anxiety management at higher breathing rates. We analyzed cardiorespiratory rhythms and blood oxygen level-dependent (BOLD) signals from the brainstem and cortex in 10 healthy fMRI participants with elevated anxiety. Results: Three subjects with slow respiratory, RRI, and neural BOLD oscillations showed 57 ± 26% negative RSA and significant anxiety reduction by 54 ± 9%. Six participants with breathing rate of ~0.3 Hz showed 41 ± 16% negative RSA and weaker anxiety reduction. They presented significant information flow from RRI to respiration and from the middle frontal cortex to the brainstem, which may result from respiration-entrained brain oscillations, indicating another anxiety management strategy. Conclusions: The two analytical approaches applied here indicate at least two different anxiety management strategies in healthy subjects.

Keywords: respiratory sinus arrhythmia; directed information flow; neural pacemaker-like activity; fMRI-related anxiety; anxiety management; causal coupling; breathing rhythm; neural BOLD oscillations; cardio-respiratory coupling; breathing-entrained oscillations

Citation: Rassler, B.; Blinowska, K.; Kaminski, M.; Pfurtscheller, G. Analysis of Respiratory Sinus Arrhythmia and Directed Information Flow between Brain and Body Indicate Different Management Strategies of fMRI-Related Anxiety. *Biomedicines* **2023**, *11*, 1028. https://doi.org/10.3390/biomedicines11041028

Academic Editors: Masaru Tanaka and Eleonóra Spekker

Received: 3 February 2023
Revised: 20 March 2023
Accepted: 22 March 2023
Published: 27 March 2023

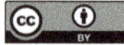

Copyright: © 2023 by the authors. Licensee MDPI, Basel, Switzerland. This article is an open access article distributed under the terms and conditions of the Creative Commons Attribution (CC BY) license (https://creativecommons.org/licenses/by/4.0/).

1. Introduction

General Background: The term "respiratory sinus arrhythmia" (RSA) denotes a physiological phenomenon based on entrainment between cardiovascular and breathing rhythms. Typical RSA is characterized by a shortening of cardiac beat-to-beat intervals (RRI), i.e., increase in heart rate (HR) during inspiration and RRI prolongation (HR decrease) during expiration [1,2]. RSA is the main part of high-frequency (HF) heart rate variability (HRV) and is often termed as HRV in synchrony with respiration [3,4]. For a long time, RSA has been considered to represent respiration-driven vagally mediated HR modulation [5], thus serving as an index of parasympathetic tone. The low-frequency (LF) component is considered to be a product of both sympathetic and parasympathetic activities [6]. Consequently, the relation of LF to HF HRV has been used as a measure of sympatho–vagal balance [7–9].

However, HRV and RSA comprise much more complex interactions between the cardiovascular, respiratory, and autonomic nervous systems [3]. Besides fluctuations in vagal activity, baroreflex mechanisms and respiratory fluctuations of intrathoracic pressure are considered to be important sources of RSA [4,10,11]. Due to the close vicinity of the central respiratory pattern generator to sympatho–excitatory neurons in the rostroventrolateral reticular nucleus, respiration exerts a marked influence upon sympathetic nerve activity [12–14]. Sympathetic depression during inspiration and an abrupt re-increase of activity during postinspiration is a typical pattern of respiratory–sympathetic coupling [12,13], which in turn, may induce modulation of HRV. A study on cardiorespiratory coupling during sympathetic activation due to graded head-up tilt showed a reduction in the direct effect of respiration on the heart rate with progressive sympathetic activation [15].

As HRV reflects the autonomic control of the heart and the autonomic balance, the magnitude of RSA is a well-accepted marker of cardiovascular diseases [7]. Chronic cardiovascular diseases such as hypertension have been described to reduce the amplitude of RRI oscillations and even to abolish RSA [16,17]. Emotional disorders such as depression or anxiety have also been shown to reduce the magnitude of RSA [18–20]. In contrast, a higher RSA magnitude was observed in healthy individuals with elevated anxiety [21]. Similarly, recent studies on fear conditioning showed increased HF HRV, indicating increased vagal activity in the response to the conditioning in contrast to a neutral stimulus [22]. These findings indicate that HRV is more than only a marker of sympatho–vagal balance. HRV is part of a complex interaction between cortical, limbic, and autonomic structures involved in adaptive functions such as emotional learning [23,24]. Accordingly, voluntary modulation of HRV including RSA such as HRV biofeedback training can be used as a therapeutic instrument [25,26]. For instance, forced (paced) resonance breathing at about 6 breaths/min, which can be applied as a relaxation technique, is accompanied by a high HRV amplitude [27,28].

The specific background of this study is the observation of phase-shifts in the respiration-related RRI variations. Recently, we found an inverse phase-relation in the cardio-respiratory coupling with HR decrease (RRI increase) during inspiration and HR increase (RRI decrease) during expiration in some participants of a functional magnetic resonance imaging (fMRI) study [29]. This type of cardio-respiratory coupling termed negative RSA (nRSA) has been observed for the first time in awake and spontaneously breathing persons and occurred predominantly in participants with high anxiety [30]. Of note, in contrast to effects of cardiovascular and other disorders as mentioned above, the magnitude of respiration-related oscillations is not reduced in nRSA. For comparison of (classical) RSA and nRSA, please see Figure 1.

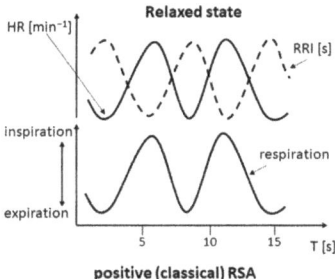 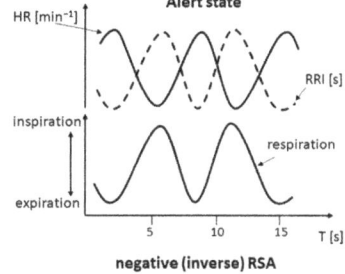

Figure 1. Cardio-respiratory phase-relations: upper curves show heart rate (HR, solid line) and cardiac beat-to-beat interval (RRI, dotted line), lower curves show respiration. Slow cardiac and respiratory waves are presented in both panels for reasons of comparability. The left panel depicts positive (classical) RSA with inspiration coinciding with increasing HR (decreasing RRI) and expiration coinciding with decreasing HR (increasing RRI). This phase-relation typically occurs in a resting and relaxed state. The right panel depicts negative (inverse) RSA with inspiration coinciding with decreasing HR (increasing RRI) and expiration coinciding with increasing HR (decreasing RRI). This phase-relation occurs rarely. In awake subjects, it has predominantly been observed in situations of elevated anxiety and during slow breathing.

Prior to our observation, nRSA has been described in anesthetized patients [31] or in persons with paced slow breathing [32]. While classical RSA means a respiration-driven modulation in HR, the rather uncommon nRSA is thought to result from a change in dominance; this means that the cardiac rhythm gains dominance over the respiratory rhythm. Using a wave-by-wave analysis, we demonstrated that nRSA was mostly associated with a transient reversal in the direction of entrainment, i.e., the RRI rhythm was the leading rhythm and entrained the respiratory rhythm for a limited period of time [30]. We hypothesized that the dominance of the RRI rhythm over the respiratory rhythm might result from the activation of a central pacemaker, which is thought to be part of an anxiety management strategy. This pacemaker predominantly acts in the 0.15 Hz range and is most probably located in the brainstem [33].

Issues addressed in the present study: In our previous studies, nRSA was predominantly observed in subjects with slow RRI oscillations and slow breathing at rates around 0.10–0.15 Hz [29,30]. A majority of our subjects, however, breathed at a rather "normal" rate (0.2–0.4 Hz, centered around 0.32 Hz; further referred to as fast breathing). In these cases, phase-coupling was also detected, but there was no clear predominance of RSA or nRSA [30]. Of note, (classical) RSA and nRSA are not the only phase-relations in cardio-respiratory coupling. Breathing and RRI oscillations may adopt any other phase-relation, which is termed "indefinite RSA" [32]. The portion of indefinite RSA was higher during breathing in the 0.2–0.4 Hz band compared to slow breathing. The prevalence of indefinite RSA impedes the analysis of the linkage between cardio-respiratory coupling and anxiety management (for a more detailed discussion, please see the Limitations section). As anxious subjects often breathe at higher rates (above 0.2 Hz) [20], the question whether signals in the HF band also allow detection of a directed information flow is of particular interest. Consequently, we extended our approach in the present study by analysis of blood-oxygen-level-dependent (BOLD) oscillations in various brain regions.

The BOLD signal is a complex signal composed of three interacting components: (i) cerebral metabolic rate of oxygen consumption (CMRO2) due to neural activation, (ii) cerebral blood flow (CBF, Mayer waves) and (iii) cerebral blood volume (CBV). Changes in BOLD signals only reflect neural activity (neural BOLD) accurately if vascular components (CBF, CBV) are not altered [34]. In contrast, the classical neurovascular coupling (NVC) reflects the close temporal and regional linkage between neural activity and cerebral blood flow (CBF) [34,35], whereby cerebral autoregulation, the intrinsic dynamic ability of cerebral vessels to maintain CBF despite fluctuations in arterial blood pressure, plays a dominant role. The evidence of such blood pressure oscillations on BOLD fluctuations is not completely clear and needs further research. In this respect, studies on the interaction of cerebrovascular and cardiovascular variability are important [36]. Neural BOLD oscillations lag behind RRI oscillations, and the time delay between the two oscillations is positive (pTD). Vascular BOLD oscillations lead before RRI oscillations, and the time delay between the two oscillations is negative (nTD) [33]. Cardiovascular and respiratory functions are involved in a multitude of interactions with cortical activities including the limbic brain areas such as the amygdala and hippocampus, regions related to regulation of emotions [23,24,37,38]. The directional interactions between the heart rate and respiration revealed that the influence is much stronger from the respiratory to the cardiac rhythm than in the opposite direction [39–43]. The direction of coupling between the heart rate and respiration may be reversed in some pathological states or during sleep [44,45].

The above-mentioned studies considered only two signals and showed directionality in cardio-respiratory interactions, which does not necessarily mean causal relations. The interaction between multiple signals including reciprocal connections is provided by means of Directed Transfer Function (DTF), which is an extension of the Granger causality principle [46] and yields causal coupling within a set of signals [47]. A recent study analyzing information flow between RRI, respiration and BOLD signals in various brain regions of interest (ROIs) in the 0.1–0.2 Hz band demonstrated that during low/no anxiety, an information flow from the cortex to the brainstem predominated while during elevated anxiety, a flow from the brainstem to the cortex was dominant. During elevated anxiety, the RRI signal received modulating input from information flow both from the cortex and from the brainstem, supporting our assumption of a neural pacemaker involved in the processing of elevated anxiety [48]. Consequently, the evidence of strong information flow from the brainstem to the RRI rhythm in the present study might explain the enhanced dominance of the RRI rhythm over the respiratory rhythm and the induction of the phase-shift typical for nRSA.

Aims of this study: The present study is designed to investigate whether detection of directed information flow is possible with signals in the HF band and whether the DTF analysis allows a more comprehensive assessment of cardio-respiratory coupling. We would expect that quantification of the directed information flow between various brain regions and cardiac and respiratory signals may extend the information provided by the analysis of phase-relations. The specific questions of this study are: (i) Can the analysis of directed information flow provide additional support for the hypothesized neural "pacemaker" by demonstrating different information flows between RRI, respiratory and BOLD signals in situations with RSA or nRSA? (ii) Can such an analysis provide information about the flow between slow RRI and fast respiratory oscillations? (iii) Can this type of analysis provide more detailed information on strategies of anxiety regulation?

2. Materials and Methods

This study was based on recordings of respiration, RRI and BOLD signals and on self-assessments of state anxiety (AS) of 10 selected participants of an fMRI study. The time course and phase-relations between RRI and respiration were analyzed wave by wave to detect the occurrence of RSA/nRSA. Synchronization between RRI and BOLD waves was assessed using phase-locking statistics. Directed Transfer Function (DTF) was applied to estimate causal coupling between respiration, RRI time courses and BOLD signals.

Study approval: All participants provided written informed consent after reading the protocol of the study, which was approved by the local Ethics Committee at the University of Graz (number: GZ. 39/75/63 ex 2013/14). Our research was performed in accordance with the ethical standards laid down in the 1964 Declaration of Helsinki.

Experimental design and participants: The present work is based on data collected in a major fMRI study that was originally designed to investigate the relations between brain oscillations in various brain regions and their relation to initiation of self-paced movements. During performance and first evaluation of the experiments, the aspect of anxiety and its relation to BOLD, RRI and respiratory oscillations received increasing attention and has become the main focus of recent studies. A detailed description of the experimental procedure in relevance to the anxiety-related studies is given [33]. In brief, each participant had to perform two identical fMRI sessions separated by a break of 50 min. AS was assessed at four different stages of the experiment.

Each session lasted about 40 min and started with a first short questionnaire to assess AS, followed by the first resting state, several movement tasks, the second resting state and the second AS questionnaire. The four resting states with their related AS values were labeled R1, R2 (first session), R3 and R4 (second session). This experimental protocol was designed to assess whether the subjective perception of anxiety remains constant during a single fMRI procedure and over an examination sequence.

In total, 23 healthy persons aged 19–34 years (12 female, 22 right-handed) participated in this experiment. They were naïve to the purpose of the study and had no former MRI experience. All of them had normal or corrected-to-normal vision and were without any record of neurological or psychiatric disorders (as assessed by self-report). From these, 10 persons with elevated anxiety were selected for the present study. A detailed description of the selection criteria is given in [30]. In brief, based on the overall mean AS values + 1 standard deviation (SD), an arbitrary threshold was defined at AS > 21. Ten participants exceeded this threshold in at least one resting state. From them, the resting states with the highest AS values were evaluated using a wave-by-wave analysis and a Directed Transfer Function calculation (for more details, see below).

Assessment of state anxiety: For assessment of anxiety, the state-trait anxiety and depression inventory (STADI; [49]) was used, which is based on the State-Trait Anxiety Inventory [50]. The STADI is an instrument constructed to assess both state and trait aspects of anxiety and depression. It allows a reasonable separation of anxiety and depression symptoms. The items were presented on a screen within the scanner and were answered via a trackball. The possible range of scores is from 10 (very low anxiety) to 40 (very high anxiety).

Recording of respiration and ECG: For the recording of ECG and respiration during BOLD image acquisition, we used the PERU (Physiological ECG/Respiration Unit), a component of the Magnetom Skyra MR system (Siemens AG Healthcare Sector, Erlangen, Germany) made for recordings of ECG and respiration inside the scanner. Data were sampled at a rate of 400 Hz. The respiratory data were acquired using a pneumatic cushion, which was attached to the participant by a respiration belt and connected to a pressure sensor on the PERU. The ECG beat-to-beat intervals (RRI) were detected using the fMRI plug-in for EEGLAB [51] and the FASTR algorithm for removal of gradient-induced artifacts. As ECG signals recorded during MRI with a high scanning rate often have a reduced quality [52], the RRI signals were re-processed using the Kubios HRV Premium Package (Kubios Ltd., Kuopio, Finland; version 3.0.2) [53].

fMRI BOLD recording and selection of ROIs: BOLD signals reflect changes in blood oxygenation and changes in CBF accompanying neural processes such as activation of a central pacemaker. Both types of changes can be detected through BOLD contrast measurements [54,55]. Besides cortical and limbic regions, BOLD signals from the brainstem (more exactly from pons/brainstem) were of particular interest in this study as two important sources for rhythmic BOLD signals are concentrated in this region. These are, on the one hand, the basilar artery, which is close to the medulla and the pons. On the other hand, important nuclei involved in cardiac control such as the solitary tract nucleus, vagal motor neurons in the nucleus ambiguus and dorsal vagal motor nucleus are localized in the medulla and the pons [56,57].

Functional images were acquired with a 3T scanner (Magnetom Skyra, Siemens AG Healthcare Sector, Erlangen, Germany) using a multiband GE-EPI sequence [58] with a simultaneous six-band acquisition with TE/TR = 34/871 ms, 52° flip angle, $2 \times 2 \times 2$ mm^3 voxel size, 66 contiguous axial slices (11×6), acquisition matrix of 90×104 and a FOV of 180×208 mm^2. Finally, the AAL atlas [59] was used to extract time courses of BOLD signals for specified regions of interest (ROIs) in the left pre-central gyrus (PCG, ROI 1), left middle frontal gyrus (MFG, ROI 7), left medial superior frontal gyrus (ROI 23), left hippocampus (ROI 37), left amygdala (ROI 41), left brainstem (ROI 93, ROI 103) and right brainstem (ROIs 96, 98, 100). For details see [48,60].

Wave-by-wave analysis of the phase-relations between respiration and RRI waves: The duration of breathing and RRI waves (period duration, PD) for the selected participants was detected period by period. A detailed description of this method is given in [29]. In brief, we detected the start of inspiration and expiration from the minima and maxima, respectively, in the respiration curve. From these, we calculated the period duration (PD) of each breath. Similarly, the PD of RRI waves was determined between two consecutive minima in the RRI curve. The phase-relations were measured as the time interval from the start of inspiration/expiration to the subsequent maximum and minimum of the RRI signal and were expressed in the percent of inspiration or expiration duration. For a detailed description of the criteria for classification as RSA or nRSA, please see [30]. Classical RSA is characterized by RRI maxima occurring in late expiration or early inspiration, and/or RRI minima in late inspiration or early expiration. In contrast, nRSA means that RRI maxima occur in late inspiration or early expiration, and RRI minima in late expiration or early inspiration. This method is an appropriate instrument to characterize frequency and phase coupling. Shifts in the phase-relation between the coupled rhythms indicate modulations of coupling and can give hints on the dominance of the rhythms.

Calculation of phase-locking between RRI and BOLD waves: The frequency-specific synchronization between RRI and BOLD waves as a putative mechanism of neural integration was analyzed by means of phase-locking statistics. We used the "Cross-wavelet and Wavelet Coherence" toolbox [61] and focused on the phase component for computing the phase-locking value (PLV). PLV is a normalized measure of how much the phase difference between two signals changes in a user-chosen time window, regardless of the actual phase difference value; for more details, see [62]. The PLV was calculated in the 0.05–0.15 Hz band between the RRI time course and the BOLD time series. The calculation procedure is based on a method reported in [63] and is described in detail in [64]. As a result, two PLV-based parameters were computed: (i) the time delay (TD), which is the phase delay converted to time; and (ii) the significant length of phase coupling (sigbin%), which is the percentage of time samples within the time series that survive a 0.05 significance threshold. A positive time delay (pTD) indicates that RRI oscillations precede BOLD oscillations and is typical for neural BOLD oscillations. A negative time delay (nTD) indicates that RRI oscillations lag behind BOLD oscillations and is typical for vascular BOLD signals.

Computing of directed coupling: The interaction between respiration, RRI time courses and BOLD signal was studied by means of Directed Transfer Function (DTF) [65], which allows to estimate causal coupling between the signals as a function of frequency. DTF is an extension of the Granger causality principle [46] to the multivariate case [66]. Granger causality measures the predictability for two time series. If the variance of the prediction error for the second time series is reduced by including past measurements from the first time series in the linear regression model, then the first time series can be said to cause the second time series. The Granger causality principle is equivalent to 2-channel Multivariate Autoregressive Model (MVAR) but it may be extended to an arbitrary number of channels [67,68]. For our study, MVAR was extended to 6 channels [47,65], four BOLD signals, respiration and RRI time courses. Epochs of 40 s were used for the analysis. We applied the full frequency version of DTF (ffDTF), which describes the causal influence of one signal on another one (the destination signal) at a certain frequency normalized in respect of inflows to the destination channel. In ffDTF, the normalization factor does not depend on frequency. The method is described in detail in [48,60]. The following bands were studied: 0.05–0.15 Hz, 0.1–0.2 Hz and 0.2–0.4 Hz.

The statistical procedure of finding significant differences in average coupling values in the chosen frequency band was based on the bootstrap approach, which is described in detail in [60]. In brief, a common pool of couplings from both cases, inflows (type 1) and outflows (type 2), for a given channel was created. From this pool were randomly selected coupling values, which were marked as type 1 or type 2. Then, the differences between drawn type 1 and type 2 values were calculated. Based on about 10,000 repetitions of this procedure, we received the empirical distribution of coupling difference values corresponding to the hypothesis of no differences between inflows and outflows from the given channel. Original values of connectivity difference lying outside an assumed confidence range of 95% of such obtained distribution were considered to represent significant differences between inflows and outflows.

3. Results

The results from wave-by-wave analysis extended by the results of the BOLD analyses (TD, sigbin%) are summarized in Table 1. The RRI oscillations presented with two dominant frequency bands centered at ~0.1 and 0.16 Hz. On average, more than 50% of all RRI periods belonged to one of these dominant frequency bands. The RRI and respiratory signals were not homogeneous. Respiration of these subjects showed three dominant frequency bands centered at ~0.1, 0.16, and 0.32 Hz. Note, 0.16 Hz and 0.32 Hz (double of 0.16 Hz) but not 0.1 Hz are parts of the binary hierarchical model of Klimesch [69]. He introduced the doubling-halving algorithm, which describes the frequency architecture of EEG rhythms during conscious cognition, which are coupled to body oscillations such as heart rate and breathing with breathing centered at harmonic frequencies of 0.08 Hz (half of 0.16 Hz), 0.16 Hz and 0.32 Hz.

Different patterns of cardio-respiratory coupling can be discriminated: three subjects (#18, #3, #11, further referred to as group 1) displayed coherent frequency components in both signals in the LF band with a predominance of nRSA. Six subjects (#24, #16, #9, #13, #14, #20, further referred to as group 2) displayed a dominant respiration with a spectral peak close to 0.32 Hz, while RRI oscillations in the LF band prevailed. These subjects presented rate ratios of 1:n between RRI and respiratory rhythms with n > 1. The preferred rate ratios were 1:2 (2 breaths per RRI wave at an RRI rate of ~0.16 Hz) and 1:3 (3 breaths per RRI wave at an RRI rate of ~0.1 Hz). Only in subject #24, fast RRI waves were most prominent, but a small spectral peak at 0.1 Hz indicated that these fast RRI waves were superimposed on a weak slow RRI wave. In three subjects from group 2, nRSA was predominant; the other three subjects showed either predominant RSA or both RSA and nRSA to a similar extent.

All these nine subjects from groups 1 and 2 exhibited "neural BOLD" oscillations, which are reflected in pTD between RRI waves and BOLD oscillations (i.e., RRI waves precede BOLD oscillations). An exception is subject #6 (further referred to as group 3) showing vascular BOLD oscillations, which are associated with nTD with RRI waves lagging behind the BOLD oscillations.

Besides RSA and nRSA, many periods presented phase-relations neither belonging to RSA nor to nRSA (termed indefinite RSA; [32]). In cases of 1:1 coupling, wave-by-wave analysis allows a reliable assessment of RSA/nRSA. However, in cases of 1:n coupling (with n > 1), a large number of breaths is not considered in the analysis, thus giving rise to some uncertainty in the assessment of the percentage of RSA/nRSA. This applies to 8 cases presented in Table 1 (all except for subjects #11 and #18).

3.1. BOLD Oscillations of Neural and Non-Neural Origin

Three different signals are related to brainstem functions, namely (i) the fluctuations of cardiac beat-to-beat interval controlled by the cardiovascular center, (ii) the respiratory rhythm associated with the pre-Bötzinger complex modulated by cortical afferences, and (iii) BOLD signals with neural and non-neural origins.

Neural BOLD oscillations are associated with rhythmically activated neural clusters with a pTD of ~2–3 s. In contrast, non-neural BOLD oscillations can be either vascular BOLD oscillations with origin in the baroreflex loop (subject #6) or respiratory artefacts caused by vessel motion. Examples of 3 subjects from group 1, all with neural BOLD oscillations, are presented in Figure 2. The figure shows averaged waves of 12 s duration (±SEM) composed of about ~10 single visually selected trials aligned to the maximum of the RR interval (RRI peak). The displayed waves are BOLD, breathing and RRI signals. All BOLD waves in line A are from the left precentral gyrus (ROI 1), the BOLD waves in line B are from the left brainstem (ROIs 103, 105), and BOLD waves in line C are from the right brainstem (ROIs 96, 100); for further details, see [33]. Breathing waves are coherent with RRI waves in the case of nRSA (subjects #11 and #18) and in opposite phase for RSA (subject #3). Note, neural BOLD waves lag behind the respiratory BOLD artefact or the RRI peak by about 2–3 s.

Table 1. Results of the wave-by-wave analysis and BOLD analysis from 10 fMRI participants (allocated to 3 groups as described in the text) with high anxiety (modified from [30]).

Subject	AS	RSA/nRSA in % of RRI Waves		Average Rate		BOLD Analysis			RRI				Respiration					
		RSA%	nRSA%	RRI [Hz]	Resp. [Hz]	TD [s]	Sigbin%	ROI	0.10 Hz Band		0.16 Hz Band		0.10 Hz Band		0.16 Hz Band		0.32 Hz Band	
									PD [s]	n [%]	PD [s]	n [%]	PD [s]	n [%]	PD [s]	n [%]	PD [s]	n [%]
Group 1																			
#18R1	28	12%	63%	0.12	0.16	2.2	36%	103	9.8	47%	6.9	40%	10.0	22%	6.5	39%	3.2	26%
#3R1	26	13%	29%	0.21	0.22	1.7	24%	93	10.5	4%	6.5	13%	—	0%	6.4	15%	3.6	39%
#11R1	25	5%	80%	0.13	0.13	2.3	70%	93	9.8	39%	6.9	54%	9.9	38%	6.9	48%	—	0%
Mean	26.3	10.0%	57.3%	0.15	0.17	2.1	43.3%		10.0	30%	6.8	35%	9.9	20%	6.6	34%	3.4	22%
SD	1.5	4.4%	26.0%	0.05	0.04	0.3	23.9%		0.4	22%	0.2	21%	0.1	19%	0.3	17%	0.3	20%
Group 2																			
#24R1	25	12%	54%	0.25	0.26	1.5	26%	93	—	0%	6.8	2%	—	0%	5.9	6%	3.4	63%
#16R4	24	18%	14%	0.22	0.33	0.8	31%	93	9.9	11%	6.4	19%	—	0%	5.9	1%	3.0	97%
#9R1	23	58%	33%	0.14	0.33	1.9	36%	93	9.9	38%	7.0	33%	—	0%	—	0%	3.0	78%
#13R2	22	47%	41%	0.10	0.35	2.0	34%	103	11.7	61%	6.9	33%	—	0%	—	0%	2.8	87%
#14R4	22	6%	58%	0.21	0.31	1.4	27%	93	9.9	20%	6.5	10%	—	0%	—	0%	3.2	88%
#20R1	22	27%	47%	0.14	0.27	2.4	47%	93	9.6	42%	6.7	24%	—	0%	6.0	2%	3.4	65%
Mean	23.0	28.0%	41.2%	0.18	0.31	1.7	33.5%		10.2	29%	6.7	21%	—	0%	5.9	1%	3.1	80%
SD	1.3	20.5%	16.0%	0.06	0.04	0.6	7.7%		0.8	22%	0.3	13%	—	0%	0.1	2%	0.2	14%
Group 3																			
#6R1	29	11%	20%	0.17	0.34	−0.5	23%	97	10.3	29%	6.7	14%	—	0%	—	0%	3.0	93%

The columns denote (from left to right): subject; anxiety score (AS); percentage of RRI waves with RSA (RSA%) and nRSA (nRSA%), respectively; average rates of RRI waves and respiration (in Hz); results of phase-coupling between BOLD oscillations in the brainstem and RRI oscillations (time delay [s] (TD), significant length of phase coupling [%] (sigbin%), ROI with the largest time delay); period duration (PD) and percentage (n) of RRI waves in the frequency bands centered at 0.10 Hz and 0.16 Hz; PD and percentage of breaths in the frequency bands centered at 0.10 Hz, 0.16 Hz, and 0.32 Hz.

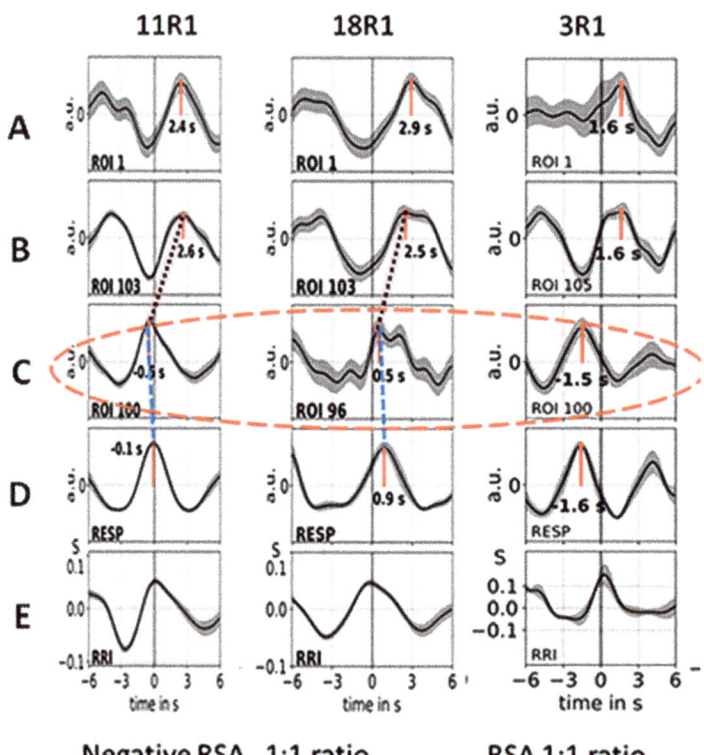

Figure 2. Examples of ~10 averaged BOLD (**A–C**), respiration (**D**) and RRI (**E**)-peak-triggered waves (mean ± SEM) of the subjects of group 1 (#11, #18, #3). Time intervals are shown from 6 s before to 6 s after the trigger. Numbers indicate the time shift in seconds between the peak and trigger. The red ellipse marks respiratory motion artefacts of the BOLD signal. The time shifts between breathing (line D) and respiratory BOLD artefacts (ROIs 96, 100; line C) are indicated by blue stippled lines, and the time shifts between respiratory BOLD artefacts and associated neural BOLD waves (ROI 103, 105; line B) are indicated by red stippled lines (only in the first two columns). The coherent breathing and RRI waves (lines D and E) in the first two subjects (#11, #18) indicate negative RSA (nRSA) while the out-of-phase behavior of breathing and RRI waves in the third column (subject #3) is characteristic for classical (positive) RSA (modified from [70]).

3.2. Cardiac RRI, Respiratory and BOLD Signals in the 0.05–0.15/0.1–0.2 Hz Band

The subjects of group 1 (#11, #18, #3) presented RRI and respiratory signals with dominance in two frequency bands centered at 0.1 Hz and at 0.16 Hz, which are assigned to the 0.05–0.15/0.1–0.2 Hz band. While BOLD waves displayed similar patterns across all subjects (examples are illustrated in Figure 2), differences were observed in RRI and breathing waves. Two subjects from group 1 (#11, #18) predominantly exhibited an in-phase (coherent) behavior of RRI and breathing waves while the other subject (#3) also showed an out-of-phase behavior over parts of the record. The latter case means that inspiration is accompanied by acceleration of the cardiac activity and expiration is associated with deceleration. This is characteristic for a positive respiratory sinus arrhythmia (pRSA or, shortly, RSA; see Figure 1). The former cases demonstrating that inspiration is accompanied by RRI increase (cardiac deceleration) and expiration by RRI decrease are characteristic for a negative RSA (nRSA; see Figure 1). The important point is that both types of patterns (negative and positive RSA) displayed the same time shifts between BOLD signals from the right and left brainstem (see Figure 2, lines B and C) and between breathing and BOLD signals (see Figure 2, lines C and D).

Besides RSA/nRSA, the wave-by-wave analysis of respiratory and RRI signals in the three frequency bands centered at 0.1 Hz, at 0.16 Hz and at 0.32 Hz provides further features of cardio-respiratory coupling, such as abrupt PD changes (termed "PD transitions") [30]. Two typical examples from #11R1 and #18R1 are presented in Figures 3 and 4. In both records, respiratory and RRI waves range in the 0.1–0.2 Hz band, and the phase relation between them indicates nRSA (Figure 3A,B and Figure 4A,B). They are associated with slow BOLD waves (PD about 6 s) in the PCG and left pons lagging behind the RRI waves, characteristic of neural BOLD oscillations. In the amygdala, waves in the different frequency bands constitute a non-sinusoidal wave resulting from a superposition of oscillations at ~0.3 Hz on a slow wave of ~0.1 Hz. The time delay between a respiratory BOLD artefact in the right pons induced by vessel (basilar artery) motion and the neural BOLD oscillations is 2–3 s corresponding to the neuro-BOLD coupling time (Figures 3B and 4B). Changes in the RRI PD are often accompanied by corresponding changes in the respiratory PD. In the cases presented here (#11R1 and #18R1), the transitions occurred first in the RRI rhythm and were followed by a transition in the respiratory rhythm (periods marked in red in Figures 3A and 4A), indicating that the RRI rhythm has entrained the respiratory rhythm, which is typical for nRSA. However, the analysis of directed information flow (Figures 3C and 4C) revealed differences between the two subjects. In #11R1, the information flow from respiration to RRI was predominant and was stronger than the opposite flow from RRI to respiration. In contrast, in #18R1, the information flow direction from RRI to respiration was clearly predominant. These are two remarkable examples showing clearly that the phase relation only shows one way in the cardio-respiratory interactions while the analysis of directed information characterizes reciprocal connections and the time variation of flow, thus providing a more differentiated representation of these processes.

3.3. Interactions of RRI, Respiratory and BOLD Signals in the 0.2–0.4 Hz Band

Group 2 of our subjects (#24, #16, #9, #13, #14, #20) presented signals in three frequency bands. While in the RRI signals, two periods were dominant (average PDs 10.2 s = 0.1 Hz and 6.7 s = 0.15 Hz), the respiratory signal predominated in the 0.2–0.4 Hz band (average PD 3.1 s = 0.32 Hz). All subjects of group 2 presented cardio-respiratory coupling with higher integer rate ratios, mainly 1:2 or 1:3, indicating that 2 or 3 breaths are coinciding with 1 RRI cycle (see Table 1). In those cases, we often observed superpositions in the slower rhythm (i.e., in the RRI rhythm) [30]. This phenomenon results when the strength of the dominant rhythm (usually, the respiratory rhythm) is not sufficient to fully entrain the other rhythm (the RRI rhythm). An example is shown in Figure 5 (#14R4). Figure 5A shows recordings from respiration and RRI waves. The vertical dotted lines show the coincidence of expiration onset with local maxima of RRI, a coherent pattern clearly indicating nRSA. The percentage of nRSA in this resting state was 58%. Frequency analysis demonstrated a clear 1:3 cardio-respiratory rate ratio with 3 breaths per one RRI cycle (Figure 5A,B). Figure 5B shows a movement artefact in the right pons coherent with respiration (lower line, left panel), slow BOLD waves in the left pons and MFG coherent with slow RRI waves (right panels) and a phase-shifted BOLD oscillation of neural origin in the amygdala (lower line, middle panel). The analysis of directed information flow confirmed this finding, showing a pronounced information flow from RRI to respiration (Figure 5C).

In contrast to the subjects from groups 1 and 2, subject #6 (group 3) showed BOLD peaks that preceded the RRI peaks by about 2 s, indicating that these BOLD oscillations were associated with dominant fluctuations in cerebral blood flow and volume (vascular BOLD) and had their origin in the baroreflex loop (Figure 6).

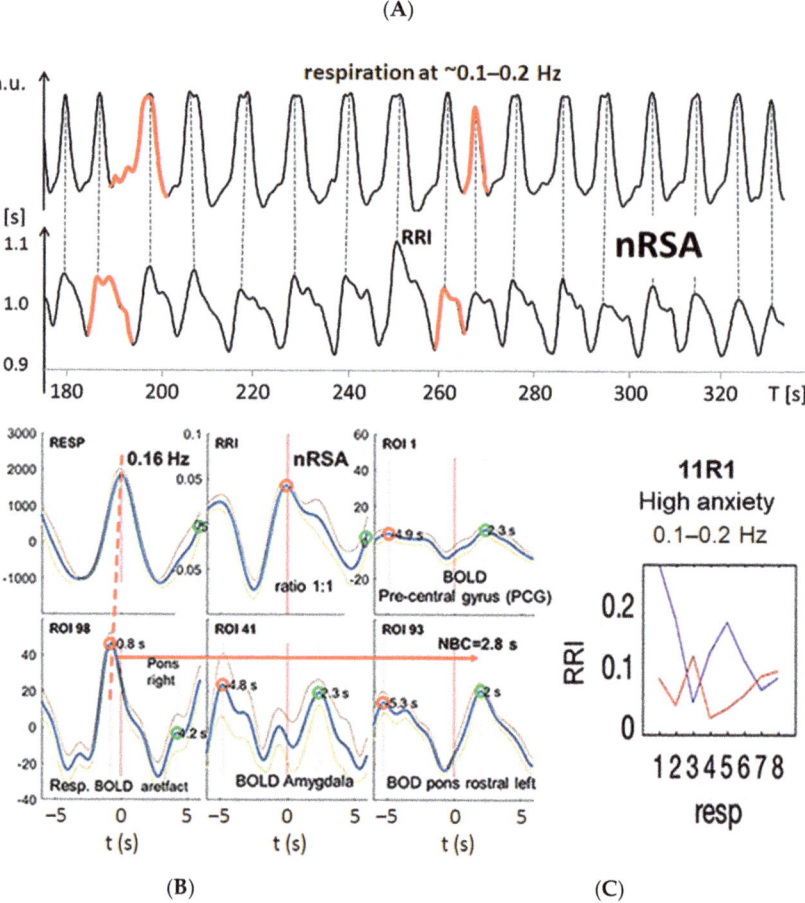

Figure 3. Example from subject #11. (**A**) Records of respiratory (upper trace) and RRI waves (lower trace); abscissa: time [s]. Some respiratory and RRI periods with PD transitions are marked in red. Note that transitions in the RRI rhythm precede changes in the respiratory rhythm by one period. (**B**) RRI peak (longest RR interval)-triggered respiratory (resp), RRI and BOLD waves from the PCG, pons and amygdala (blue and gray lines: mean ± SEM). The red and green circles have been automatically inserted by the computer program and mark local maxima on the negative and positive time scale, respectively. The coherence of respiratory and RRI waves indicates nRSA (upper line, left and middle panels). The vascular BOLD artefact in the right pons (lower line, left panel) slightly precedes respiration (red stippled line). The red horizontal arrow indicates the neural-BOLD coupling time (NBC) between the vessel motion artefact and the neural BOLD component. Note the non-sinusoidal oscillation in the amygdala (lower line, middle panel). (**C**) Information flow between RRI and respiration, blue lines indicate flow from respiration to RRI, red lines indicate flow from RRI to respiration. The numbers 1–8 on the abscissas represent consecutive time windows of the recording.

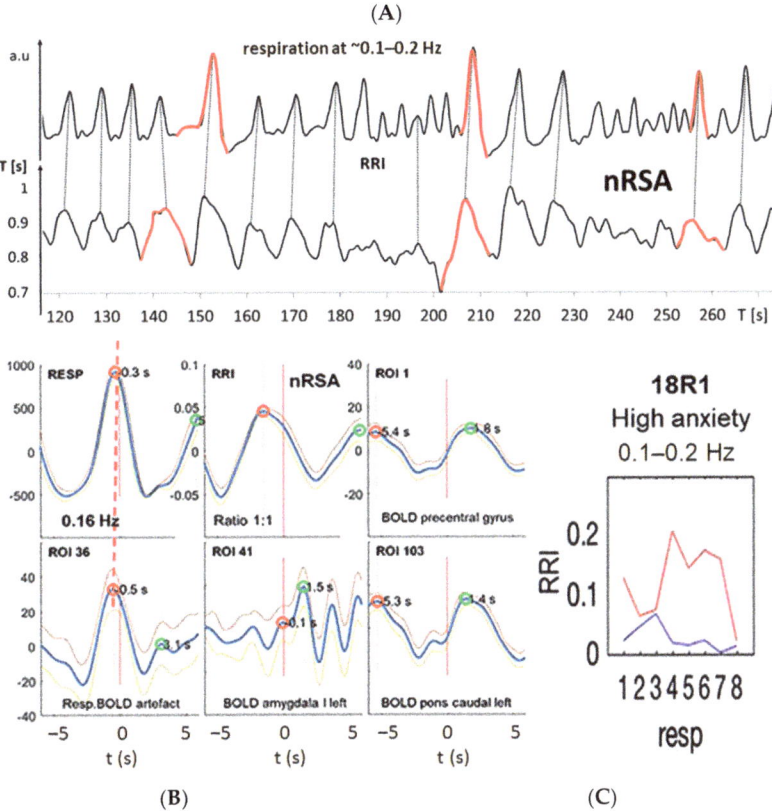

Figure 4. Example from subject #18. (**A**) Records of respiratory (upper trace) and RRI waves (lower trace); abscissa: time [s]. Some respiratory and RRI periods with PD transitions are marked in red. Note that transitions in the RRI rhythm precede the changes in the respiratory rhythm. (**B**) RRI peak (longest RR interval)-triggered respiratory (resp), RRI and slow BOLD waves (mean ± SEM; more details see text). Note the fast oscillation in the amygdala (lower line, middle panel). (**C**) Information flow is predominant from RRI to respiration; for further explanations, see Figure 3.

3.4. Dominant Information Flow between Cardiac (RRI), Respiratory and BOLD Oscillations in the 0.1–0.2 Hz and 0.2–0.4 Hz Bands

We found heterogenous patterns of information flow between cardiac (RRI), respiratory and BOLD oscillations among the 10 subjects with high anxiety in the fMRI scanner. In seven subjects (groups 2 and 3), respiration was dominant in the HF band (0.2–0.4 Hz), which corresponds to a "normal" respiratory rate at rest. In three subjects (group 1), respiration was dominant in the 0.1–0.2 Hz band, which is rather seldom during unconscious spontaneous breathing but is typically for conscious breathing such as resonance breathing [27]. It is noteworthy that all subjects except one (#6R1) displayed neural BOLD oscillations with RRI waves preceding BOLD waves (pTD). In addition, we observed, in most of the subjects, a clear predominance of information flow from the RRI to the respiratory rhythm, as it was expected during elevated anxiety. Coupling properties such as a predominant information flow from the RRI to the respiratory signal and neural BOLD oscillations with pTD to RRI waves are typically accompanied by a nRSA coupling pattern, i.e., a coherence between respiratory and RRI rhythms.

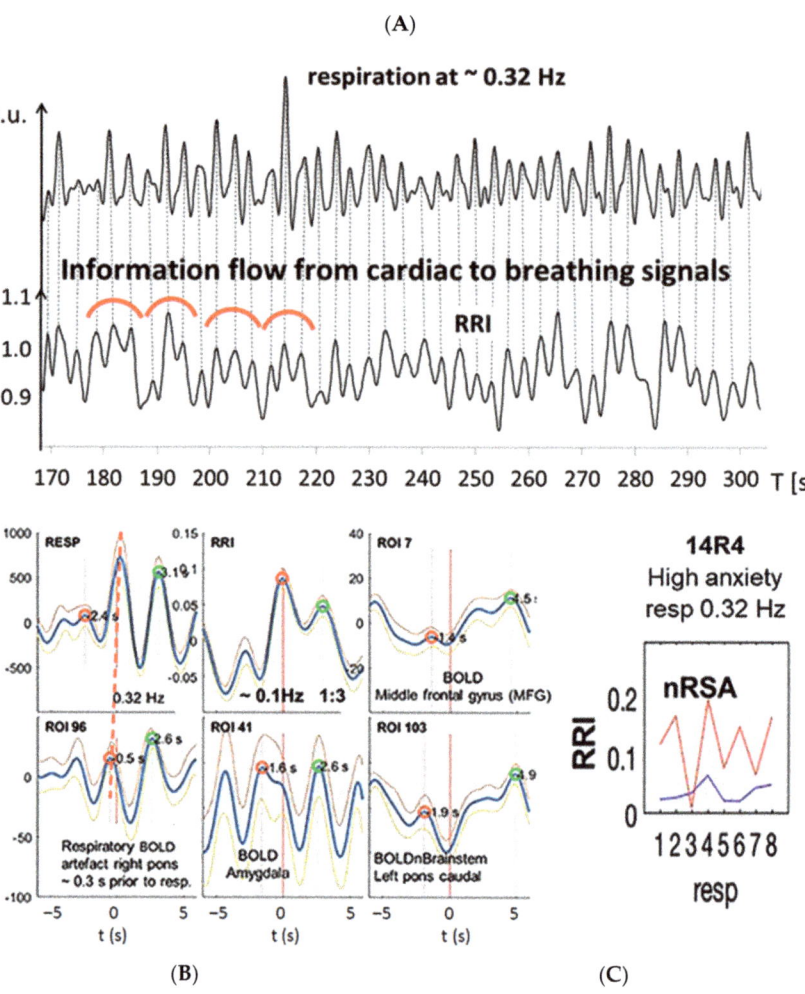

Figure 5. Example from subject #14 with dominant fast respiration in the 0.2–0.4 Hz band. (**A**) Records of respiratory and RRI waves. Some RRI periods with 1:3 coupling are marked with red semi-circles, indicating superposition of fast wavelets at ~0.3 Hz originating from the respiratory rhythm on slow RRI waves at ~0.1 Hz. (**B**) RRI peak (longest RR interval)-triggered respiratory (resp), RRI and slow BOLD waves (mean ± SEM; more details, see text). (**C**) The information flow diagram indicates a predominant flow from RRI to respiration. For further explanations, see Figure 3.

Previous DTF studies in subjects with prevailing anxiety revealed a rhythmic neural source (pacemaker) in the brainstem operating in the frequency range 0.1–0.2 Hz as a driving force for RRI signals [48]. We wondered whether a similar information flow can be demonstrated using DTF analysis in the 0.2–0.4 Hz band, indicating that modulations of cardio-respiratory coupling observed in subjects with high anxiety are present across wide ranges of respiratory and RRI frequencies. The DTF data from the subcluster of 6 subjects (group 2) were averaged and statistically compared via a bootstrap approach (Figure 7). Characteristic for these subjects is a predominant respiration in the 0.2–0.4 Hz frequency band (fast respiration). Most prominent was a significant top-down information flow from the MFG to the brain stem, the RRI and the respiratory rhythm (Figure 7A,B). Of note, there is a small information flow from respiration to the cortical and brainstem ROIs as well as to RRI. In contrast, the information flow from RRI to respiration was significantly greater than that from respiration to RRI ($p = 0.01$). These results clearly indicate that in situations of elevated anxiety, a significant information flow from RRI to respiration is not only demonstrable in the LF and IMF bands but also in the HF band. It may account for the reversal of the cardio-respiratory entrainment with a reduced dominance of the respiratory rhythm over the RRI rhythm in situations of elevated anxiety.

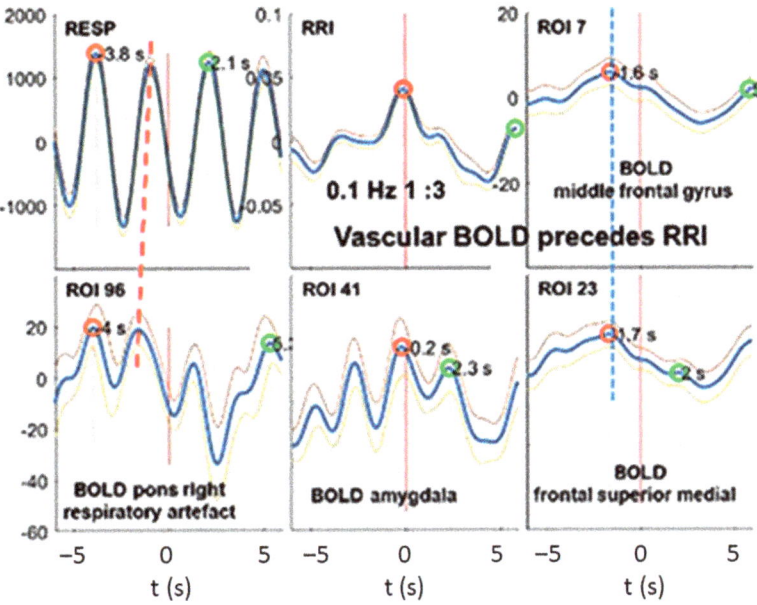

Figure 6. Example from subject #6 with dominant fast respiration in the 0.2–0.4 Hz band (for more detailed explanation, please see Figure 3). The RRI peak-triggered vascular BOLD waves were derived from MFG as depicted in the upper middle and right panels. The blue stippled vertical line indicates the maxima of slow BOLD waves about ~2 s before the RRI peak (longest RR interval), this means, a negative time delay indicating the vascular origin of the BOLD waves. Note the ~0.32 Hz oscillations in the amygdala (lower middle panel).

3.5. Management of Anxiety

All participants analyzed in this study showed high anxiety at least in the first session in the scanner. While their average AS in session R1 was 24 ± 4.1, it decreased by session R4 to 16 ± 5.4. However, there were considerable differences in the success of reducing anxiety (Figure 8). While the subjects in group 1 reduced their AS from R1 to R4 by more than 50% (ranging from 48–64%; $p = 0.016$, paired t test), the change of AS was widely scattering in groups 2 and 3 ($p = 0.20$, paired t test): two subjects in group 2 (#20 and #24) reduced their AS clearly (by 36 and 60%, respectively). Of note, nRSA prevailed in these two participants (see Table 1). Subject #6 (group 3) showed a similar reduction in AS. However, in two subjects (#9 and #14), AS remained almost unchanged throughout the whole experiment, while in two other subjects (#13 and #16), AS even increased over the two-hour fMRI session. Across all 10 participants, there was no significant correlation between the percentage of nRSA and reduction of AS ($r = 0.32$, $p = 0.37$).

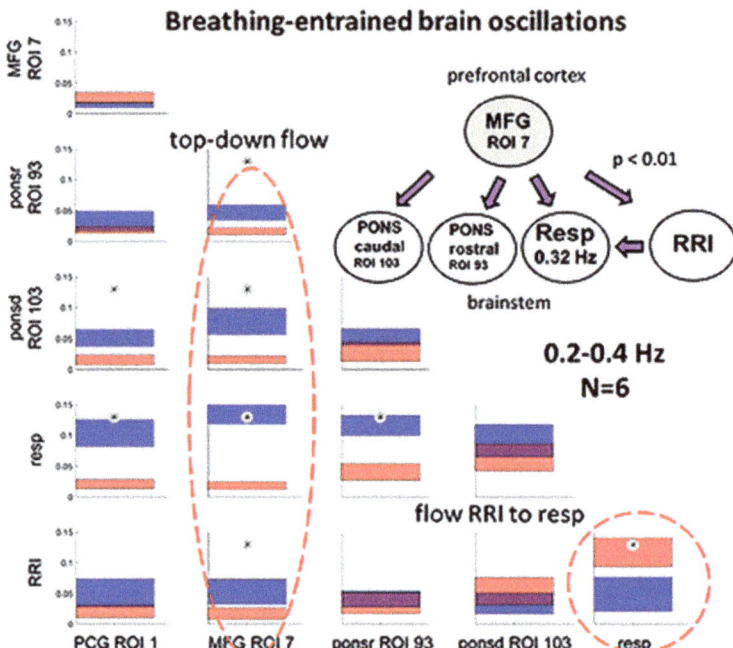

Figure 7. Directed coupling strengths for group 2 (n = 6) with high anxiety and predominant respiration in the 0.2–0.4 Hz frequency band. Each box shows the strength of coupling on the vertical scale. The width of bars is proportional to the mean error. The blue color shows the flow from the signal marked below the given column to the signal marked on the left, and the red color shows the flow from the signal marked on the left to the signal marked below. Violet areas mark an overlap of the two flow directions. Significant differences between couplings of inflow and outflow are marked by asterisks ($p < 0.05$). Red stippled ellipses mark the dominant downward flow (on the left) and the information flow from RRI to respiratory signal (on the right). The insert in the right upper corner indicates a diagram with the most important downward flows. Less pronounced flows, especially upward flows, are not shown.

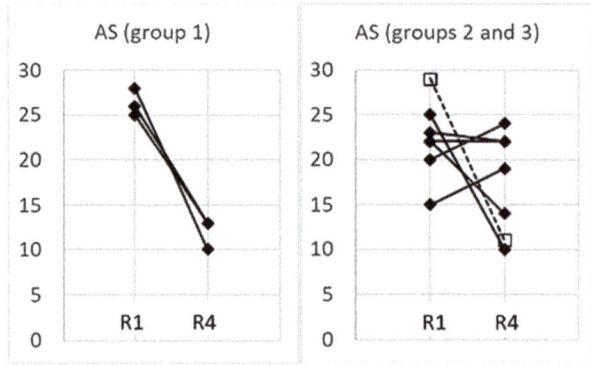

Figure 8. AS values obtained from all 10 subjects in sessions R1 and R4. In the interest of greater clarity, the subjects of group 1 are presented in the left panel and the subjects of groups 2 and 3 in the right panel. Subject #6 (group 3) is marked as ☐- - -☐.

To summarize, the results show that cardio-respiratory phase-relations may indicate different entrainment processes between brain and body rhythms involved in regulation of anxiety. However, the percentage of RSA/nRSA as an indicator of anxiety or anxiety management contains some uncertainty, especially in the HF band. Our results show that the directed information flow allows a more comprehensive assessment of the interplay between brain and body rhythms in a wide frequency range. Slow breathing seems to be an important component of successful anxiety management, presumably via the activation of a central pacemaker in the brainstem operating in the 0.15–0.16 Hz range. At higher breathing rates, respiration-entrained oscillations in different brain areas indicate that more pacemakers operating at different frequencies may be involved in anxiety management.

4. Discussion

The interactions between respiratory, RRI and BOLD signals from different brain regions provide insights into the strategies of anxiety management. In particular, the direction of information flow indicates different types of interaction between the involved processes and brain regions. All subjects presented in this study were characterized by high anxiety in at least one of four sessions within a two-hour fMRI examination. The results indicate that these subjects used different strategies to manage their anxiety. Some of these subjects showed high AS values in the first session and a decrease of AS up to the last session. In four subjects, however, AS did not decrease or even increased throughout the sessions, indicating a less successful anxiety managing process. The main and most evident difference between the subjects was their breathing rate: While seven subjects (groups 2 and 3) breathed at "normal" breathing rates (0.32 Hz on average), three subjects (group 1) presented slow breathing with prevailing breathing rates in the 0.05–0.15 Hz band (see Table 1). The groups further differed by the predominant directions of information flow and their success in anxiety management.

4.1. Different Cardio-Respiratory Coupling during High Anxiety

4.1.1. Slow Breathing during High Anxiety (Group 1)

Group 1 consisting of subjects #18, #3 and #11 showed RRI and respiratory oscillations in the LF/IMF band with a predominant 1:1 rate ratio. RRI and respiratory waves were either in-phase (nRSA) or out-of-phase (RSA), but the portion of nRSA was higher than that of RSA in all three subjects (see Table 1). All three subjects presented their highest AS values in session R1 and significantly reduced their AS by more than 50% on average up to session R4 (see Figure 8).

Noteworthy, nRSA is not associated with a change in magnitude of RSA. Cardiovascular or emotional disorders are usually associated with a reduction in the magnitude of RSA, i.e., reduced cardiorespiratory coupling [16–18,20,23]. Likewise, sympathetic activation induced by graded postural challenge diminished cardiorespiratory coupling [15]. In contrast, all patterns of respiration-related RRI oscillations observed in this and in previous studies showed no indication of reduced cardiovascular coupling [29,30,70].

nRSA was typically observed in subjects breathing at a lower rate than the "normal" resting breathing rate [29,31,32]. Besides slow respiration, the common feature of the three subjects in group 1 was coherent neural BOLD oscillations in the PFC and brainstem centered at ~0.16 Hz and ~0.1 Hz, respectively (Figures 3 and 4), indicating activation of a pacemaker in the brainstem. The BOLD peaks were clearly delayed from the largest RRI interval (RRI peak) by 2–3 s characteristic for an associated neural BOLD component. An interesting counterexample is subject #6, which is discussed below.

Figures 3 and 4 exhibit characteristic examples of RRI peak-triggered averaged RRI, breathing and BOLD waves. Both figures have in common that they represent subjects with nRSA showing slow neural BOLD waves in the brainstem and PCG as well as slow BOLD waves with superimposed fast wavelets in the amygdala (ROI 41). However, there exists an interesting difference. Subject #18, on the one hand, presented a strong information flow from RRI to the respiratory signal (Figure 4C) and from the MFG to respiration and brainstem (not shown). On the other hand, in subject #11, the information flow from respiration to RRI was dominant (Figure 3C) and also the flow from brainstem to the PCG (not shown). It is speculated that in the former case (#18R1), nasal breathing was predominant, while in the latter case (#11R1), a second possible pathway was active. This second pathway is thought to originate from the preBötzinger complex and to project to the suprapontine nuclei (via the locus coeruleus in the pons and olfactory nuclei [71] as well as to the central medial thalamus, which is directly connected to the limbic and sensorimotor cortical areas [72]. The nasal route of breathing seems to have particular importance for breathing-entrained oscillations [37,73–75] as is discussed in more detail below. Further research is necessary to specifically study the importance of nasal breathing for the management of anxiety.

4.1.2. Fast Breathing during High Anxiety (Groups 2 and 3)

Group 2 consists of six subjects, which presented respiratory oscillations in the HF band. In all except one (subject #24), RRI oscillations were predominant in the 0.1–0.2 Hz band. In four subjects of this group, AS values did not decrease or even increased from session R1 to session R4 (see Figure 8).

All six subjects in group 2 displayed delayed slow BOLD oscillations in the left PFC and the left brainstem, similar to that observed in group 1. Typically, RRI oscillations and respiration were coupled at higher integer rate ratios such as 1:2 or 1:3 (for an example, see Figure 5). Despite these high-integer rate ratios, there was also tight phase-coupling. This is in accordance with observations from motor-respiratory coupling studies demonstrating that a near-integer rate ratio favors stable entrainment [76]. Only in three subjects, the portion of nRSA was clearly higher than the portion of RSA; in the others, RSA and nRSA had a similar incidence or RSA even prevailed (see Table 1).

The most interesting part in this group is the highly significant information flow from MFG to the brainstem, to respiration and to RRI signals in the 0.2–0.4 Hz band (see Figure 7). Such a directed flow is characteristic for brain rhythms in the 0.1–0.2 Hz band entrained by nasal respiration and was recently reported and discussed [48]. The present results demonstrate that respiratory entrainment of brain rhythms is not confined to the 0.1–0.2 Hz band but also exists in the 0.2–0.4 Hz band.

Subject #6 (group 3) represents a particular case, as they were the only subject with high anxiety and vascular BOLD oscillations. This participant showed slow RRI and fast respiratory oscillations but no slow BOLD oscillations after slow RRI oscillations (Figure 6). The implications of this specific observation are discussed below.

4.2. Coupling of Respiration with Heart and Brain Oscillatory Activity

4.2.1. Phase-Shifts in Respiration-Related RRI Oscillations and Activation of a Central Pacemaker

The RRI increase is never an isolated process and is always accompanied by a simultaneous desynchronization of EEG alpha and/or beta rhythms. One example of the common RRI increase and EEG desynchronization is the Orienting Reflex [77,78], another the decision-making process [79]. Changes in EEG activity are associated with metabolic processes and a causal BOLD response [80]. As in the case of nRSA, the increase of RRIs coincides with inspiration (activation of the preBötzinger complex), the corresponding BOLD response is of large magnitude. Dominant slow BOLD oscillations in the brainstem, therefore, point more to nRSA than to RSA.

Among cardio-respiratory interactions, the respiratory modulation of the cardiac RRI (RSA) is certainly the most prominent one [5,11,39]. For classical RSA, it is widely accepted that the respiratory rhythm is the leading one entraining the fluctuations of RRI [2,17,30]. However, this is not the only phase-relation induced by cardio-respiratory coupling. A detailed analysis of cardio-respiratory phase-relations demonstrated an inverse phase-relation, termed negative RSA (nRSA) and many phase-relations summarized as indefinite RSA [32]. Such phase-shifts are thought to result from a change in the direction of entrainment between the cardiac and the respiratory rhythm. The wave-by-wave analysis is an appropriate instrument to characterize frequency and phase coupling [29]. It allows to differentiate changes in rate ratios, which may result from simple rate changes, from true modulations of coupling as may be indicated by shifts in the phase-relation between the coupled rhythms. These modulations can give hints on the dominance of the rhythms. Using a wave-by-wave analysis, we recently demonstrated that nRSA was mostly associated with a change in dominance, i.e., the RRI rhythm was the leading rhythm and entrained the respiratory rhythm [30]. This was confirmed by the present results of the DTF analysis revealing a significant information flow from the RRI to the respiratory rhythm (see Figure 7). However, only few of our subjects showed prevailing nRSA in the recorded sessions. Many subjects presented both RSA and nRSA at similar percentages (see Table 1), indicating that such a switching in dominance is a rather occasional event.

As nRSA is an untypical coupling pattern, it is unclear which factors may promote the change of dominance and the switching in the cardio-respiratory phase-relation from the common RSA pattern to the inverse nRSA pattern. The activation of an additional neural rhythm integrated in the cardio-respiratory coupling might account for the supposed change of dominance. Such phenomena have often been reported in studies on motor-respiratory coupling [76,81–83]. Usually, coupling between two or more concomitant rhythms is based on a mutual interaction. This means that the dominance can fluctuate, so that each of the concomitant rhythmic processes can take the lead for a limited interval of time. If three or more oscillators are coupled, synchronization between two oscillators (e.g., acoustic pacing of limb rhythms or synchronous activity of several muscle groups) increases their frequency- and phase-locking effects onto a third one (e.g., respiration) and stabilizes coupling [81,84–86]. In a previous study, we investigated PLV-derived time delays between slow RRI oscillations and slow BOLD signals in the frequency range of 0.10–0.15 Hz and showed that neural BOLD oscillations lagging behind the RRI waves indicate activation of a central pacemaker [33]. Such a pacemaker activity located in the reticular formation of the brainstem operating in the frequency range around 0.15 Hz has been proposed by Perlitz and co-workers [87]. This "0.15-Hz rhythm" that was observed both in men and dogs was synchronized with all cardiovascular-respiratory oscillations. Of note, this synchronization is not confined to 1:1 coupling but also includes higher integer rate ratios [87]. This one or a similar rhythm might be candidates reflecting pacemaker-like processes activated during emotional regulation and anxiety management, which may account for a switching in dominance. The assumption that activation of a central pacemaker-like mechanism is involved in the management of scanner-related anxiety is supported by stable phase-coupling between respiratory and RRI oscillations at 1:1 or at higher integer rate ratios and by the occurrence of slow neural BOLD oscillations in nine of ten subjects of the present study. Another support, in the reverse direction, comes from subject #6 presenting slow RRI oscillations and vascular BOLD oscillations, but no slow neural BOLD oscillations. If no pacemaker in the brainstem is activated, no associated BOLD oscillations can be expected in the brainstem or in the cortex. Moreover, a DTF analysis recently revealed a significant information flow in the 0.1–0.2 Hz band from the pons to the precentral cortex and to the RRI signal. This flow was interpreted to result from the activation of a rhythmic neural source in the brain stem operating at about 0.15 Hz (such as Perlitz' "0.15-Hz rhythm") [48]. However, the nature of the hypothesized pacemaker or pacemakers cannot be identified from the present data. In particular, neural processes involved in autonomic regulation would be candidates of interest. A recent study on causal relations among heart period, systolic arterial pressure and respiration and their interactions with autonomic control showed that bidirectional interactions between cardiac and respiratory rhythms were not modified by parasympathetic or sympathetic blockade [88].

4.2.2. Respiration-Entrained Brain Oscillations and Possible Strategies of Anxiety Management

The respiratory rhythm provides a continuous rhythmic modulation of cortical neuronal activity that, in turn, modulates autonomic, sensorimotor, cognitive and emotional processes [17,84,89,90]. Respiration-entrained oscillations in neural activity are ubiquitous in the brain. They have mostly been described in rodents, e.g., in the parietal and in the frontal cortex [91,92], but also in large areas of the human cortex [75,90,93]. Of note, most of these observations in humans were mostly made during nasal breathing, indicating a particular role of the olfactory tract [37,73–75]. Nasal breathing induces rhythmical bursting of olfactory receptor neurons, which in turn entrains activity of the olfactory bulb and the piriform cortex [75]. Moreover, respiration can entrain the activity of various cortical and subcortical structures such as the prefrontal cortex, amygdala and hippocampus [37,91,93], thus forming a wide-spread network of respiration-modulated brain oscillation across all major frequency bands [73]. Nasal respiration significantly modulated cortical excitability, and these changes were followed by respiration-locked changes in perceptual sensitivity [74]. A comparison of oral and nasal breathing revealed a significant influence of the nasal but not the oral respiratory phase on the performance of emotion and memory tasks, which were closely related to the function of the amygdala and hippocampus [37], thus suggesting a role of the nasal route of breathing in emotional regulation.

As healthy awake subjects predominantly breathe through their nose, it is likely that nasal breathing might also be preferred in the subjects of the present study. We would therefore assume that respiration-entrained oscillations in cortical and limbic areas are involved in the strategies of anxiety management. Upward flows from respiration to cortical and pontine ROIs as well as to RRI have been observed in the present study even though they seemed unimportant in comparison to the highly predominant downward flows from MFG to the brainstem and to RRI and respiration (see Figure 7). We would speculate that one or more pacemakers operating in a frequency range centered at ~0.10 Hz and/or ~0.16 Hz are activated through nasal breathing. These pacemakers may primarily entrain the RRI rhythm, and the coupled rhythms then entrain the rhythm generated by the medullary respiratory neurons. This means a reduced dominance of the respiratory rhythm over the RRI rhythm that favors a shift in the phase-relation towards nRSA. Alternatively, the pacemaker rhythm primarily entrains the medullary respiratory rhythm, which subsequently entrains rhythms in other parts of the brain such as in the middle frontal cortex and in the brainstem. In this case, respiration also entrains the RRI rhythm, which may stabilize (classical) RSA. The results suggest that activation of one or more pacemakers operating especially in the 0.1–0.2 Hz band may be an important mechanism of managing high anxiety. The particular case of subject 6 presenting no neural BOLD waves indicates that activation of such a pacemaker is not the only way of successful anxiety processing.

In turn, the reduction of anxiety over the total fMRI experiment varied widely among the 9 subjects with neural BOLD oscillations where activation of a pacemaker can be assumed. Another important mechanism for successfully managing anxiety is slow breathing as can be concluded from the comparison between groups 1 and 2. Since hundreds of years, slow breathing has been used in various human societies, particularly in eastern cultures, for strategies of calming down, relaxing and emotional processing such as in yoga, qigong or other types of meditation (for a review, see [94]). Resonance breathing at about 6 breaths/min as used in biofeedback training has been reported to increase the amplitude of heart rate variability, which is considered to contribute to stress reduction and emotional regulation [26,27]. Nasal breathing is an essential component of such breathing techniques [95,96].

4.3. Limitations and Future Directions

This study has several limitations. A major limitation is that measurement of respiration did not allow to differentiate between nasal and oral breathing. The nasal route of breathing, especially the olfactory tract, seems to have particular importance for entrainment of brain rhythms to respiration [37,73–75]. We have good reason to suppose that our subjects mainly performed nasal breathing as healthy awake subjects prefer to breathe through their nose, but we cannot estimate whether and to which extent oral breathing may have contributed to their breathing pattern. For accurate assessment of the proposed mechanisms, a comparative study with nasal and oral breathing is necessary.

A further limitation of the study is that assessment of anxiety was only based on questionnaires for AS values. This was mainly due to the original intention of the fMRI study. At the time of planning the experiment, the main interest was directed on the initiation of self-paced movements and their relation to 0.1 Hz brain oscillations. The question of scanner-related anxiety came into focus during the experiments and the evaluation period. Therefore, no further psychophysiological measure of anxiety such as the skin conductance response was included.

The original intention of the fMRI experiment as described above may also account for the lack of collecting more data, reflecting autonomic regulation and autonomic functions. For instance, examination of further respiratory parameters such as tidal volume, ventilation or end-tidal partial pressure of CO_2 might indicate a possible hyperventilation, which, in turn, affects CBF. Continuous blood pressure measurements would provide more information on the relation of the baroreflex pathway with the RSA patterns observed in this study. In addition, those parameters might corroborate the information obtained by the AS values.

Many chronic cardiovascular diseases are associated with affection of HRV, in particular, with a change in HRV magnitude even up to abolishment of RSA [7,16,17]. Reduced HRV magnitude is also characteristic for emotional dysregulation [20,23] and for sympathetic activation [15]. In the present study, we focused on the phase-relationship between respiratory and RRI rhythms and did not explicitly analyze the amplitude of respiration-related RRI oscillations. This is a limitation as the amplitude of HRV may give additional information, e.g., on the sympathetic or vagal activation in the processing of anxiety. Future studies on interactions between heart, respiration and brain signals should include analyses of HRV magnitude.

Previously, we have applied a wave-by-wave analysis to characterize the coupling between respiration and RRI oscillations. Using this method, we were able to exactly assess the phase-relations between these rhythms and to identify nRSA, preferably in subjects with slow breathing and slow RRI waves [29]. The specific cardio-respiratory phase-relations (RSA or nRSA) may be masked when the respiratory rate considerably differs from the rate of RRI oscillations as reflected in a predominance of 1:2, 1:3 or even higher cardio-respiratory rate ratios. The main problem with high breathing rates and higher-integer cardio-respiratory rate ratios is that the number of cardiac periods per breath decreases at higher breathing rates, thus complicating the assessment of RRI changes during inspiration or expiration. In addition, only every second or third breath is included in the analysis of phase-relations between respiratory and RRI oscillations. As a result, the number of evaluated periods was reduced, and the percentage of indefinite RSA increased while the portion of positive or negative RSA types decreased.

The wave-by-wave analysis allows a precise and reliable assessment of cardio-respiratory phase relations if (a) the period durations (PD) of RRI waves and breathing cycles are similar, i.e., the rate ratio between RRI and breathing waves is about 1:1, and (b) both rhythms are slow (below ~0.2 Hz), that means, in the low-frequency (LF) and intermediate-frequency (IMF) bands. With respiratory and/or RRI waves at higher rates, detection of nRSA according to wave-by-wave analysis contains a degree of uncertainty and has only limited significance. The results of this study demonstrated that the combination with causal coupling analysis outweighs this disadvantage and provides additional and more detailed information, in particular in the HF band. The slight discrepancies between the results of the two analysis methods can easily be explained by the different meanings of the results: The directed information flow characterizes the cause while the phase-relationship characterizes the consequence of the modulation in the coupling between cardio-respiratory and brain rhythms.

5. Conclusions

Previous studies on participants of fMRI examinations showed that persons with elevated anxiety presented a rather unusual cardio-respiratory coupling pattern characterized by an inverse phase-relation (compared to the normal RSA), termed as nRSA [29,70]. We had hypothesized that a "central pacemaker", which is involved in emotional regulation and activated in situations of elevated anxiety, would entrain the RRI rhythm and thus modulate cardio-respiratory coupling [30]. The present results revealed a prevalence of neural BOLD oscillations in the brain stem, supporting this assumption. In addition, the DTF analyses revealed a strong directed information flow from the RRI rhythm to the respiratory rhythm, thus providing additional support to this hypothesis. Moreover, DTF analysis data indicated that respiration-entrained brain oscillations are involved in strategies of anxiety regulation. However, further research is necessary to prove this assumption.

Author Contributions: Conceptualization, B.R. and G.P.; methodology, data processing, statistics, K.B., M.K. and B.R.; writing—original draft preparation, B.R.; writing—review and editing, K.B. and G.P.; visualization, G.P., K.B. and B.R. All authors have read and agreed to the published version of the manuscript.

Funding: This research received no external funding.

Institutional Review Board Statement: The study was conducted in accordance with the Declaration of Helsinki, and approved by the local Ethics Committee at the University of Graz (number: GZ. 39/75/63 ex 2013/14).

Informed Consent Statement: Written informed consent was obtained from all subjects involved in the study.

Data Availability Statement: Not applicable.

Acknowledgments: We like to thank David Fink for support in data acquisition, Clemens Brunner for support in data processing and Andreas Schwerdtfeger for evaluations of state anxiety (all of them from University of Graz). The authors acknowledge support from the German Research Foundation (DFG) and Universität Leipzig within the program of Open Access Publishing.

Conflicts of Interest: The authors declare no conflict of interest.

References

1. Eckberg, D.L. Human sinus arrhythmia as an index of vagal cardiac outflow. *J. Appl. Physiol.* **1983**, *54*, 961–966. [CrossRef]
2. Hayano, J.; Yasuma, F.; Okada, A.; Mukai, S.; Fujinami, T. Respiratory sinus arrhythmia. A phenomenon improving pulmonary gas exchange and circulatory efficiency. *Circulation* **1996**, *94*, 842–847. [CrossRef] [PubMed]
3. Grossman, P.; Taylor, E.W. Toward understanding respiratory sinus arrhythmia: Relations to cardiac vagal tone, evolution and biobehavioral functions. *Biol. Psychol.* **2007**, *74*, 263–285. [CrossRef] [PubMed]
4. Yasuma, F.; Hayano, J. Respiratory sinus arrhythmia: Why does the heartbeat synchronize with respiratory rhythm? *Chest* **2004**, *125*, 683–690. [CrossRef]
5. Karemaker, J.M. Counterpoint: Respiratory sinus arrhythmia is due to the baroreflex mechanism. *J. Appl. Physiol.* **2009**, *106*, 1742–1743. [CrossRef]
6. Akselrod, S.; Gordon, D.; Ubel, F.; Shannon, D.; Berger, A.; Cohen, R.J. Power spectrum analysis of heart rate fluctuation: A quantitative probe of beat-to-beat cardiovascular control. *Science* **1981**, *213*, 220–222. [CrossRef] [PubMed]
7. Task Force of the European Society of Cardiology and the North American Society of Pacing and Electrophysiology. Heart rate variability: Standards of measurement, physiological interpretation and clinical use. *Circulation* **1996**, *93*, 1043–1065. [CrossRef]
8. Pagani, M.; Lombardi, F.; Guzzetti, S.; Rimoldi, O.; Furlan, R.; Pizzinelli, P.; Sandrone, G.; Malfatto, G.; Dell'Orto, S.; Piccaluga, E.; et al. Power spectral analysis of heart rate and arterial pressure variabilities as a marker of sympatho-vagal interaction in man and conscious dog. *Circ. Res.* **1986**, *59*, 178–193. [CrossRef] [PubMed]
9. Malliani, A.; Pagani, M.; Lombardi, F.; Cerutti, S. Cardiovascular neural regulation explored in the frequency domain. *Circulation* **1991**, *84*, 482–492. [CrossRef]
10. Eckberg, D.L. The human respiratory gate. *J. Physiol.* **2003**, *548*, 339–352. [CrossRef]
11. Eckberg, D.L. Point:counterpoint: Respiratory sinus arrhythmia is due to a central mechanism vs. respiratory sinus arrhythmia is due to the baroreflex mechanism. *J. Appl. Physiol.* **2009**, *106*, 1740–1742. [CrossRef] [PubMed]
12. Haselton, J.R.; Guyenet, P.G. Central respiratory modulation of medullary sympathoexcitatory neurons in rat. *Am. J. Physiol.* **1989**, *256*, R739–R750. [CrossRef] [PubMed]

13. Häbler, H.J.; Jänig, W.; Krummel, M.; Peters, O.A. Respiratory modulation of the activity in postganglionic neurons supplying skeletal muscle and skin of the rat hindlimb. *J. Neurophysiol.* **1993**, *70*, 920–930. [CrossRef] [PubMed]
14. Mandel, D.A.; Schreihofer, A.M. Central respiratory modulation of barosensitive neurones in rat caudal ventrolateral medulla. *J. Physiol.* **2006**, *572*, 881–896. [CrossRef]
15. Porta, A.; Bassani, T.; Bari, V.; Tobaldini, E.; Takahashi, A.C.; Catai, A.M.; Montano, N. Model-based assessment of baroreflex and cardiopulmonary couplings during graded head-up tilt. *Comput. Biol. Med.* **2012**, *42*, 298–305. [CrossRef] [PubMed]
16. Machado, B.H.; Zoccal, D.B.; Moraes, D.J.A. Neurogenic hypertension and the secrets of respiration. *Am. J. Physiol. Regul. Integr. Comp. Physiol.* **2017**, *312*, R864–R872. [CrossRef] [PubMed]
17. Menuet, C.; Connelly, A.A.; Bassi, J.K.; Melo, M.R.; Le, S.; Kamar, J.; Kumar, N.N.; McDougall, S.J.; McMullan, S.; Allen, A.M. PreBötzinger complex neurons drive respiratory modulation of blood pressure and heart rate. *eLife* **2020**, *9*, e57288. [CrossRef]
18. Thayer, J.F.; Friedman, B.H.; Borkovec, T.D. Autonomic characteristics of generalized anxiety disorder and worry. *Biol. Psychiatry* **1996**, *39*, 255–266. [CrossRef]
19. Watkins, L.L.; Grossman, P.; Krishnan, R.; Sherwood, A. Anxiety and vagal control of heart rate. *Psychosom. Med.* **1998**, *60*, 498–502. [CrossRef]
20. Licht, C.M.; de Geus, E.J.; van Dyck, R.; Penninx, B.W. Association between anxiety disorders and heart rate variability in The Netherlands Study of Depression and Anxiety (NESDA). *Psychosom. Med.* **2009**, *71*, 508–518. [CrossRef]
21. Jönsson, P. Respiratory sinus arrhythmia as a function of state anxiety in healthy individuals. *Int. J. Psychophysiol.* **2007**, *63*, 48–54. [CrossRef] [PubMed]
22. Battaglia, S.; Orsolini, S.; Borgomaneri, S.; Barbieri, R.; Diciotti, S.; di Pellegrino, G. Characterizing cardiac autonomic dynamics of fear learning in humans. *Psychophysiology* **2022**, *59*, e14122. [CrossRef] [PubMed]
23. Cattaneo, L.A.; Franquillo, A.C.; Grecucci, A.; Beccia, L.; Caretti, V.; Dadomo, H. Is Low Heart Rate Variability Associated with Emotional Dysregulation, Psychopathological Dimensions, and Prefrontal Dysfunctions? An Integrative View. *J. Pers. Med.* **2021**, *11*, 872. [CrossRef] [PubMed]
24. Battaglia, S.; Thayer, J.F. Functional interplay between central and autonomic nervous systems in human fear conditioning. *Trends Neurosci.* **2022**, *45*, 504–506. [CrossRef] [PubMed]
25. Shaffer, F.; Ginsberg, J.P. An Overview of Heart Rate Variability Metrics and Norms. *Front. Public Health* **2017**, *5*, 258. [CrossRef] [PubMed]
26. Steffen, P.R.; Austin, T.; DeBarros, A.; Brown, T. The Impact of Resonance Frequency Breathing on Measures of Heart Rate Variability, Blood Pressure, and Mood. *Front. Public Health* **2017**, *5*, 222. [CrossRef]
27. Lehrer, P. How does heart rate variability biofeedback work? Resonance, the baroreflex, and other mechanisms. *Biofeedback* **2013**, *41*, 26–31. [CrossRef]
28. Mather, M.; Thayer, J.F. How heart rate variability affects emotion regulation brain networks. *Curr. Opin. Behav. Sci.* **2018**, *19*, 98–104. [CrossRef] [PubMed]
29. Rassler, B.; Schwerdtfeger, A.; Aigner, C.S.; Pfurtscheller, G. Switch-off" of respiratory sinus arrhythmia can occur in a minority of subjects during functional magnetic resonance imaging (fMRI). *Front. Physiol.* **2018**, *9*, 1688. [CrossRef]
30. Rassler, B.; Schwerdtfeger, A.R.; Schwarz, G.; Pfurtscheller, G. Negative respiratory sinus arrhythmia (nRSA) in the MRI-scanner—A physiologic phenomenon observed during elevated anxiety in healthy persons. *Physiol. Behav.* **2022**, *245*, 113676. [CrossRef]
31. Yli-Hankala, A.; Porkkala, T.; Kaukinen, S.; Häkkinen, V.; Jäntti, V. Respiratory sinus arrhythmia is reversed during positive pressure ventilation. *Acta Physiol. Scand.* **1991**, *141*, 399–407. [CrossRef] [PubMed]
32. Carvalho, N.C.; Beda, A.; de Abreu, M.G.; Spieth, P.M.; Granja-Filho, P.; Jandre, F.C.; Giannella-Neto, A. Comparison of objective methods to classify the pattern of respiratory sinus arrhythmia during mechanical ventilation and paced spontaneous breathing. *Physiol. Meas.* **2009**, *30*, 1151–1162. [CrossRef] [PubMed]
33. Pfurtscheller, G.; Schwerdtfeger, A.; Rassler, B.; Andrade, A.; Schwarz, G.; Klimesch, W. Verification of a central pacemaker in brain stem by phase-coupling analysis between HR interval- and BOLD-oscillations in the 0.10–0.15 Hz frequency band. *Front. Neurosci.* **2020**, *14*, 922. [CrossRef] [PubMed]
34. Murphy, K.; Birn, R.M.; Bandettini, P.A. Resting-state fMRI confounds and cleanup. *Neuroimage* **2013**, *80*, 349–359. [CrossRef]
35. Huneau, C.; Benali, H.; Chabriat, H. Investigating Human Neurovascular Coupling Using Functional Neuroimaging: A Critical Review of Dynamic Models. *Front. Neurosci.* **2015**, *9*, 467. [CrossRef]
36. Bari, V.; De Maria, B.; Mazzucco, C.E.; Rossato, G.; Tonon, D.; Nollo, G.; Faes, L.; Porta, A. Cerebrovascular and cardiovascular variability interactions investigated through conditional joint transfer entropy in subjects prone to postural syncope. *Physiol. Meas.* **2017**, *38*, 976–991. [CrossRef]
37. Zelano, C.; Jiang, H.; Zhou, G.; Arora, N.; Schuele, S.; Rosenow, J.; Gottfried, J.A. Nasal Respiration Entrains Human Limbic Oscillations and Modulates Cognitive Function. *J. Neurosci.* **2016**, *36*, 12448–12467. [CrossRef]
38. Valenza, G.; Passamonti, L.; Duggento, A.; Toschi, N.; Barbieri, R. Uncovering complex central autonomic networks at rest: A functional magnetic resonance imaging study on complex cardiovascular oscillations. *J. R. Soc. Interface* **2020**, *17*, 20190878. [CrossRef]
39. Faes, L.; Porta, A.; Cucino, R.; Cerutti, S.; Antolini, R.; Nollo, G. Causal transfer function analysis to describe closed loop interactions between cardiovascular and cardiorespiratory variability signals. *Biol. Cybern.* **2004**, *90*, 390–399. [CrossRef]

40. Faes, L.; Nollo, G.; Porta, A. Non-uniform multivariate embedding to assess the information transfer in cardiovascular and cardiorespiratory variability series. *Comput. Biol. Med.* **2011**, *42*, 290–297. [CrossRef]
41. Porta, A.; Bassani, T.; Bari, V.; Pinna, G.D.; Maestri, R.; Guzzetti, S. Accounting for respiration is necessary to reliably infer Granger causality from cardiovascular variability series. *IEEE Trans. Biomed. Eng.* **2012**, *59*, 832–841. [CrossRef] [PubMed]
42. Mrowka, R.; Cimponeriu, L.; Patzak, A.; Rosenblum, M.G. Directionality of coupling of physiological subsystems: Age-related changes of cardiorespiratory interaction during different sleep stages in babies. *Am. J. Physiol. Regul. Integr. Comp. Physiol.* **2003**, *285*, R1395–R1401. [CrossRef] [PubMed]
43. Shiogai, Y.; Stefanovska, A.; McClintock, P.V.E. Nonlinear dynamics of cardiovascular ageing. *Phys. Rep.* **2010**, *488*, 51–110. [CrossRef]
44. Bhattacharya, J.; Pereda, E.; Petsche, H. Effective detection of coupling in short and noisy bivariate data. *IEEE Trans. Syst. Man. Cybern. B Cybern.* **2003**, *33*, 85–95. [CrossRef]
45. Borovkova, E.I.; Prokhorov, M.D.; Kiselev, A.R.; Hramkov, A.N.; Mironov, S.A.; Agaltsov, M.V.; Ponomarenko, V.I.; Karavaev, A.S.; Drapkina, O.M.; Penzel, T. Directional couplings between the respiration and parasympathetic control of the heart rate during sleep and wakefulness in healthy subjects at different ages. *Front. Netw. Physiol.* **2022**, *2*, 942700. [CrossRef] [PubMed]
46. Granger, C.W.J. Investigating causal relations by econometric models and cross-spectral methods. *Econometrica* **1969**, *37*, 424. [CrossRef]
47. Lachert, P.; Zygierewicz, J.; Janusek, D.; Pulawski, P.; Sawosz, P.; Kacprzak, M.; Liebert, A.; Blinowska, K.J. Causal Coupling Between Electrophysiological Signals, Cerebral Hemodynamics and Systemic Blood Supply Oscillations in Mayer Wave Frequency Range. *Int. J. Neural Syst.* **2019**, *29*, 1850033. [CrossRef]
48. Pfurtscheller, G.; Blinowska, K.J.; Kaminski, M.; Rassler, B.; Klimesch, W. Processing of fMRI-related anxiety and information flow between brain and body revealed a preponderance of oscillations at 0.15/0.16 Hz. *Sci. Rep.* **2022**, *12*, 9117. [CrossRef]
49. Laux, L.; Hock, M.; Bergner-Koether, R.; Hodapp, V.; Renner, K.H.; Merzbacher, G. *Das State-Trait-Angst-Depressions-Inventar [The State-Trait Anxiety-Depression Inventory]*; Hogrefe: Goettingen, Germany, 2013.
50. Spielberger, C.D.; Gorssuch, R.L.; Lushene, P.R.; Vagg, P.R.; Jacobs, G. *Manual for the State-Trait Anxiety Inventory*; Consulting Psychologists Press Inc.: Palo Alto, CA, USA, 2009.
51. Niazy, R.K.; Beckmann, C.F.; Iannetti, G.D.; Brady, J.M.; Smith, S.M. Removal of fMRI environment artifacts from EEG data using optimal basis sets. *Neuroimage* **2005**, *28*, 720–737. [CrossRef]
52. Kugel, H.; Bremer, C.; Peschel, M.; Fischbach, R.; Lenzen, H.; Tombach, B.; Van Aken, H.; Heindel, W. Hazardous situation in the MR bore: Induction in ECG leads causes fire. *Eur. Radiol.* **2003**, *13*, 690–694. [CrossRef]
53. Tarvainen, M.P.; Niskanen, J.-P.; Lipponen, J.A.; Ranta-Aho, P.O.; Karjalainen, P.A. Kubios HRV—Heart rate variability analysis software. *Comput. Methods Programs Biomed.* **2014**, *113*, 210–220. [CrossRef]
54. Obrig, H.; Neufang, M.; Wenzel, R.; Kohl, M.; Steinbrink, J.; Einhäupl, K.; Villringer, A. Spontaneous low frequency oscillations of ccerebral hemodynamics and metabolism in human adults. *Neuroimage* **2000**, *12*, 623–639. [CrossRef]
55. Buxton, R.B.; Uludag, K.; Dubowitz, D.J.; Liu, T.T. Modeling the hemodynamic response to brain activation. *Neuroimage* **2004**, *23*, 220–233. [CrossRef]
56. Verberne, A.J.M.; Owens, N.C. Cortical modulation of the cardiovascular system. *Progr. Neurobiol.* **1998**, *54*, 149–168. [CrossRef]
57. Thayer, J.F.; Lane, R.D. Claude Bernard and the heart-brain connection: Further elaboration of a model of neurovisceral integration. *Neurosci. Biobehav. Rev.* **2009**, *33*, 81–88. [CrossRef] [PubMed]
58. Moeller, S.; Yacoub, E.; Olman, C.A.; Auerbach, E.; Strupp, J.; Harel, N.; Uğurbil, K. Multiband multislice GE-EPI at 7 Tesla, with 16-fold acceleration using partial parallel imaging with application to high spatial and temporal whole-brain fMRI. *Magn. Reson. Med.* **2010**, *63*, 1144–1153. [CrossRef] [PubMed]
59. Tzourio-Mazoyer, N.; Landeau, B.; Papathanassiou, D.; Crivello, F.; Etard, O.; Delcroix, N.; Mazoyer, B.; Joliot, M. Automated anatomical labeling of activations in SPM using a macroscopic anatomical parcellation of the MNI MRI single-subject brain. *Neuroimage* **2002**, *15*, 273–289. [CrossRef]
60. Pfurtscheller, G.; Blinowska, K.J.; Kaminski, M.; Schwerdtfeger, A.R.; Rassler, B.; Schwarz, G.; Klimesch, W. Processing of fMRI-related anxiety and bi-directional information flow between prefrontal cortex and brainstem. *Sci. Rep.* **2021**, *11*, 22348. [CrossRef] [PubMed]
61. Grinsted, A.; Moore, J.C.; Jevrejeva, S. Application of the cross wavelet transform and wavelet coherence to geophysical time series. *Nonlinear Process. Geophys.* **2004**, *11*, 561–566. [CrossRef]
62. Lachaux, J.; Rodriguez, E.; Martinerie, J.; Varela, F.J. Measuring phase synchrony in brain signals. *Hum. Brain Mapp.* **1999**, *208*, 194–208. [CrossRef]
63. Hurtado, J.M.; Rubchinsky, L.L.; Sigvardt, K.A. Statistical method for detection of phase-locking episodes in neural oscillations. *J. Neurophysiol.* **2004**, *91*, 1883–1898. [CrossRef]
64. Pfurtscheller, G.; Schwerdtfeger, A.; Seither-Preisler, A.; Brunner, C.; Aigner, C.S.; Brito, J.; Carmo, M.P.; Andrade, A. Brain-heart communication: Evidence for "central pacemaker" oscillations with a dominant frequency at 0.1 Hz in the cingulum. *Clin. Neurophysiol.* **2017**, *128*, 183–193. [CrossRef]
65. Kaminski, M.J.; Blinowska, K.J. A new method of the description of the information flow in the brain structures. *Biol. Cybern.* **1991**, *65*, 203–210. [CrossRef] [PubMed]

66. Blinowska, K.J.; Kuś, R.; Kamiński, M. Granger causality and information flow in multivariate processes. *Phys. Rev. E Stat. Nonlin. Soft Matter Phys.* **2004**, *70*, 050902. [CrossRef] [PubMed]
67. Geweke, J. Measurement of Linear Dependence and Feedback between Multiple Time Series. *J. Am. Stat. Assoc.* **1982**, *77*, 304–313. [CrossRef]
68. Schulz, S.; Adochiei, F.C.; Edu, I.R.; Schroeder, R.; Costin, H.; Bär, K.J.; Voss, A. Cardiovascular and cardiorespiratory coupling analyses: A review. *Philos. Trans. R. Soc. A* **2013**, *37*, 20120191. [CrossRef] [PubMed]
69. Klimesch, W. The frequency architecture of brain and body oscillations: An analysis. *Eur. J. Neurosci.* **2018**, *48*, 2431–2453. [CrossRef]
70. Pfurtscheller, G.; Rassler, B.; Schwerdtfeger, A.; Klimesch, W.; Andrade, A.; Schwarz, G.; Thayer, J.F. "Switch-off" of respiratory sinus arrhythmia may be associated with the activation of an oscillatory source (pacemaker) in the brain stem. *Front. Physiol.* **2019**, *10*, 939. [CrossRef]
71. Del Negro, C.A.; Funk, G.D.; Feldman, J.L. Breathing matters. *Nat. Rev. Neurosci.* **2018**, *19*, 351–367. [CrossRef]
72. Yang, C.F.; Feldman, J.L. Efferent projections of excitatory and inhibitory preBötzinger Complex neurons. *J. Comp. Neurol.* **2018**, *526*, 1389–1402. [CrossRef]
73. Kluger, D.S.; Gross, J. Respiration modulates oscillatory neural network activity at rest. *PLoS Biol.* **2021**, *19*, e3001457. [CrossRef] [PubMed]
74. Kluger, D.S.; Balestrieri, E.; Busch, N.A.; Gross, J. Respiration aligns perception with neural excitability. *eLife* **2021**, *10*, e70907. [CrossRef] [PubMed]
75. Watanabe, T.; Itagaki, A.; Hashizume, A.; Takahashi, A.; Ishizaka, R.; Ozaki, I. Observation of respiration-entrained brain oscillations with scalp EEG. *Neurosci. Lett.* **2023**, *797*, 137079. [CrossRef] [PubMed]
76. Ebert, D.; Rassler, B.; Hefter, H. Coordination between breathing and forearm movements during sinusoidal tracking. *Eur. J. Appl. Physiol.* **2000**, *81*, 288–296. [CrossRef] [PubMed]
77. Sokolov, E.N. *Perception and the Conditioned Reflex*; Pergamon: Oxford, UK, 1963.
78. Barry, R.J.; Rushby, J.A. An orienting reflex perspective on anteriorisation of the P3 of the event-related potential. *Exp. Brain Res.* **2006**, *173*, 539–545. [CrossRef]
79. Pfurtscheller, G.; Solis-Escalante, T.; Barry, R.J.; Klobassa, D.S.; Neuper, C.; Müller-Putz, G.R. Brisk heart rate and EEG changes during execution and withholding of cue-paced foot motor imagery. *Front. Hum. Neurosci.* **2013**, *7*, 379. [CrossRef]
80. Logothetis, N.K.; Pauls, J.; Augath, M.; Trinath, T.; Oeltermann, A. Neurophysiological investigation of the basis of the fMRI signal. *Nature* **2001**, *412*, 150–157. [CrossRef]
81. Rassler, B.; Kohl, J. Coordination-related changes in the rhythms of breathing and walking in humans. *Eur. J. Appl. Physiol.* **2000**, *82*, 280–288. [CrossRef]
82. McDermott, W.J.; Van Emmerik, R.E.; Hamill, J. Running training and adaptive strategies of locomotor-respiratory coordination. *Eur. J. Appl. Physiol.* **2003**, *89*, 435–444. [CrossRef]
83. O'Halloran, J.; Hamill, J.; McDermott, W.J.; Remelius, J.G.; Van Emmerik, R.E. Locomotor-respiratory coupling patterns and oxygen consumption during walking above and below preferred stride frequency. *Eur. J. Appl. Physiol.* **2012**, *112*, 929–940. [CrossRef]
84. Hoffmann, C.P.; Torregrosa, G.; Bardy, B.G. Sound stabilizes locomotor-respiratory coupling and reduces energy cost. *PLoS ONE* **2012**, *7*, e45206. [CrossRef]
85. Rassler, B.; Waurick, S.; Ebert, D. Einfluss zentralnervoser ¨ Koordination im Sinne v. HOLSTs auf die Steuerung von Atem- und Extremit¨ atenmotorik des Menschen [Effect of central coordination in the sense of v. Holst on the control of breathing and limb movements in humans]. *Biol. Cybern.* **1990**, *63*, 457–462. [CrossRef] [PubMed]
86. Bernasconi, P.; Kohl, J. Analysis of co-ordination between breathing and exercise rhythms in man. *J. Physiol.* **1993**, *471*, 693–706. [CrossRef] [PubMed]
87. Perlitz, V.; Lambertz, M.; Cotuk, B.; Grebe, R.; Vandenhouten, R.; Flatten, G.; Petzold, E.R.; Schmid-Schönbein, H.; Langhorst, P. Cardiovascular rhythms in the 0.15-Hz band: Common origin of identical phenomena in man and dog in the reticular formation of the brain stem? *Eur. J. Physiol.* **2004**, *448*, 579–591. [CrossRef]
88. Porta, A.; Castiglioni, P.; Di Rienzo, M.; Bassani, T.; Bari, V.; Faes, L.; Nollo, G.; Cividjan, A.; Quintin, L. Cardiovascular control and time domain Granger causality: Insights from selective autonomic blockade. *Phil. Trans. R. Soc. A* **2013**, *371*, 20120161. [CrossRef] [PubMed]
89. Rassler, B.; Raabe, J. Co-ordination of breathing with rhythmic head and eye movements and with passive turnings of the body. *Eur. J. Appl. Physiol.* **2003**, *90*, 125–130. [CrossRef]
90. Heck, D.H.; McAfee, S.S.; Liu, Y.; Babajani-Feremi, A.; Rezaie, R.; Freeman, W.J.; Wheless, J.W.; Papanicolaou, A.C.; Ruszinkó, M.; Sokolov, Y.; et al. Breathing as a Fundamental Rhythm of Brain Function. *Front. Neural Circuits* **2017**, *10*, 115. [CrossRef]
91. Tort, A.B.L.; Brankačk, J.; Draguhn, A. Respiration-Entrained Brain Rhythms Are Global but Often Overlooked. *Trends Neurosci.* **2018**, *41*, 186–197. [CrossRef]
92. Jung, F.; Yanovsky, Y.; Brankačk, J.; Tort, A.B.L.; Draguhn, A. Respiratory entrainment of units in the mouse parietal cortex depends on vigilance state. *Pflugers Arch.* **2023**, *475*, 65–76. [CrossRef]
93. Herrero, J.L.; Khuvis, S.; Yeagle, E.; Cerf, M.; Mehta, A.D. Breathing above the brain stem: Volitional control and attentional modulation in humans. *J. Neurophysiol.* **2018**, *119*, 145–159. [CrossRef] [PubMed]

94. Zaccaro, A.; Piarulli, A.; Laurino, M.; Garbella, E.; Menicucci, D.; Neri, B.; Gemignani, A. How Breath-Control Can Change Your Life: A Systematic Review on Psycho-Physiological Correlates of Slow Breathing. *Front. Hum. Neurosci.* **2018**, *12*, 353. [CrossRef] [PubMed]
95. Stancák, A., Jr.; Kuna, M. EEG changes during forced alternate nostril breathing. *Int. J. Psychophysiol.* **1994**, *18*, 75–79. [CrossRef] [PubMed]
96. Telles, S.; Verma, S.; Sharma, S.K.; Gupta, R.K.; Balkrishna, A. Alternate-Nostril Yoga Breathing Reduced Blood Pressure While Increasing Performance in a Vigilance Test. *Med. Sci. Monit. Basic Res.* **2017**, *23*, 392–398. [CrossRef] [PubMed]

Disclaimer/Publisher's Note: The statements, opinions and data contained in all publications are solely those of the individual author(s) and contributor(s) and not of MDPI and/or the editor(s). MDPI and/or the editor(s) disclaim responsibility for any injury to people or property resulting from any ideas, methods, instructions or products referred to in the content.

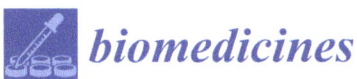

Review

Unraveling the Thread of Aphasia Rehabilitation: A Translational Cognitive Perspective

Georgios Papageorgiou [1,*], Dimitrios Kasselimis [1,2], Nikolaos Laskaris [1,3] and Constantin Potagas [1]

[1] Neuropsychology and Language Disorders Unit, 1st Department of Neurology, Eginition Hospital, National and Kapodistrian University of Athens, 11528 Athens, Greece
[2] Department of Psychology, Panteion University of Social and Political Sciences, 17671 Athens, Greece
[3] Department of Industrial Design and Production Engineering, School of Engineering, University of West Attica, 12241 Athens, Greece
* Correspondence: georgipapageorgiou@gmail.com; Tel.: +30-2107289307; Fax: +30-2107216474

Abstract: Translational neuroscience is a multidisciplinary field that aims to bridge the gap between basic science and clinical practice. Regarding aphasia rehabilitation, there are still several unresolved issues related to the neural mechanisms that optimize language treatment. Although there are studies providing indications toward a translational approach to the remediation of acquired language disorders, the incorporation of fundamental neuroplasticity principles into this field is still in progress. From that aspect, in this narrative review, we discuss some key neuroplasticity principles, which have been elucidated through animal studies and which could eventually be applied in the context of aphasia treatment. This translational approach could be further strengthened by the implementation of intervention strategies that incorporate the idea that language is supported by domain-general mechanisms, which highlights the impact of non-linguistic factors in post-stroke language recovery. Here, we highlight that translational research in aphasia has the potential to advance our knowledge of brain–language relationships. We further argue that advances in this field could lead to improvement in the remediation of acquired language disturbances by remodeling the rationale of aphasia–therapy approaches. Arguably, the complex anatomy and phenomenology of aphasia dictate the need for a multidisciplinary approach with one of its main pillars being translational research.

Keywords: translational neuroscience; neuroplasticity; aphasia; rehabilitation; stroke; language impairment; cognitive recovery; brain; animals; language

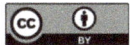

1. Introduction

The principles that govern language rehabilitation remain a perpetual topic of interest in the field of aphasia [1]. In the short history of language treatment, there have been several approaches to the study of aphasia rehabilitation. Most of them usually focus on language per se, whether it is the exact aphasic profile, the type and/or severity of observed language disturbances, the underlying—and supposedly impaired—language mechanisms, or techniques to enhance verbal behavior and overall communication ability. (For a review of these approaches, see [2]). This is probably derived from the fact that for more than a century, the Wernicke–Lichtheim model defined not only the neural and functional substrate of language [3] but also the ideas and strategies concerning aphasia rehabilitation [1].

In recent years, an emerging alternative perspective, based on comparative anatomy, neuroimaging, and lesion studies, has contradicted this functional organization dogma. This theoretical perspective states that the so-called "language network" may have evolved before the emergence of language as a neural substrate of a domain-general processing mechanism [3]. Thus, language faculty could be viewed as the product of natural selection based on physiological and cognitive pre-adaptations, such as perisylvian networks or white-matter pathways that are also present in animals [4], which may appear, prima facie, to be specialized for discrete functions such as syntax but actually support other, more fundamental cognitive domains, such as working memory (for a relevant short discussion, see [5]).

For example, it has been argued that Broca's area, a traditionally labeled "language" region that has primarily been associated with speech production, is a "supra-modal hierarchical processor", even in non-verbal tasks (see [6]). It has been demonstrated that Broca's area is engaged in abstract sequencing [7] as well as in the processing of other types of information related to complex motor sequences, music, or mathematics [8] (for a review of the involvement of Broca's area in several non-language processes, see [9]). There is also evidence, derived from healthy brain functioning, of the involvement of perisylvian "language" regions in a broad spectrum of executive functions. Brodmann area 45 has been shown to be involved in selective retrieval [10], while Brodmann area 46 and inferior parietal cortices have been associated with monitoring within working memory and manipulation, respectively [11,12].

In a similar context, there have been studies showing that the dorsal or ventral streams that are associated with language are critical in other, more "basic" cognitive functions. For example, the third branch of the superior longitudinal fasciculus which connects prefrontal, premotor and parietal areas (SLF III) is involved in phonological processing, but it is also assumed to control orofacial action, even in non-verbal tasks [13]. On the other hand, the extreme capsule fasciculus, which is also present in the macaque monkey [14], has been associated with semantic language processing, while there are studies that support its role in the actively controlled retrieval of information [15].

Lesion studies on aphasia have also shown that patients with acquired language disturbances commonly face difficulties in other cognitive domains, such as short-term memory, working memory [16,17], or other executive functions (for a review, see [18]). Overall, an aphasia-producing lesion will inevitably result in deficits in cognitive domains other than language, and these deficits have been shown to be related to the severity of language. This notion is further supported by lesion studies that do not focus on aphasia per se but investigate lesion loci that affect language-related areas. It should be noted that the latter term is not used a strict sense here, and thus it is not limited to the traditional regions identified as "Broca's" and "Wernicke's" areas but rather extends to a quite broad perisylvian region that includes cortices or even white matter pathways, which have been associated with various aspects of language processing, as indicated by brain-imaging studies (for a review, see [19]). In this context, there have been studies showing that such perisylvian lesion sites may affect several cognitive skills. For example, Baldo and Dronkers [20] showed that damage to the inferior parietal cortex and the inferior frontal cortex may differentially affect different components of working memory tasks. Leff et al. [21] argued that the superior temporal gyrus in the left hemisphere is a shared neural substrate for both auditory comprehension and short-term memory. Furthermore, Chapados and Petrides [22] highlighted the importance of the ventrolateral prefrontal cortex for selective retrieval. This notion was further supported by a recent study which showed that a lesion specifically affecting fundamental components of the ventral "language" stream, including pars triangularis and the temporo-frontal extreme capsule fasciculus, has detrimental effects on lexico-semantic processing and active selective controlled retrieval [23].

Regarding these advances that delve even more deeply into the neurobiology of language and, ultimately, raise doubt about the traditional dogma of the neural organization of language, there has been, in recent years, an ongoing debate regarding how (or even if) findings from basic neuroscience studies can be exploited in order to optimize language treatment [24]. In this vein, neuroscience research has revealed a universal characteristic of human and animal brain—neuroplasticity—which potentially serves as a bridge between basic research and clinical practice [25,26]. This emerging field, i.e., cognitive neurorehabilitation, is founded on a set of specific neural principles that could probably be translated and applied to human recovery from language and cognitive deficits [27].

This translational approach in rehabilitation inevitably leads to two major questions. The first question is whether clinicians specialized in the rehabilitation of cognitive disorders, and particularly aphasia, can manipulate the principles of neuroplasticity in order to maximize language treatment, based on findings from animal research. The second question is broadly related to the possible links between language and other cognitive domains. Animal studies usually examine sensory and motor functions, but there are also sparse data on cognitive functions such as object recognition or spatial memory [28]. From that perspective, it is essential to take into account the idea that the grounding evolutionary foundations for language to root were probably other domain-general cognitive mechanisms [3]. Consequently, the second question is formulated as such: are there studies with stroke-induced aphasia patients which designate the significance of non-linguistic functions in language rehabilitation? In the following sections of this paper, we will attempt to describe a potential translational framework in aphasia rehabilitation (see Figure 1).

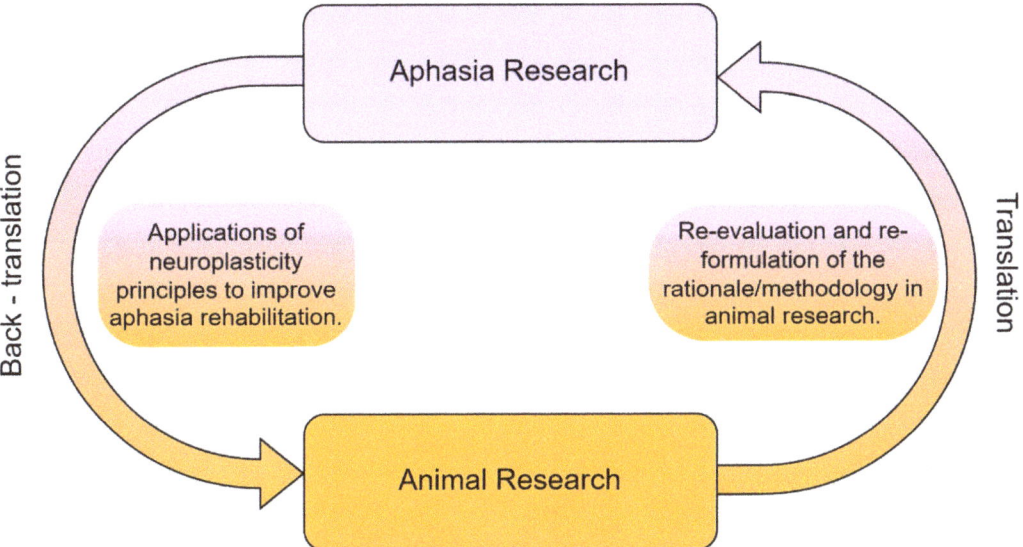

Figure 1. The reciprocal relationship between animal and aphasia research.

2. Neuroplasticity in Animals and Aphasia Research

Several animal studies in the broader field of evolutionary biology confirm that mammalian species demonstrate differences but also substantial similarities in cerebral organization and function [29]. Based on this line of research, a fundamental attribute of the brain has emerged, i.e., neuroplasticity. This term refers to the neurons' intrinsic capacity to reorganize their structure and function in response to environmental stimuli and injuries [30]. It is well documented that humans have a larger cortical surface area compared to other animals; however, this is not the primary impetus of brain plasticity [29]. In their seminal paper, Rockel et al. [31] compared specific properties of cortical neurons such as number and density, in cat, macaque, rat and human. They concluded that the core difference across the aforementioned species was not the distribution of neurons in each section but instead the pattern of synaptic connections among brain areas. Based on that notion, it has been theorized that the ability to 'sculpt' these connections is the cornerstone of neuroplasticity and, more interestingly, the underlying mechanisms of this neural modification are parallel between humans and animals [32]. This hypothesis has formulated the basis of translating results from animal research to humans [25]. In general, neuroplasticity is a dynamic process underlying normal development or learning, and it includes various atrophic and trophic processes, such as neurogenesis, synaptogenesis, and the removal of unused synapses [33]. In this context, neuroscientific research has suggested that the refinement and alteration of behavior via neuroplasticity is primarily influenced by a wide variety of stimuli and experience [34]. Similar studies have indicated structural alterations in brain areas following cognitive training in animals and humans [35,36]. As Turkstra and colleagues [26] have highlighted, 'there is an ongoing process of modification in both directions: experience to brain and brain to experience' (p. 604). On the grounds of this interaction, it has been argued that structural mechanisms underlying experience-dependent plasticity in the cortex, such as axonal sprouting or the growth of new dendritic spines, could be manipulated toward the reorganization of cognitive functions and language following stroke [36]. Thus, the study of the principal rules governing neuroplasticity in the intact or the injured brain of both animals and humans could provide valuable guidelines for understanding how the neural circuits are remodeled following stroke either during the course of recovery or in the context of rehabilitation.

In the case of aphasia, there is accumulating evidence suggesting that spontaneous neuroplastic brain changes following stroke could result in language reorganization [36]. In general, neuroimaging studies indicate that the compensation for impaired language functions relies on the increased activation of residual undamaged left hemispheric areas or the recruitment of homologous right hemispheric areas [37]. For instance, Fridriksson [38] showed a correlation between improved naming performance and increased cortical activation in left undamaged areas in untreated post-stroke aphasia. On the other hand, patients with aphasia (PWAs) have been shown to exhibit a right-lateralized activation pattern during a silent word-generation task, which is a pattern similar to that of left hemispheric regions of healthy right-handed individuals [39]. It should be however noted that right hemisphere changes have also been reported to be maladaptive, and increased activation in those areas could be associated with impaired performance [40].

The involvement of neuroplasticity in language reorganization has been addressed not only as an important aspect of spontaneous recovery but also in the context of rehabilitation research. Although sparse, there are functional imaging studies which have demonstrated brain changes as a result of treatment programs. Thompson et al. [41] have shown that training in producing specific sentence structures may result in increased right-hemisphere activity during verb production in PWAs; the sites of such increased activation were different from those usually identified in neurologically intact individuals. Therefore, these results provided indications of remapping language functions to previously uninvolved brain regions, such as the superior parietal cortex. Furthermore, in a study by Fridriksson [42], twenty-six left stroke survivors received an intense aphasia treatment focusing on object naming. The results showed that even though damage to the left middle temporal lobe and the temporal–occipital junction had a negative effect on performance, increased brain activation in the anterior and posterior regions of the left hemisphere was correlated with improved outcomes. There are also findings highlighting treatment-induced activity changes in brain connectivity patterns involving language-related tracts, such as the arcuate fasciculus [43]; however, this line of evidence is still inconclusive [44].

Apart from functional changes, there have also been sparse reports of structural brain alterations following language rehabilitation. One study found an increase in the number of fibers and volume of the right arcuate fasciculus after melodic intonation therapy in PWAs [45]. It has also been shown that an improvement of word retrieval may be associated with increased structural integrity of the left arcuate fasciculus [24]. Furthermore, improved naming performance has been associated with different patterns of gray matter density in specific right hemisphere areas, such as the precentral gyrus or the temporal lobe [44]. A study by Allendorfer et al. [46] reported increased axonal density in left frontal areas following transcranial magnetic stimulation over the left hemisphere; nevertheless, more research is required to clarify the effect of gray and white matter changes on specific language domains.

In summary, a surge of basic and neuroimaging research indicates that neuroplasticity is the cornerstone of cognition and language recovery after brain damage. However, only recent studies have focused on specific principles of neuroplasticity that could be manipulated in order to maximize language treatment (Figure 2) [30].

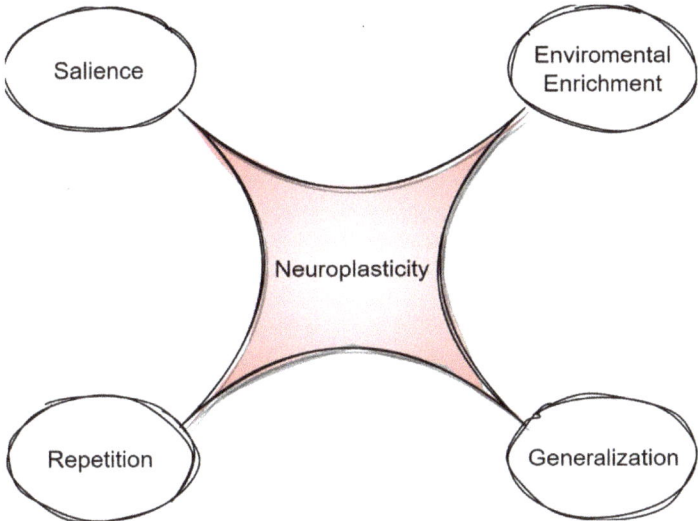

Figure 2. Principles of neuroplasticity.

3. Generalization, Environmental Enrichment, and Salience in Rehabilitation

In the last few decades, animal research has suggested that specific rehabilitation principles promote neuroplasticity and functional recovery [30,47]. Sparse experiments have demonstrated that treatment focused on one particular function can generalize to the improvement of untrained behavior in animals [48]. For example, Liu et al. [49] have shown that cognitive training in rats via a T-shaped maze may improve memory after a 4-week program; that improvement was accompanied by enhanced functional activity of the hippocampus and the medial–prefrontal cortex. In a similar context, there has been evidence of increased dendritic patterns in both hemispheres of rats following sensory-motor intervention during a skilled one-paw reaching task, which was also 'transferred' to reaching with two paws [50]. Other researchers have proposed that such generalization could be influenced by the complexity and richness of training surroundings [51]. In animal research, environmental enrichment generally refers to a more challenging environment (e.g., group housing, toys, diverse food), and it facilitates neurogenesis and synaptic plasticity [52]. It has been also argued that a more complex intervention environment may affect memory and learning. Hamm et al. [53] have shown that the training of rats in an enriched environment may result in better performance regarding spatial memory, while other studies have highlighted the recovery of motor coordination [54]. Moreover, enriched environments are considered to promote salience, which is an important factor of neuroplasticity [30]. Salience is the perceived value or relevance of the experience to the individual [27] and has been associated with motivation and attention in animals [55]. Animal research using auditory tunes has demonstrated that there could be an alteration and reorganization of auditory maps in rats when training is salience based [56].

Based on the aphasia literature, the generalization of language treatment has been a perennial issue for clinicians [57]. The implications for language reorganization is that training a specific language modality could influence the neural capacity to improve in other untrained language behaviors [30]. Several studies have examined generalization effects in other language functions when rehabilitating confrontation or picture naming (for a review, see [58]). Hillis and colleagues [59] have reported significantly better semantic and comprehension performance following naming rehabilitation, although there are approaches which doubt the methodological processes that lead to generalization gains [60]. In the domain of syntax and speech production, the training of sentences could result in generalization gains of untrained sentences when they exhibit similar grammatical and semantic properties [61]. On the other hand, the importance of salience has not been systematically studied in the field of aphasia rehabilitation. However, it is well known that PWA may demonstrate a lack of motivation in daily activities and even depression, especially when language disturbances are severe [1]. A recent study that could shed light on this subject is that of Janssen et al. [62]. The authors designed an enriched environment in a rehabilitation setting with stroke patients. The primary outcome was that patients in the enriched environment had higher engagement compared to the control group (rehabilitated in a non-enriched environment), and they also demonstrated improvement in cognitive functions. The principle of salience in aphasia should be further investigated with intervention protocols that promote motivation and are meaningful for the participant [24].

4. *Repetitio Est Mater Studiorum* or "Repetition Influences Recovery"

There are animal studies which support the idea that the training and acquisition of a learned behavior after brain injury is not sufficient for the reorganization of function [63]. Research on the principles that facilitate neuroplasticity highlights repetition and intensity as key elements for the maintenance of neural changes in the brain [64]. For instance, Monfils and Teskey [65] have reported that an increase in synaptic strength and number can be observed in rats only after several days of training. In addition, a motor map reorganization can be achieved in rats after an intense and repetitive training program [63]. However, there is still no gold standard concerning the number or the duration of trials that animals should undertake in order to achieve improved functional outcomes [24,25]. Microstimulation and functional mapping studies have also shown that repetitive exercise can influence the activity of neural circuits (for a review, see [66]). Repetitive motor training combined with brain stimulation could lead to functional improvements by reducing activity in specific brain areas [67]. It is noteworthy that repetition and intensity, although theoretically distinct principles of neuroplasticity, are often not separated in animal studies [24,68]. However, some studies have proposed that exaggerated intensity and repetition of training in rehabilitation could lead to tissue loss and reduced functional gains [69].

Based on these animal studies, aphasiologists have examined the issue of intensity in language treatment [70]. Greater intensity of rehabilitation, when reported, is shown to have positive functional outcomes for PWA in naming [71] or spoken language [72]. In a similar vein, there are studies which have reported an improvement of language following treatment of 8.8 h per week for 11.2 weeks [73], while others do not confirm such a positive effect [70]. It has also been noted that intensity may have positive effects on language-related functional and structural reorganization: Meinzer et al. [74] have shown increased activation in perilesional areas in PWA after an intensive 2-week training program, while Schlaug, Marchina, and Norton [45] have reported increased volume of the arcuate fasciculus after a longer intensive rehabilitation program.

In summary, the existing studies on humans, although scarce, have provided indications about the benefits of intensity; however, similarly to animal research, the specifics of such programs are yet to be fully understood [70]. Future studies should provide guidelines for the optimized duration of intervention protocols, focusing on specific language domains of PWA.

5. Rehabilitation of Cognitive Functions and Its Reflection to Language

It has already been established that sensory-motor and memory functions in animals can be improved following neurorehabilitation protocols [34]. Until the field of translational research expands further, researchers can only formulate theories about possible parallels between humans and other animals concerning the structural and functional mechanisms involved in rehabilitation [25,27]. Within this context, the notion that language is supported by 'basic' cognitive domains (e.g., action, memory, etc.) has led scholars to investigate if the rehabilitation of non-linguistic functions also present in animals can optimize language treatment. This idea is supported by researchers who explore the critical aspect of cognitive mechanisms in the rehabilitation of language in humans [75].

Over the years, the elucidation of the brain–language relationship has proven to be a Sisyphean task, which is mainly due to the lack of a robust consensus for creating an accurate and comprehensive functional neuroanatomy model [76]. This nebulous picture has also affected recovery studies which primarily focus on impaired language modalities and their neural substrates and eventually ignore or underestimate the impact of non-linguistic factors on the behavioral manifestation of aphasia [77].

The idea that other cognitive mechanisms, which are obviously present in animals, can contribute to the structural and functional reshaping of neural networks supporting language is not new [78]. In recent years, there has been growing support of the notion that PWA exploit various cognitive functions for language processes, including—but not limited to—short-term or working memory [79,80], attention [81,82] or other executive functions [83], and praxis [84].

This rationale has paved the way for the investigation of the presumable interrelation between attention and language recovery in PWA. Perhaps the most intriguing observation supporting this relationship is that the majority of these training studies have shown that subcomponents of attention, e.g., sustained or divided, may affect access to lexical representations [85]. Helm-Estabrooks, Connor, and Albert [86] have developed a rehabilitation program consisting of different non-verbal simple or complex attention alteration tasks. Their results have shown a significant improvement as well as generalization effects on auditory comprehension and visual analytic reasoning. There have been also findings indicating neural changes in attention pathways following language treatment [87], with increased connectivity on parietal regions of the default mode network associated with naming gains. Beyond the attention domain, early lesion studies have revealed that short-term (STM) and working memory (WM) may share common neural substrates with language [20]. This notion has been further supported by subsequent studies which have shown that it is an aphasia-producing lesion—rather than any left-lateralized lesion—that leads to STM/WM deficits [88]. In this framework, one could arguably ask whether language recovery outcomes may be affected by training verbal STM and/or WM. For instance, in their case study, Koenig-Bruhin and Studer-Eichenberger [89] reported an improvement in the delayed recall of nouns and sentences following intervention in STM and WM. It has been also suggested that reduced memory span, which is usually accessed by repetition tasks, is strongly correlated with lexical deficits and increased aphasia severity [16]. Another piece of evidence that further fortifies the argument that non-linguistic functions are of essence is that there have been studies highlighting the prognostic value of cognitive factors in language recovery [90]. For example, Gilmore, Meir, Johnson and Kiran [91] have reported that WM, inhibition and processing speed predicted language improvement in PWA, following naming and sentence comprehension rehabilitation, whereas visual STM was associated with the maintenance of naming gains after a 12-week no-treatment phase.

6. Discussion

As stated before, the short history of aphasia rehabilitation [1] has demonstrated that treatment strategies in general have been significantly influenced by the presumed neurobiological model for language of a particular time period, while neuroplasticity has been highlighted as an important rehabilitation factor only recently. The Wernicke–Lichtheim paradigm has been severely doubted by more recent theoretical accounts based on accumulating research evidence derived from studies involving patients with aphasia, but it has not yet been completely replaced [76] by other, more concrete, and modern language models which focus on neural language networks [92]. In this context, as has been thoroughly described in the previous section, it is undeniable that aphasiologists have only recently started to focus on the impact of fundamental cognitive functions in language therapy [78]. However, it is also undeniable that we have yet to delineate an integrated framework of aphasia rehabilitation. This could be attributed to limited research focus on the neural bases of spared, non-linguistic functions and the implementation of neuroplasticity principles (derived from animal studies) as well as their interaction with recovery variables which are essential in therapy strategies.

In general, post-stroke aphasia studies have examined the impact of clinical and demographic factors on language recovery, which are theorized to differentially affect brain plasticity [93]. In the past few years, there have been several inconsistencies concerning the influence of demographic factors such as age, sex and educational level on language spontaneous recovery or rehabilitation induced by intervention programs not only in the chronic but also in the acute or subacute phase (for a review, see [94]). It is generally accepted that younger brains have greater plasticity and ultimately a greater capacity for recovery [50]. Accordingly, it has been assumed that younger patients are more likely to recover than older patients [95]. However, more recent studies have not found a significant association between age and recovery (see for example [96]). Future research is thus required in order to thoroughly investigate and hopefully clarify the specifics of the process by which older adults with acquired aphasia demonstrate different patterns of recovery and reorganization compared to younger patients, and also how age interacts with other predictors of recovery, such as motivation or personality traits [24]. On the other hand, most researchers have confirmed an inverse relationship between recovery and lesion size, while lesion location has been shown to be rather more critical [97,98]. The degree of white-matter integrity, in both the left and right hemisphere, has also been documented to affect language rehabilitation [24]. Diffusion tensor imaging techniques have revealed that the disruption of specific white matter tracts of the left cerebral hemisphere such as the arcuate fasciculus or the superior longitudinal fasciculus may lead to speech production impairment [59]. However, there is still limited data regarding how rehabilitation methods can 'reformulate', structurally or functionally, specific white matter pathways. In sum, it is crucial to understand how aphasia-producing lesions may affect other cognitive domains (keeping in mind that language-related neural networks are not language specific and may be involved in other aspects of cognition), how neuroplasticity principles (repetition, environmental enrichment, generalization) may mediate observable post-stroke language recovery, and how neuroplastic mechanisms may interact with demographic, lesional, cognitive, or other variables [27].

Despite the interrelation between language and other cognitive domains, there have been sparse studies exploiting the key elements which facilitate brain plasticity in specific language modalities, such as word finding or auditory comprehension in the translational field (for a review, see [99]). In addition, the available findings regarding the impact of neuroplasticity in the enhancement of non-linguistic factors are still very limited. Thus, more data are needed in order to create efficient intervention protocols that focus on specific language domains. There have been some recent efforts, such as Semantic Feature Analysis or Phonomotor Treatment, which target the mental lexicon and phonological speech sounds, respectively; however, this line of research is still in its infancy [100,101]. Although the clinical relevance of rehabilitating specific functions is undoubted, the complexity of language material in aphasia treatment has also been shown to be beneficial in several domains such as syntax or lexical semantic impairments [61]. There have also been studies which explore the effect of non-language behaviors in aphasia recovery. For example, there have been promising results which demonstrate that rhythm and melodic intonation may lead to structural changes in the right hemisphere [45], while intention treatment has been reported to improve word retrieval following left-hand movements [102]. However, this is a field which has not been sufficiently studied. Given the potential to improve recovery outcomes with non-invasive and cognitively oriented methods, further research is required; such research attempts could focus on the neuroplasticity-induced structural and functional brain changes.

As the field of neurorehabilitation progressively unfolds, more and more researchers are recognizing the importance of the key parameters of neuroplasticity and the critical need for the design of a neurobiological approach to aphasia therapies [27]. Animal models allow analysis of brain injuries and strokes at a molecular level and may thus provide insight to the core mechanisms of functional recovery [26].

In the context of this ongoing effort, researchers have developed stroke models; however, these are limited to motor recovery [103]. In this translational continuum, future animal studies should be more reflective of human cognitive deficits and recovery, while clinicians and aphasiologists could apply concepts derived from basic neuroscience more systematically [36]. In relation to the latter issue, throughout the history of post-stroke aphasia rehabilitation, important variables that facilitate neuroplasticity, such as intensity or timing of treatment [99], were often disregarded or characterized by a significant degree of variability among patients [1]. It has been recently reported that a higher intensity of treatment protocols may induce neuroplasticity, which eventually may lead to improved language outcomes [104]. Moreover, the issue of the timing of therapy deliverance has been revealed to be critical for rehabilitation protocols, since early intervention could be either beneficial or maladaptive [105]. However, more research is necessary to understand the interaction between intensity and timing of rehabilitation across different stages of recovery as well as the optimization of neural mechanisms which respond to treatment schedules.

Except for neuroimaging advances, which in the last decades can identify structural and functional changes following language treatment, the rise of neuromodulation technologies such as transcranial direct current stimulation and repetitive transcranial magnetic stimulation has allowed the immediate manipulation of training-induced neuroplasticity [44]. This effect can be achieved by facilitating activity in brain regions or by suppressing maladaptive neural processes [106] and is also combined with behavior treatment [44]. These stimulation methods have also been applied to modulate specific language domains, such as naming, even before intervention, with quite promising results [44,107]. Recent meta-analyses have suggested that the aforementioned neurostimulation techniques may also be associated with the timing of intervention, as positive treatment outcomes have been indicated in both subacute and chronic patients with aphasia [44]. However, there is still a lack of consensus with regard to the optimal choice of neuromodulation method depending on the possible implications posed by lesion size or location [108].

Even though scholars working on language rehabilitation have achieved a significant theoretical and practical development, translational aphasia research is still at its origins. Overall, the present review aimed to highlight basic principles stemming from the evidence available in the animal and human literature, in a translational framework, focused on aphasia rehabilitation. However, translational research is not a panacea and still remains rather challenging regarding not only aphasia rehabilitation but also other fields of neuroscience (for a review, see [109]). We are aware of the main impediment to this aim, i.e., the major difficulty of translating findings from animal studies to human patients with aphasia. This difficulty can be attributed to obvious reasons: brain differences between human and non-human mammals and, most importantly, the uniqueness of language in *Homo sapiens*. However, we argue that there are possible reciprocal gains from this effort: the field of aphasiology could benefit from basic neuroscience and, in turn, animal research could be inspired from the field of language treatment, thus forming a new translational direction in aphasia rehabilitation.

7. Conclusions

This study has highlighted findings derived from animal and aphasia research that could influence future studies in developing neurorehabilitation approaches emphasizing the improvement of cognitive factors and their reflection on language modalities based on neuroplasticity optimization. From a contemporary neuropsychological perspective, we argue that people with aphasia should not be treated as "aphasics" but as stroke patients with prominent language difficulties as well as significant deficits in other cognitive domains, which, in turn, may contribute to—or even be the root of—their language impairment. More and more researchers are recognizing the need for a holistic approach in aphasia rehabilitation; however, further progress is required in deciphering common parallels between animals and humans. This rationale, combined with treatment protocols that focus on the enhancement of neuroplasticity, via specific neural principles, and their association with language and non-language domains, could provide an innovative, neurobiological, and multi-modality foundation for aphasia rehabilitation.

Author Contributions: Conceptualization: G.P., D.K. and C.P.; Research design and literature search: G.P. and D.K.; Drafting the manuscript: G.P., D.K. and N.L.; Critically reviewing the manuscript for important intellectual content: C.P.; Supervision: C.P. and D.K. All authors have read and agreed to the published version of the manuscript.

Funding: This study was supported by the Hellenic Foundation for Research and. Innovation (H.F.R.I.) under the "First Call for H.F.R.I. Research Projects to support Faculty members and Researchers and the procurement of high-cost research equipment grant" (Project Number 4081). We also acknowledge the financial contribution of the Dean of the School of Medicine through the Special Account for Research Grants of the University of Athens.

Conflicts of Interest: The authors declare no conflict of interest.

References

1. Basso, A. *Aphasia and Its Therapy*; Oxford University Press: New York, NY, USA, 2003.
2. Kasselimis, D.S.; Potagas, C. Language Disorders, Treatment and Remediation of James Wright. In *Encyclopedia of the Social & Behavioral Sciences*, 2nd ed.; Elsevier: Oxford, UK, 2015; pp. 329–336.
3. Rijntjes, M.; Weiller, C.; Bormann, T.; Musso, M. The dual loop model: Its relation to language and other modalities. *Front. Evol. Neurosci.* **2012**, *4*, 9. [CrossRef] [PubMed]
4. Barbeau, E.B.; Descoteaux, M.; Petrides, M. Dissociating the white matter tracts connecting the temporo-parietal cortical region with frontal cortex using diffusion tractography. *Sci. Rep.* **2020**, *10*, 8186. [CrossRef]
5. Kasselimis, D.; Angelopoulou, G.; Simos, P.; Petrides, M.; Peppas, C.; Velonakis, G.; Potagas, C. Working memory impairment in aphasia: The issue of stimulus modality. *J. Neurolinguistics* **2018**, *48*, 104–116. [CrossRef]
6. Tettamanti, M.; Weniger, D. Broca's area: A supramodal hierarchical processor? *Cortex* **2006**, *42*, 491–494. [CrossRef] [PubMed]
7. Hoen, M.; Pachot-Clouard, M.; Segebarth, C.; Dominey, P.F. When Broca experiences the Janus syndrome: An ER-fMRI study comparing sentence comprehension and cognitive sequence processing. *Cortex* **2006**, *42*, 605–623. [CrossRef] [PubMed]
8. Schubotz, R.I.; Fiebach, C.J. Integrative models of Broca's Area and the Ventral Premotor. *Cortex* **2006**, *42*, 461–463. [CrossRef]
9. Fadiga, L.; Craighero, L.; Roy, A. Broca's region: A speech area? In *Broca's Region*; Grodzinsky, Y., Ed.; Oxford University Press: Oxford, UK, 2006; pp. 137–152.
10. Kostopoulos, P.; Petrides, M. Selective memory retrieval of auditory what and auditory where involves the ventrolateral prefrontal cortex. *Proc. Natl. Acad. Sci. USA* **2016**, *113*, 1919–1924. [CrossRef]
11. Champod, A.S.; Petrides, M. Dissociation within the frontoparietal network in verbal working memory: A parametric functional magnetic resonance imaging study. *J. Neuro. Sci.* **2010**, *30*, 3849–3866. [CrossRef]
12. Champod, A.S.; Petrides, M. Dissociable Roles of the Posterior Parietal and the Prefrontal Cortex in Manipulation and Monitoring Processes. *Proc. Natl. Acad. Sci. USA* **2007**, *104*, 14837–14842. [CrossRef]
13. Janelle, F.; Iorio-Morin, C.; D'amour, S.; Fortin, D. Superior Longitudinal Fasciculus: A Review of the Anatomical Descriptions with Functional Correlates. *Front. Neurol.* **2022**, *13*, 794618. [CrossRef]
14. Petrides, M.; Pandya, D.N. Association fiber pathways to the frontal cortex from the superior temporal region in the rhesus monkey. *J. Comp. Neurol.* **1988**, *273*, 52–66. [CrossRef]
15. Petrides, M.; Pandya, D.N. Comparative cytoarchitectonic analysis of the human and the macaque ventrolateral prefrontal cortex and corticocortical connection patterns in the monkey. *Eur. J. Neurosci.* **2002**, *16*, 291–310. [CrossRef] [PubMed]
16. Martin, N.; Ayala, J. Measurements of auditory-verbal STM span in aphasia: Effects of item, task, and lexical impairment. *Brain Lang.* **2004**, *89*, 463–483. [CrossRef] [PubMed]
17. Minkina, I.; Salis, C.; Martin, N. Short-term and working memory deficits in aphasia: Current issues in theory, evidence, and treatment. *J. Neuroling.* **2018**, *48*, 1–3. [CrossRef]
18. Fonseca, J.; Ferreira, J.J.; Martins, I.P. Cognitive performance in aphasia due to stroke: A systematic review. *Int. J. Disabil. Hum. Dev.* **2016**, *16*, 127–139. [CrossRef]
19. Price, C.J. A review and synthesis of the first 20 years of PET and fMRI studies of heard speech, spoken language and reading. *Neuroimage* **2012**, *62*, 816–847. [CrossRef]

20. Baldo, J.V.; Dronkers, N.F. The role of inferior parietal and inferior frontal cortex in working memory. *Neuropsychology* **2006**, *20*, 529. [CrossRef]
21. Leff, A.P.; Schofield, T.M.; Crinion, J.T.; Seghier, M.L.; Grogan, A.; Green, D.W.; Price, C.J. The left superior temporal gyrus is a shared substrate for auditory short-term memory and speech comprehension: Evidence from 210 patients with stroke. *Brain* **2009**, *132*, 3401–3410. [CrossRef]
22. Chapados, C.; Petrides, M. Ventrolateral and dorsomedial frontal cortex lesions impair mnemonic context retrieval. *Proc. R. Soc. B Nat. Environ.* **2015**, *282*, 1801. [CrossRef]
23. Kourtidou, E.; Kasselimis, D.; Angelopoulou, G.; Karavasilis, E.; Velonakis, G.; Kelekis, N.; Petrides, M. Specific disruption of the ventral anterior temporo-frontal network reveals key implications for language comprehension and cognition. *Commun. Biol.* **2022**, *5*, 1077. [CrossRef]
24. Kiran, S.; Thompson, C.K. Neuroplasticity of Language Networks in Aphasia: Advances, Updates, and Future Challenges. *Front. Neurol.* **2019**, *10*, 295. [CrossRef]
25. Keefe, K.A. Applying basic neuroscience to aphasia therapy: What the animals are tellingus. *Am. J. Speech Lang. Pathol.* **1995**, *4*, 88–93. [CrossRef]
26. Turkstra, L.S.; Holland, A.L.; Bays, G.A. The neuroscience of recovery and rehabilitation:What have we learned from animal research? *Arch. Phys. Med. Rehabil.* **2003**, *84*, 604–612. [CrossRef]
27. Raymer, A.M.; Holland, A.; Kendall, D.; Maher, L.M.; Martin, N.; Murray, L.; Gonzalez Rothi, L.J. Translational research in aphasia: From neuroscience to neurorehabilitation. *J. Speech Lang. Hear. Res.* **2007**, *50*, S259–S275. [CrossRef] [PubMed]
28. Dahlqvist, P.; Rönnbäck, A.; Bergström, S.A.; Söderström, I.; Olsson, T. Environmental enrichment reverses learning impairment in the Morris water maze after focal cerebral ischemia in rats. *Eur. J. Neurosci.* **2004**, *19*, 2288–2298. [CrossRef]
29. Kaas, J. *Evolution of Nervous Systems*; Elsevier: New York, NY, USA, 2006.
30. Kleim, J.A.; Jones, T.A. Principles of experience-dependent neural plasticity: Implications for rehabilitation after brain damage. of speech, language, and hearing research. *J. Speech Lang. Hear. Res.* **2008**, *51*, S225–S239. [CrossRef] [PubMed]
31. Rockel, A.J.; Hiorns, R.W.; Powell, T.P. The basic uniformity in structure of the neocortex. *Brain* **1980**, *103*, 221–244. [CrossRef] [PubMed]
32. Buonomano, D.V.; Merzenich, M.M. Cortical plasticity: From synapses to maps. *Ann. Rev. Neurosci.* **1998**, *21*, 149–186. [CrossRef] [PubMed]
33. Farokhi-Sisakht, F.; Farhoudi, M.; Sadigh-Eteghad, S.; Mahmoudi, J.; Mohaddes, G. Cognitive Rehabilitation Improves Ischemic Stroke-Induced Cognitive Impairment: Role of Growth Factors. *J. Stroke Cerebrovasc. Dis.* **2019**, *28*, 104299. [CrossRef]
34. Kleim, J.A. Neural plasticity and neurorehabilitation: Teaching the new brain old tricks. *J. Commun. Disord.* **2011**, *44*, 521–528. [CrossRef]
35. Valenzuela, M.J.; Jones, M.; Wen, W.; Rae, C.; Graham, S.; Shnier, R.; Sachdev, P. Memory training alters hippocampal neurochemistry in healthy elderly. *Neuroreport* **2003**, *14*, 1333–1337. [CrossRef]
36. Berlucchi, G. Brain plasticity and cognitive neurorehabilitation. *Neuropsychol. Rehabil.* **2011**, *21*, 560–578. [CrossRef]
37. Thompson, C.K. Neuroplasticity: Evidence from aphasia. *J. Commun. Disord.* **2000**, *33*, 357–366. [CrossRef]
38. Fridriksson, J. Preservation and modulation of specific left hemisphere regions is vital for treated recovery from anomia in stroke. *J. Neurosci.* **2010**, *30*, 11558–11564. [CrossRef] [PubMed]
39. Staudt, M.; Lidzba, K.; Grodd, W.; Wildgruber, D.; Erb, M.; Krägeloh-Mann, I. Right-hemispheric organization of language following early left-sided brain lesions: Functional MRI topography. *NeuroImage* **2002**, *16*, 954–967. [CrossRef]
40. Martin, P.I.; Naeser, M.A.; Ho, M.; Treglia, E.; Kaplan, E.; Baker, E.H.; Pascual-Leone, A. Research with transcranial magnetic stimulation in the treatment of aphasia. *Curr. Neurol. Neurosci. Rep.* **2009**, *9*, 451. [CrossRef] [PubMed]
41. Thompson, C.K.; Riley, E.A.; den Ouden, D.B.; Meltzer-Asscher, A.; Lukic, S. Training verb argument structure production in agrammatic aphasia: Behavioral and neural recovery patterns. *Cortex* **2013**, *49*, 2358–2376. [CrossRef]
42. Fridriksson, J.; Morrow-Odom, L.; Moser, D.; Fridriksson, A.; Baylis, G. Neural recruitment associated with anomia treatment in aphasia. *Neuroimage* **2006**, *32*, 1403–1412. [CrossRef]
43. Kiran, S.; Meier, E.L.; Kapse, K.J.; Glynn, P.A. Changes in task-based effective connectivity in language networks following rehabilitation in post-stroke patients with aphasia. *Front. Hum. Neurosci.* **2015**, *9*, 316. [CrossRef]
44. Crosson, B.; Rodriguez, A.D.; Copland, D.; Fridriksson, J.; Krishnamurthy, L.C.; Meinzer, M.; Raymer, A.M.; Krishnamurthy, V.; Leff, A.P. Neuroplasticity and aphasia treatments: New approaches for an old problem. *J. Neurol. Neurosurg. Psychiatry* **2019**, *90*, 1147–1155. [CrossRef]
45. Schlaug, G.; Marchina, S.; Norton, A. Evidence for plasticity in white-matter tracts of patients with chronic Broca's aphasia undergoing intense intonation-based speech therapy. *Ann. N. Y. Acad. Sci.* **2009**, *1169*, 385–394. [CrossRef] [PubMed]
46. Allendorfer, J.B.; Storrs, J.M.; Szaflarski, J.P. Changes in white matter integrity follow excitatory rTMS treatment of post-stroke aphasia. *Restor. Neurol. Neurosci.* **2012**, *30*, 103–113. [CrossRef] [PubMed]
47. Kandel, E.R. Cellular Mechanisms of Learning and the Biological Basis of Individuality. In *Principles of Neuroscience*; Kandel, E.R., Schwartz, J.H., Eds.; Elsevier Science Publishers: New York, NY, USA, 1985.

48. Jenkins, W.M.; Merzenich, M.M.; Recanzone, G. Neocortical representational dynamics in adult primates: Implications for neuropsychology. *Neuropsychologia* **1990**, *28*, 573–584. [CrossRef]
49. Liu, W.; Li, J.; Li, L.; Zhang, Y.; Yang, M.; Liang, S.; Li, L.; Dai, Y.; Chen, L.; Jia, W.; et al. Enhanced Medial Prefrontal Cortex and Hippocampal Activity Improves Memory Generalization in APP/PS1 Mice: A Multimodal Animal MRI Study. *Front. Cell. Neurosci.* **2022**, *16*, 848967. [CrossRef]
50. Kolb, B. *Brain Plasticity and Behavior*; Lawrence Erlbaum Associates: Mahwah, NJ, USA, 1995.
51. York, A.; Breedlove, S.M.; Diamond, M.A. Increase in granule cell neurogenesis following exposure to enriched environments. *Neurosci. Abstr.* **1989**, *15*, 602.
52. Zentall, T.R. Effect of Environmental Enrichment on the Brain and on Learning and Cognition by Animals. *Animals* **2021**, *11*, 973. [CrossRef] [PubMed]
53. Hamm, R.J.; Temple, M.D.; Pike, B.R.; O'Dell, D.M.; Buck, D.L.; Lyeth, B.G. Working memory deficits following traumatic brain injury in the rat. *J. Neurotrauma* **1996**, *13*, 317–323. [CrossRef]
54. Vasn Dellen, A.; Blakemore, C.; Deacon, R.; York, D.; Hannan, A.J. Delaying the onset of Huntington's in mice. *Nature* **2000**, *404*, 721–722. [CrossRef]
55. Han, P.P.; Han, Y.; Shen, X.Y.; Gao, Z.K.; Bi, X. Enriched environment-induced neuroplasticity in ischemic stroke and its underlying mechanisms. *Front. Cell Neurosci.* **2023**, *17*, 1210361. [CrossRef]
56. Weinberger, N.M. Specific long-term memory traces in primary auditory cortex. *Nat. Rev. Neurosci.* **2004**, *5*, 279–290. [CrossRef]
57. Kiran, S.; Thompson, C.K. The role of semantic complexity in treatment of naming deficits: Training semantic categories in fluent aphasia by controlling exemplar typicality. *J. Speech Lang. Hear. Res.* **2003**, *46*, 773–787. [CrossRef] [PubMed]
58. Nickels, L. Therapy for naming disorders: Revisiting, revising, and reviewing. *Aphasiology* **2002**, *16*, 935–979. [CrossRef]
59. Hillis, A.E.; Beh, Y.Y.; Sebastian, R.; Breining, B.; Tippett, D.C.; Wright, A.; Saxena, S.; Rorden, C.; Bonilha, L.; Basilakos, A.; et al. Predicting recovery in acute poststroke aphasia. *Ann. Neurol.* **2018**, *83*, 612–622. [CrossRef] [PubMed]
60. Howard, D. Cognitive Neuropsychology and Aphasia Therapy: The Case of Word Retrieval. In *Acquired Neurogenic Communication Disorders: A Clinical Perspective*; Papathanasiou, I., Ed.; Whurr: London, UK, 2000.
61. Thompson, C.K.; Shapiro, L.P. Complexity in treatment of syntactic deficits. *Am. J. Speech Lang. Pathol.* **2007**, *16*, 30–42. [CrossRef]
62. Janssen, H.; Ada, L.; Middleton, S.; Pollack, M.; Nilsson, M.; Churilov, L.; Blennerhassett, J.; Faux, S.; New, P.; McCluskey, A.; et al. Altering the rehabilitation environment to improve stroke survivor activity: A Phase II trial. *Int. J. Stroke* **2022**, *17*, 299–307. [CrossRef]
63. Kleim, J.A.; Bruneau, R.; VandenBerg, P.; MacDonald, E.; Mulrooney, R.; Pocock, D. Motor cortex stimulation enhances motor recovery and reduces peri-infarct dysfunction following ischemic insult. *Neurol. Res.* **2003**, *25*, 789–793. [CrossRef] [PubMed]
64. Kilgard, M.P.; Merzenich, M.M. Cortical map reorganization enabled by nucleus basalis activity. *Science* **1998**, *279*, 1714–1718. [CrossRef]
65. Monfils, M.H.; Teskey, G.C. Skilled-learning-induced potentiation in rat sensorimotor cortex: A transient form of behavioural long-term potentiation. *Neuroscience* **2004**, *125*, 329–336. [CrossRef]
66. Xing, Y.; Bai, Y. A Review of Exercise-Induced Neuroplasticity in Ischemic Stroke: Pathology and Mechanisms. *Mol. Neurobiol.* **2020**, *57*, 4218–4231. [CrossRef]
67. Koganemaru, S.; Sawamoto, N.; Aso, T.; Sagara, A.; Ikkaku, T.; Shimada, K.; Kanematsu, M.; Takahashi, R.; Domen, K.; Fu-kuyama, H.; et al. Task-specific brain reorganization during motor recovery induced by a hybrid-rehabilitation combining training with brain stimulation after stroke. *Neurosci. Res.* **2015**, *92*, 29–38. [CrossRef]
68. Luke, L.M.; Allred, R.P.; Jones, T.A. Unilateral ischemic sensorimotor cortical damage induces contralesional synaptogenesis and enhances skilled reaching with the ipsilateral forelimb in adult male rats. *Synapse* **2004**, *54*, 187–199. [CrossRef] [PubMed]
69. Kozlowski, D.A.; James, D.C.; Schallert, T. Use-dependent exaggeration of neuronal injury after unilateral sensorimotor cortex lesions. *J. Neurosci.* **1996**, *16*, 4776–4786. [CrossRef] [PubMed]
70. Cherney, L.R.; Patterson, J.P.; Raymer, A.M. Intensity of aphasia therapy: Evidence and efficacy. *Curr. Neurol. Neurosci. Rep.* **2011**, *11*, 560–569. [CrossRef]
71. Sage, K.; Snell, C.; Lambon Ralph, M.A. How intensive does anomia therapy for people with aphasia need to be? *Neuropsychol. Rehabil.* **2011**, *21*, 26–41. [CrossRef]
72. Pulvermüller, F.; Neininger, B.; Elbert, T.; Mohr, B.; Rockstroh, B.; Koebbel, P.; Taub, E. Constraint-induced therapy of chronic aphasia after stroke. *Stroke* **2001**, *32*, 1621–1626. [CrossRef]
73. Bhogal, S.K.; Teasell, R.; Speechley, M. Intensity of aphasia therapy, impact on recovery. *Stroke* **2003**, *34*, 987–993. [CrossRef]
74. Meinzer, M.; Flaisch, T.; Breitenstein, C.; Wienbruch, C.; Elbert, T.; Rockstroh, B. Functional re-recruitment of dysfunctional brain areas predicts language recovery in chronic aphasia. *NeuroImage* **2008**, *39*, 2038–2046. [CrossRef] [PubMed]
75. Badre, D.; Wagner, A.D. Left ventrolateral prefrontal cortex and the cognitive control of memory. *Neuropsychologia* **2007**, *45*, 2883–2901. [CrossRef]
76. Tremblay, P.; Dick, A.S. Broca and Wernicke are dead, or moving past the classic model of language neurobiology. *Brain Lang.* **2016**, *162*, 60–71. [CrossRef]

77. Rapp, B.; Caplan, D.; Edwards, S.; Visch-Brink, E.; Thompson, C.K. Neuroimaging in aphasia treatment research: Issues of experimental design for relating cognitive to neural changes. *Neuroimage* **2013**, *73*, 200–207. [CrossRef]
78. Gainotti, G. Old and recent approaches to the problem of non-verbal conceptual disorders in aphasic patients. *Cortex* **2014**, *53*, 78–89. [CrossRef] [PubMed]
79. Allen, C.M.; Martin, R.C.; Martin, N. Relations between Short-term Memory Deficits, Semantic Processing, and Executive Function. *Aphasiology* **2012**, *26*, 428–461. [CrossRef] [PubMed]
80. Lang, C.J.; Quitz, A. Verbal and nonverbal memory impairment in aphasia. *J. Neurol.* **2012**, *259*, 1655–1661. [CrossRef] [PubMed]
81. Murray, L.L.; Keeton, R.J.; Karcher, L. Treating attention in mild aphasia: Evaluation of attention process training-II. *J. Commun. Disord.* **2006**, *39*, 37–61. [CrossRef]
82. Lesniak, M.; Bak, T.; Czepiel, W.; Seniow, J.; Czlonkowska, A. Frequency and prognostic value of cognitive disorders in stroke patients. *Dement. Geriatr. Cogn. Disord.* **2008**, *26*, 356–363. [CrossRef] [PubMed]
83. Purdy, M. Executive function ability in persons with aphasia. *Aphasiology* **2002**, *16*, 549–557. [CrossRef]
84. Sekine, K.; Rose, M.L. The relationship of aphasia type and gesture production in people with aphasia. *Am. J. Speech Lang. Pathol.* **2013**, *22*, 662–672. [CrossRef]
85. Murray, L.L.; Holland, A.L.; Beeson, P.M. Auditory processing in individuals with mild aphasia: A study of resource allocation. *J. Speech Lang. Hear. Res.* **1997**, *40*, 792–808. [CrossRef]
86. Helm-Estabrooks, N.; Connor, L.T.; Albert, M.L. Training attention to improve auditory comprehension in aphasia. *Brain Lang.* **2000**, *74*, 469–472. [CrossRef]
87. Marrelec, G.; Bellec, P.; Krainik, A.; Duffau, H.; Pélégrini-Issac, M.; Lehéricy, S.; Benali, H.; Doyon, J. Regions, systems, and the brain: Hierarchical measures of functional integration in fMRI. *Med. Image Anal.* **2008**, *12*, 484–496. [CrossRef]
88. Kasselimis, D.S.; Simos, P.G.; Economou, A.; Peppas, C.; Evdokimidis, I.; Potagas, C. Are memory deficits dependent on the presence of aphasia in left brain damaged patients? *Neuropsychologia* **2013**, *51*, 1773–1776. [CrossRef] [PubMed]
89. Koenig-Bruhin, M.; Studer-Eichenberger, F. Therapy of short-term memory disorders in fluent aphasia: A single case study. *Aphasiology* **2007**, *21*, 448–458. [CrossRef]
90. Friedmann, N.; Gvion, A. Sentence comprehension and working memory limitation in aphasia: A dissociation between semantic-syntactic and phonological reactivation. *Brain Lang.* **2003**, *86*, 23–39. [CrossRef]
91. Gilmore, N.; Meier, E.L.; Johnson, J.P.; Kiran, S. Nonlinguistic Cognitive Factors Predict Treatment-Induced Recovery in Chronic Poststroke Aphasia. *Arch. Phys. Med. Rehabil.* **2019**, *100*, 1251–1258. [CrossRef]
92. Blumstein, S.E.; Amso, D. Dynamic Functional Organization of Language: Insights from Functional Neuroimaging. *Perspect Psychol Sci.* **2013**, *8*, 44–48. [CrossRef]
93. Watila, M.M.; Balarabe, S.A. Factors predicting post-stroke aphasia recovery. *J. Neurol. Sci.* **2015**, *12*, 352. [CrossRef]
94. Lazar, R.M.; Antoniello, D. Variability in recovery from aphasia. *Curr. Neurol. Neurosci. Rep.* **2008**, *8*, 497–502. [CrossRef]
95. Laska, A.C.; Hellblom, A.; Murray, V.; Kahan, T.; Von Arbin, M. Aphasia in acute stroke and relation to outcome. *J. Intern. Med.* **2001**, *249*, 413–422. [CrossRef]
96. Inatomi, Y.; Yonehara, T.; Omiya, S.; Hashimoto, Y.; Hirano, T.; Uchino, M. Aphasia during the acute phase in ischemic stroke. *Cerebrovasc. Dis.* **2008**, *25*, 316–323. [CrossRef] [PubMed]
97. Mazzoni, M.; Vista, M.; Pardossi, L.; Avila, L.; Bianchi, F.; Moretti, P. Spontaneous evolution of aphasia after ischaemic stroke. *Aphasiology* **2007**, *6*, 387–396. [CrossRef]
98. Maas, M.B.; Lev, M.H.; Ay, H.; Singhal, A.B.; Greer, D.M.; Smith, W.S.; Harris, G.J.; Halpern, E.F.; Koroshetz, W.J.; Furie, K.L. The prognosis for aphasia in stroke. *J. Stroke Cerebrovasc. Dis.* **2012**, *21*, 350–357. [CrossRef]
99. Kasselimis, D.; Papageorgiou, G.; Angelopoulou, G.; Tsolakopoulos, D.; Potagas, C. Translational Neuroscience of Aphasia and Adult Language Rehabilitation. In *Neuroscience of Speech and Language Disorders*; Argyropoulos, G., Ed.; Contemporary Clinical Neuroscience Series; Springer: Berlin, Germany, 2020; pp. 5–20.
100. Boyle, M. Semantic feature analysis treatment for aphasic word retrieval impairments: What's in a name? *Top. Stroke Rehabil.* **2010**, *17*, 411–412. [CrossRef]
101. Kendall, D.L.; Oelke, M.; Brookshire, C.E.; Nadeau, S.E. The influence of phonomotor treatment on word retrieval abilities in 26 individuals with chronic aphasia: An open trial. *J. Speech Language Hear. Res.* **2015**, *58*, 798–812. [CrossRef] [PubMed]
102. Benjamin, M.L.; Towler, S.; Garcia, A.; Park, H.; Sudhyadhom, A.; Harnish, S.; McGregor, K.M.; Zlatar, Z.; Reilly, J.J.; Rosenbek, J.C.; et al. A behavioral manipulation engages right frontal cortex during aphasia therapy. *Neurorehab. Neural Rep.* **2014**, *28*, 545–553. [CrossRef]
103. Dromerick, A.W.; Edwardson, M.A.; Edwards, D.F.; Giannetti, M.L.; Barth, J.; Brady, K.P.; Chan, E.; Tan, M.T.; Tamboli, I.; Chia, R.; et al. Critical periods after stroke study: Translating animal stroke recovery experiments into a clinical trial. *Front. Hum. Neurosci.* **2015**, *9*, 231. [CrossRef] [PubMed]
104. Dignam, J.; Copland, D.; McKinnon, E.; Burfein, P.; O'Brien, K.; Farrell, A.; Rodriguez, A.D. Intensive Versus Distributed Aphasia Therapy: A Nonrandomized, Parallel-Group, Dosage-Controlled Study. *Stroke* **2015**, *46*, 2206–2211. [CrossRef]
105. Woodlee, M.T.; Schallert, T. The interplay between behavior and neurodegeneration in rat models of Parkinson's disease and stroke. *Restor. Neurol. Neurosci.* **2004**, *22*, 153–161. [PubMed]

106. Kapoor, A. Repetitive transcranial magnetic stimulation therapy for post-stroke non-fluent aphasia: A critical review. *Top. Stroke Rehabil.* **2017**, *24*, 547–553. [CrossRef]
107. Shah, P.P.; Szaflarski, J.P.; Allendorfer, J.; Hamilton, R.H. Induction of neuroplasticity and recovery in post-stroke aphasia by non-invasive brain stimulation. *Front. Hum. Neurosci.* **2013**, *7*, 888. [CrossRef]
108. Dmochowski, J.P.; Datta, A.; Huang, Y.; Richardson, J.D.; Bikson, M.; Fridriksson, J.; Parra, L.C. Targeted transcranial direct current stimulation for rehabilitation after stroke. *Neuroimage* **2013**, *75*, 12–19. [CrossRef]
109. Lourbopoulos, A.; Mourouzis, I.; Xinaris, C.; Zerva, N.; Filippakis, K.; Pavlopoulos, A.; Pantos, C. Translational Block in Stroke: A Constructive and "Out-of-the-Box" Reappraisal. *Front. Neurosci.* **2021**, *15*, 652403. [CrossRef] [PubMed]

Disclaimer/Publisher's Note: The statements, opinions and data contained in all publications are solely those of the individual author(s) and contributor(s) and not of MDPI and/or the editor(s). MDPI and/or the editor(s) disclaim responsibility for any injury to people or property resulting from any ideas, methods, instructions or products referred to in the content.

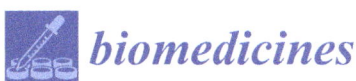

Article

PET/MRI in the Presurgical Evaluation of Patients with Epilepsy: A Concordance Analysis

Katalin Borbély [1,*], Miklós Emri [2,3], István Kenessey [4,5], Márton Tóth [6], Júlia Singer [7], Péter Barsi [8], Zsolt Vajda [9], Endre Pál [10], Zoltán Tóth [2], Thomas Beyer [11], Tamás Dóczi [12], Gábor Bajzik [9], Dániel Fabó [13], József Janszky [6], Zsófia Jordán [13], Dániel Fajtai [2], Anna Kelemen [13], Vera Juhos [14], Max Wintermark [15], Ferenc Nagy [16], Mariann Moizs [2,16], Dávid Nagy [13], János Lückl [2,16,†] and Imre Repa [2,16,†]

1. PET/CT Outpatient Department, National Institute of Oncology, H1122 Budapest, Hungary
2. Medicopus Healthcare Provider and Public Nonprofit Ltd., Somogy County Moritz Kaposi Teaching Hospital, H7400 Kaposvár, Hungary; emri.miklos@med.unideb.hu (M.E.); toth.zoltan@sic.medicopus.hu (Z.T.); daniel.fajtai@sic.medicopus.hu (D.F.); moizs.mariann@kmmk.hu (M.M.); janos.luckl@sic.ke.hu (J.L.); repa.imre@sic.medicopus.hu (I.R.)
3. Division of Nuclear Medicine and Translational Imaging, Department of Medical Imaging, Faculty of Medicine, University of Debrecen, H4032 Debrecen, Hungary
4. National Cancer Registry, National Institute of Oncology, H1122 Budapest, Hungary; kenessey.istvan@oncol.hu
5. Department of Pathology, Forensic and Insurance Medicine, Semmelweis University, H1091 Budapest, Hungary
6. Department of Neurology, Medical School, University of Pécs, H7623 Pécs, Hungary; toth.marton@pte.hu (M.T.); janszky.jozsef@pte.hu (J.J.)
7. Accelsiors Ltd., H1222 Budapest, Hungary; j.singer@accelsiors.com
8. Neuroradiology Department, Semmelweis University, H1083 Budapest, Hungary; barsi.peter@semmelweis-univ.hu
9. Dr. József Baka Diagnostic, Radiation Oncology, Research and Teaching Center, Somogy County Moritz Kaposi Teaching Hospital, H7400 Kaposvár, Hungary; vajda.zsolt@sic.medicopus.hu (Z.V.); bajzik.gabor@sic.medicopus.hu (G.B.)
10. Department of Pathology, Medical School, University of Pécs, H7623 Pécs, Hungary; pal.endre@pte.hu
11. QIMP Team, Center for Medical Physics and Biomedical Engineering, Medical University of Vienna, 1090 Vienna, Austria; thomas.beyer@meduniwien.ac.at
12. Department of Neurosurgery, Medical School, University of Pécs, H7623 Pécs, Hungary; doczi.tamas@pte.hu
13. Department of Neurology and Neurosurgery, National Institute of Mental Health, Neurology and Neurosurgery, H1145 Budapest, Hungary; fabo@mail.oiti.hu (D.F.); jordan.zsofia@mail.oiti.hu (Z.J.); kelemen.anna@oiti.hu (A.K.); nagy.david.gergo@mail.oiti.hu (D.N.)
14. Epihope Non-Profit Kft, H1026 Budapest, Hungary; epilepszia.juhos@gmail.com
15. Department of Neuroradiology, MD Anderson, Houston, TX 77030, USA; max.wintermark@gmail.com
16. Department of Neurology, Somogy County Moritz Kaposi Teaching Hospital, H7400 Kaposvár, Hungary; nagy.ferenc2@kmmk.hu
* Correspondence: katalin.borbely@oncol.hu; Tel.: +36-1224-8600 (ext. 3468)
† These authors contributed equally to this work.

Abstract: The aim of our prospective study was to evaluate the clinical impact of hybrid [^{18}F]-fluorodeoxyglucose positron emission tomography/magnetic resonance imaging ([^{18}F]-FDG PET/MRI) on the decision workflow of epileptic patients with discordant electroclinical and MRI data. A novel mathematical model was introduced for a clinical concordance calculation supporting the classification of our patients by subgroups of clinical decisions. Fifty-nine epileptic patients with discordant clinical and diagnostic results or MRI negativity were included in this study. The diagnostic value of the PET/MRI was compared to other modalities of presurgical evaluation (e.g., electroclinical data, PET, and MRI). The results of the population-level statistical analysis of the introduced data fusion technique and concordance analysis demonstrated that this model could be the basis for the development of a more accurate clinical decision support parameter in the future. Therefore, making the establishment of "invasive" (operable and implantable) and "not eligible for any further invasive procedures" groups could be much more exact. Our results confirmed the relevance of PET/MRI with the diagnostic algorithm of presurgical evaluation. The introduction of a concordance analysis could be of high importance in clinical and surgical decision-making in the management of epileptic patients. Our study

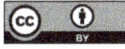

corroborated previous findings regarding the advantages of hybrid PET/MRI technology over MRI and electroclinical data.

Keywords: epilepsy surgery; medically refractory focal epilepsy; presurgical evaluation; MRI-negative patients; discordant electroclinical and MRI data; metabolic PET; hybrid [^{18}F]-FDG PET/MRI; preoperative workflow; concordance analysis; epilepsy team

1. Introduction

The precise localization of epileptic foci and mapping the relation to the eloquent cortical areas is a prerequisite for the successful presurgical evaluation of patients with pharmacoresistant focal epilepsy [1,2]. Long-term scalp video-electroencephalography (VEEG) monitoring to record ictal EEG and seizure, semiology, neuropsychological assessment, magnetic resonance imaging (MRI), interictal [^{18}F]-fluoro-deoxyglucose ([^{18}F]-FDG) positron emission tomography (PET) imaging are relevant constituents of this workflow [3–6]. The epileptic patients with concordant electroclinical data may have a chance at seizure freedom in approximately 30–90% of cases [7–9]. In the rest of the patients, MRI findings appeared to be normal or discordant with VEEG and clinical data, and they may benefit from intracranial EEG (icEEG) recordings for the localization of the seizure onset zone [7,8,10]. [^{18}F]-FDG PET mapping holds promise for evaluating both temporal [11–14] and extra-temporal lobe epilepsy [15].

Clinical decision-making is particularly challenging in patients with discordant neuroimaging and electroclinical data, with MRI-negative results, or with the occurrence of multiple epileptic foci. Furthermore, the complexity of electroclinical and neuroimaging data challenges presurgical decision-making [2,6,14,16].

The optimal presurgical diagnostic work-up of epilepsy patients remains a subject of debate, despite significant advances in diagnostic imaging techniques, such as MRI and PET imaging and, distinctively, hybrid PET/MRI [3–5,17–28].

The aim of our prospective study was to evaluate the clinical impact of hybrid [^{18}F]-FDG PET/MRI on the presurgical evaluation of patients with pharmacoresistant epilepsy and to introduce a mathematical model from the multi-modality tests that may facilitate the development of artificial intelligence for the analysis of different concordance patterns.

2. Materials and Methods

2.1. Subjects

This prospective study was approved by the Scientific Research Ethics Committee of the Medical Research Council (008899/2016/OTIG) and carried out in accordance with the Declaration of Helsinki of the World Medical Association. Seventy patients with refractory focal epilepsy underwent a full electroclinical presurgical evaluation between June 2016 and December 2017. The inclusion criteria were: (i) pharmacoresistant focal epilepsy, (ii) MRI scans with discordant results or without noticeable morphologic epileptogenic lesion, (iii) VEEG monitoring in each patient, and (iv) age of 18–65 years. Exclusion criteria included: (i) standard contraindications for MRI examinations, (ii) acute non-epileptic neurological disorder, (iii) acute infection, and (iv) serious comorbidities. Ten of these patients were excluded from further analysis after the multidisciplinary team revealed multifocal or diffuse pathological alterations (encephalitis $n = 7$, vasculitis $n = 2$, and hydrocephalus $n = 1$). One more patient was removed from the current analysis because of compromised image quality. The median age of the remaining 59 patients was 33 years (range: 18–57 years), and the cohort contained 35 male and 24 female patients.

2.2. Patient Preparation

All epileptic patients were hospitalized for adaptation a day prior to the study, and a standard neurological examination, electrocardiography (ECG), and routine laboratory tests were performed. Written consent was obtained from all participants. Dual-modality [^{18}F]-

FDG PET/MR imaging was performed the next day. The standardized patient preparation for the PET examination was performed according to the European guideline of 2009 [29]. Briefly, supervision of a 2 h duration and VEEG monitoring (in 10–20 EEG Placement) were performed before the intravenous tracer administration. VEEG monitoring covered the whole uptake period of the tracer to ensure the interictal state. PET/MRI acquisition started 60 min after the injection.

2.3. PET/MRI Acquisition

All PET/MRI acquisitions were performed on a Biograph mMR scanner (Siemens Healthineers, Erlangen, Germany). The detailed dedicated seizure protocol of MRI acquisition is summarized in Table 1. In order to provide a complete temporally and spatially correlated PET dataset, a 20 min and 35 min list-mode 3D PET acquisition was performed simultaneously for each patient. Vendor-provided UTE sequence was used for PET attenuation correction (AC) purposes, and MR-based attenuation maps were generated automatically. Static image reconstruction was performed both for 20 min and 35 min. AC and non-AC transaxial slices were generated. For PET image reconstruction, the OP-OSEM method was applied, including PSF correction (3 iterations, 21 subsets, 4 mm full-width at half-maximum (FWHM) Gaussian filtering, and $344 \times 344 \times 127$ imaging matrix). µMaps were checked for potential artifacts, and the completed PET raw data were archived for further evaluation. For the current assessment, a 20 min static PET image dataset was used.

Table 1. Dedicated MRI epilepsy protocol.

MR Sequence	TR (ms)	TE (ms)	FA	Slice Thickness	Imaging Matrix	Voxel Size	TA
Axial T2 UTE (MRAC)	11.94	TE1:0.07, TE:2:2.46	10			$1.6 \times 1.6 \times 1.6$ mm	1:38
Sagittal MPRAGE	2300	2.98	9	1.2 mm	240×256	$1.0 \times 1.0 \times 1.2$	9:14
Axial T2 TSE	6000	106	150	4 mm	358×448	$0.5 \times 0.5 \times 4$ mm	4:08
Coronal T2 TSE HR	6770	89	150	3 mm	307×384	$0.5 \times 0.5 \times 3$ mm	3:04
Coronal FLAIR HR	9000	128	120	3 mm	192×256	$0.9 \times 0.9 \times 3$ mm	5:44
Axial DTI	3600	95	-	4 mm	128×128	$1.7 \times 1.7 \times 4$ mm	3:59
Axial T2 HEMO	620	19.9	20	4 mm	205×256	$0.4 \times 0.4 \times 4$ mm	2:09
SagittalT2 SPC 3D	3200	409	120	1.0 mm	261×256	$0.5 \times 0.5 \times 1$ mm	4:43
Sagittal T2 FLAIR 3D	5000	395	120	1.0 mm	261×256	$0.5 \times 0.5 \times 1$ mm	5:52
Resting state fMRI	2580	30	90	3 mm	74×74	$3 \times 3 \times 3$ mm	10:54
GRE Field Mapping	400	4.92/7.38	60	3 mm	64×64	$3.4 \times 3.4 \times 3$	0:54
Axial ASL	3060.4	17	90	5 mm	64×64	$3.6 \times 3.6 \times 5$ mm	5:14

2.4. Image Processing

An in-house image processing pipeline was applied to transform all individual images into the MNI152 atlas space prior to the regional analysis of the [^{18}F]-FDG PET images using Statistical Parametric Mapping (SPM). At the beginning of this procedure, we used the "recon-all" pipeline of FreeSurfer software (version 7.0) for the segmentation of T1-

MPRAGE images [30–32]. The produced segmented T1-MPRAGE images were used for correcting the misalignment of PET/MR image pairs, global voxel intensity scaling, and calculating the transformations required by the spatial normalization. In the latter case, we applied the FSL software package (version 6.0) [33] and the Advanced Normalization Tools software (version 2.3.5) [34] for calculating the rigid body, 12-parameter affine, and non-linear transformations. After the transformations of the [^{18}F]-FDG PET images into the MNI152 space, to eliminate the inter-subject variability of the measured global-brain metabolism according to the standard PET-SPM method, we set the average of the within-brain mask voxel-values of the PET images to 50 [35]. Finally, on the normalized [^{18}F]-FDG PET images, we applied a 10 mm and 2 mm 3D Gaussian kernel-based smoothing for the SPM and the regional analysis, respectively.

We used the spatially standardized, globally normalized, and smoothed [^{18}F]-FDG PET data and the spatially standardized T1-MPRAGE and T2-FLAIR images for calculating 15 quantitative image-processing parameters for all patients with four image-processing methods (Table 2). The quantitative image-processing parameters were evaluated by VOI (volume of interest) analysis, asymmetry index calculations, SPM analysis, and MAP07 analysis using the spatially standardized, globally normalized, and smoothed [^{18}F]-FDG PET, and the spatially standardized T1-MPRAGE and T2-FLAIR images.

Table 2. Evaluated quantitative [^{18}F]-FDG PET image-processing parameters.

Image Processing Data	Description of PET Data	Source
voi.min	minimal [^{18}F]-FDG uptake value	
voi.max	maximal [^{18}F]-FDG uptake value	
voi.mean	average of mean values according to Harvard-Oxford Cortical and Subcortical atlases (HOVOI)	
voi.median	median of HOVOI medians values	
voi.sd	maximal HOVOI based standard deviation	the globally normalized and spatially standardized [^{18}F]-FDG PET image
ai.min	minimum of the asymmetry of minimal HOVOI's [^{18}F]-FDG values	
ai.max	maximum of the asymmetry of maximal HOVOI's [^{18}F]-FDG values	
ai.mean	the maximum value of the asymmetry of HOVOI's [^{18}F]-FDG value means	
ai.median	the maximum value of the asymmetry of HOVOI's [^{18}F]-FDG value medians	
ai.sd	the maximum value of the asymmetry of standard deviations of HOVOI's [^{18}F]-FDG values	
spm.max	highest Student-t value in the HOVOI region	SPM generated Student-t map
spm.vol	the relative volume of hypometabolic area (thresholded by uncorrected $p < 0.001$) in the HOVOI region	
map.max	maximum z-value in the HOVOI region	Combined z-score image produced by MAP07
map.mean	maximum value of the HOVOI's mean z-values in the HOVOI's region	

During this study, two regional systems in the MNI152 space were applied: the Harvard-Oxford Cortical and Subcortical Atlas (HOVOI), containing 124 (96 cortical and 28 subcortical) regions suitable for regional analysis, and the 14 regions, combined from HOVOI's regions, used in electroclinical data evaluation (EPIREG system) [36]. All quantitative image-processing parameters were converted into these regions for the purpose of statistical and concordance analysis.

The minimum, maximum, mean, median, and standard deviation (voi.min, voi.max, voi.mean, voi.median, and voi.sd) of the regional [^{18}F]-FDG values for all HOVOI regions were estimated in the VOI analysis procedure of the [^{18}F]-FDG PET images. The VOI parameters of the overlapping HOVOI regions were used for the regional characterization of the EPIREG system by selecting the minimal value in the case of the voi.min parameter and maximum values in the other cases (Table 2). The maximum values were applied to ensure that the highest average, median, and standard deviation HOVOI data were used to characterize the appropriate EPIREG area, thus preserving the regional variability of the [^{18}F]-FDG PET and composite z-score images.

An asymmetry index (AI) calculation of the [^{18}F]-FDG PET images was used on symmetric regions of the HOVOI system by applying the formula AI = $100 \times 2 \times (L - R)/(L + R)$, where L and R represent the mean intensity values (ai.mean) of the corresponding left and right regions of the HOVOI system. Additionally, using a similar formula, the asymmetry of the maximum, median, and standard deviation (ai.max, ai.median, and ai.sd) were evaluated using a similar formula (Table 2).

An HOVOI-based regional analysis of the Student-t maps was performed by the SPM12 software [37]. A Student-t map was created for each patient using the statistical comparison of their [^{18}F]-FDG PET image and the reference metabolic PET image database from our lab, which was built from a previously recorded data pool of 19 cases showing normal PET/MRI patterns. The maximum of the Student-t values and the volume of the hypometabolic region were deployed for characterizing the regional properties of the Student-t maps, sorted by an uncorrected $p < 0.001$ as a threshold (spm.max, spm.vol) (Table 2).

An HOVOI-based regional analysis of the "Composite z-score" images was performed by MAP07. Morphometric analyses were applied to the T1-MPRAGE and T2-FLAIR MRI data sets of the patients using the MAP07 software [38]. The maximum, mean, median, and standard deviation estimates (map.max, map.mean, map.median, and map.sd) were used for characterizing the regional properties of the "Composite z-score" images (Table 2).

The visual analysis of the PET images was performed and analyzed by the authors, KB and ZT, and the MRI images by the authors PB and ZV.

2.5. Clinical Data

Electroclinical information and the results of the visual analysis of the PET and MRI images were extracted from patient documentation. Additional PET/MRI investigations were applied for the EPILOBE region-based statistical and concordance analysis (Table 3). According to the possible therapeutic options (resective surgery, neuromodulation, and new antiepileptic drugs), the experts of the epilepsy team (EPI team) categorized the patients by two methods using clinical decision (CD): "Grouping Method 1" (CD1): eligible for resective surgery (without icEEG investigation) and defined as "operable" (7 patients), considered for icEEG exploration and defined as "implantable" (38 patients), or not eligible for any further invasive procedures and defined as "inoperable" (14 patients). During the "Grouping Method 2" (CD2), the simplification of categorization was performed for "inoperable" (14 patients) vs. "eligible for invasive treatment" (45 patients) groups.

Table 3. EPILOBE region-wide electroclinical and expert-based imaging data recorded during the study.

Diagnostic Parameters	Description	Value
Semiology	Possible localization considered by semiology in the given EPILOBE region.	0.0: certainly not 0.3: slightly possible 0.6: possible 1.0: the most likely
iiEEG.mfl	Occurrence of interictal EEG activity in the given EPILOBE region (most frequent localization).	0: no 1: yes
iiEEG	Occurrence of interictal EEG activity in the given EPILOBE region.	0: no 1: yes
iEEG.mfl	Possible ictal EEG activity in the given EPILOBE region (most frequent localization).	0.0: certainly not 0.3: slightly possible 0.6: possible 1.0: the most likely
iEEG	Possible ictal EEG activity in the given EPILOBE region.	0.0: certainly not 0.3: slightly possible 0.6: possible 1.0: the most likely
MRI1	Specific epileptogenic MRI lesions found by radiologist experts (before this study).	0: no 1: yes
MRI2	Possible specific epileptogenic MRI lesions found by radiologist experts (during this study).	0.0: certainly not 0.5: possible 1.0: exist
PETvis	Visual PET findings detected by nuclear medicine experts (during this study).	0: no abnormal pattern 0.5: possible 1.0: the most likely

2.6. Statistical Comparison of Electroclinical and Image Processing Data

Non-normal distribution of the investigated variables was confirmed by the Shapiro–Wilk test. Hence, to assess the relationship between these data and the categorical clinical parameters, non-parametric Mann–Whitney or pairwise Wilcoxon tests were performed. After the statistical analysis, p-values were adjusted to control the False Discovery Rate (FDR) [39], and significant relations were selected by the corrected $p < 0.05$ criteria. All statistical analyses were performed by R version 3.6.3. (The R Foundation).

2.7. Concordance of the Clinical Data

Using the EPILOBE region-wide electroclinical (Semiology, interictal EEG-iiEEG, and ictal EEG-iEEG) and expert-based imaging data (MRI1, MRI2, and PET.vis), we constructed a localization observation matrix according to the 14 brain regions and the six diagnostic parameters. We excluded the most frequent iiEEG (iiEEG.mfl) and the most frequent iEEG (iEEG.mfl) localization parameters to avoid the over-representation of the ictal and interictal EEG observations. This type of data fusion is suitable for interobserver-analysis regarding different diagnostic procedures, including the independent observations and different regions of EPIREG. Gwet's AC1 statistics was chosen for the agreement analysis since it was demonstrated to be insensitive to small differences [40,41].

Gwet's AC1 parameters helped to assess the agreement between different ratings, thus enabling the definition of a new parameter for clinical data concordance (CDC). For our study, the value of the CDC was between 0 and 1, whereby 0 meant "full discordance" and 1 stood for "full concordance." The performance of the CDC parameters was assessed by means of patient categories, similar to the expert-made clinical decisions-based classification ("eligible for resective surgery," "considered for icEEG," "not eligible for any further invasive procedures"). Eight CDC values (electroclinical data (EC), EC + MRI1, EC + MRI2, EC + PET, EC + PET + MRI2, EC + MRI1 + PET + MRI2, EC + MRI1 + MRI2, and EC + MRI1 + PET) were assessed, applying two types of patient classifications (CD1 and CD2).

3. Results

3.1. Quantitative PET and MRI Analysis

Examples of the results of the presurgical evaluation tests with pathologic findings and the corresponding circular plots of the presurgical data demonstrating different patterns of concordance are shown in Figure 1A–D.

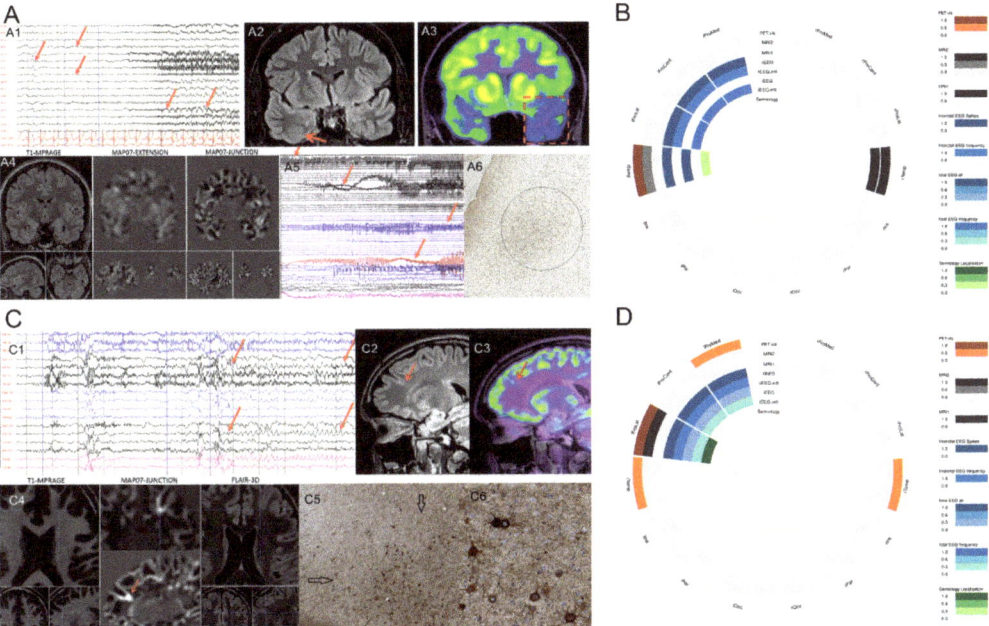

Figure 1. Examples of the results of presurgical evaluation tests proved by pathologic findings. (**A**) A drug-resistant epileptic patient with atypical temporal lobe seizures. (**A1**) Video-EEG monitoring. During her stereotype seizures, left frontotemporal seizure activity was seen (marked with arrows). (**A2**) A cranial MRI showed an FCD2 in the right collateral sulcus (arrow), while (**A3**) [^{18}F]-FDG PET/MRI presented a PET hypometabolism in the left temporal lobe (square). (**A4**) The junction map from the MAP07 analysis did not reveal any lesion in the temporal regions. (**A5**) An iEEG monitor was performed because of discordant results. Habitual seizures were registered, and the intervention was conclusive, resulting in a left temporal pole resection (resected region marked with dashed red box) with an Engel I/a outcome (24 months of seizure-free period). (**A6**) Histopathology (NeuN stain) proved an FCD1 in the left temporal pole with irregularly arranged neurons. (**B**) The circular plot refers to the electro-clinical data and imaging modalities of the patient in panel A. (**C**) A drug-resistant epileptic patient with hypermotor seizures. (**C1**) Video-EEG monitoring showed short, stereotype seizures, with left frontal seizure activity (between the arrows). Before the hybrid [^{18}F]-FDG PET/MRI study, all MRI investigations were negative. (**C2**) The cranial MRI showed an FCD 2 connected to the left superior frontal sulcus, which was in concordance with (**C3**) [^{18}F]-FDG PET/MRI presented a PET hypometabolic pattern. (**C4**) The junction map of MAP07 analysis also detected the lesion (red arrow). Epilepsy surgery with intraoperative electrophysiology was performed targeting this lesion, with an Engel I/a outcome (24 months of follow-up). (**C5**) Histopathology identified an FCD 2a with dysmorphic neurons (arrows; the region is shown in higher magnification in (**C6**) characterized by a lack of anatomical orientation and accumulation of neurofilaments (SMI32, neurofilament immunohistochemistry). (**D**) The circular plot refers to the electro-clinical data and imaging modalities of the patient in panel C. The patterns of presurgical evaluation tests and electroclinical data demonstrated a wide variety of discordances.

The statistical analysis resulted in 28 significant (FDR-corrected $p < 0.05$) regional associations between the image processing data and clinical data (Table 4). Visual PET investigations (PET.vis) of the regional data correlated with the metabolic-PET asymmetry parameters and the maximal Student-t value of the SPM analysis. The visually localized lesions in the MRI component of the PET/MRI (MRI2) measurements correlated with the PET asymmetry indexes; however, they did not correlate with the MAP07 data. The interictal EEG (iiEEG) localization significantly correlated with the VOI analysis data and the MAP07 regional maximum values, while the iiEEG.mfl localization presented a statistically significant association with the SPM-detected relative volume of hypometabolism. Semiology- or iEEG-based localization did not show any significant association with the image processing data.

Table 4. Association between interictal EEG, MRI2, and [^{18}F]-FDG PET localization, and [^{18}F]-FDG PET image processing data (performed by pairwise Wilcoxon test with FDR adjustment) l: left; r: right; FroMed: frontomedial; FroLat: frontolateral; FroCent: frontocentral; Temp: temporal; Par: parietal; Occ: occipital; Ins: insular.

Source	Image Processing Data	EPILOBE Region	p-Value	FDR Adjusted p-Value	Meaning in the Detected Lesion
iiEEG	ai.max	lTemp	0.0039	0.0467	lower asymmetry index
	map.max	rTemp	0.0014	0.0172	higher z-score
	voi.mean	rFroLat	0.0020	0.0245	
	voi.median	rFroLat	<0.0001	0.0086	lower [^{18}F]-FDG
	voi.sd	rFroLat	<0.0001	0.0025	
iiEEG.mfl	spm.vol	rTemp	0.0040	0.0396	larger SPM hypometabolism area
MRI2	ai.median	rTemp	0.0013	0.0179	
	ai.mean	rTemp	0.0016	0.0225	
		lFroMed	0.0065	0.0276	
		lOcc	0.0166	0.0465	
PET.vis	ai.max	lTemp	0.0012	0.0081	
		rIns	0.0076	0.0267	
		rTemp	0.0004	0.0057	
		lTemp	<0.0001	0.0004	
	ai.median	rFroLat	0.0041	0.0145	
		rIns	0.0012	0.0083	lower asymmetry index
		rTemp	0.0037	0.0145	
		lFroLat	0.0091	0.0254	
		lTemp	0.0002	0.0031	
	ai.mean	rFroLat	0.0067	0.0234	
		rIns	0.0013	0.0060	
		rTemp	0.0006	0.0044	
	ai.sd	lTemp	0.0005	0.0068	
		rFroLat	0.0055	0.0382	
	spm.max	lTemp	<0.0001	0.0012	higher Student-t value
	spm.vol	lTemp	<0.0001	0.0016	larger SPM hypometabolism area
		rTemp	<0.0001	0.0019	

The iiEEG and iiEEG.mfl activity localization significantly correlated with the [^{18}F]-FDG regional maximum value asymmetry, the [^{18}F]-FDG regional mean, median, and standard deviation, the MAP07 generated "composite z-score" maximum, and the SPM-based estimation of the hypometabolic region of the temporal and frontolateral lobes.

We found that the asymmetry score of the regions was highly correlated with the visually identified lesions, mostly in the temporal and the frontal lobes. Despite the low amount of the cardinality of the normative [^{18}F]-FDG PET database ($n = 19$), we could demonstrate that the results of SPM analysis, in the cases of temporal lobe hypometabolism, correlated with the visual findings.

3.2. Concordance Analysis

The eight concordance parameters in the CD1-type classification statistical analysis by FDR-corrected *p*-values revealed that neither CDC variant could significantly separate the group pairs (Figure 2). However, a tendency was present; in the case of PET-related CDCs, the "inoperable" group showed a borderline significant difference compared to the "operable" or "implantable" groups. In contrast, when the "operable" and "implantable" groups were integrated into the "invasive" group (CD2 classification), only CDC variants containing PET were able to statistically differentiate between the "invasive" and "inoperable" categories (Figure 3A). Figure 3B illustrates the clinical decision differentiation capabilities of the introduced eight CDC parameters by the *p*-values of the Mann–Whitney applied on the CDC-CD2 analysis tests (controlled for FDR).

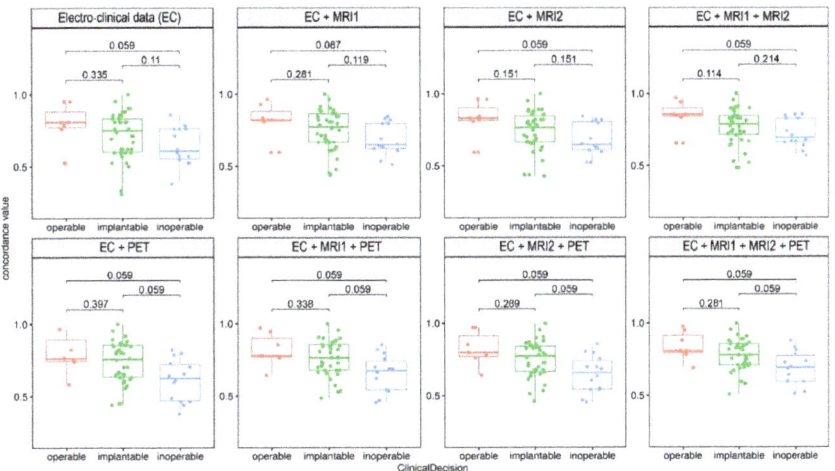

Figure 2. Clinical data concordance (CDC) of "Grouping Method 1." Boxplots of the eight CDCs grouped by three-way clinical decisions. PET-related measurements showed a slight, but not significant, difference between the "inoperable" versus the "operable" or the "implantable" groups, while PET-independent methods showed relatively less accuracy. Analyzed by Mann–Whitney tests with FDR-correction, *p*-values are shown on the intervals in the charts.

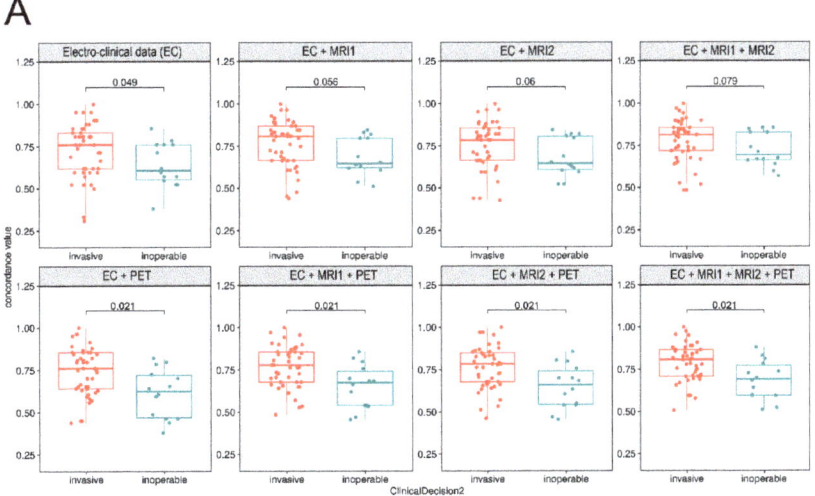

Figure 3. *Cont.*

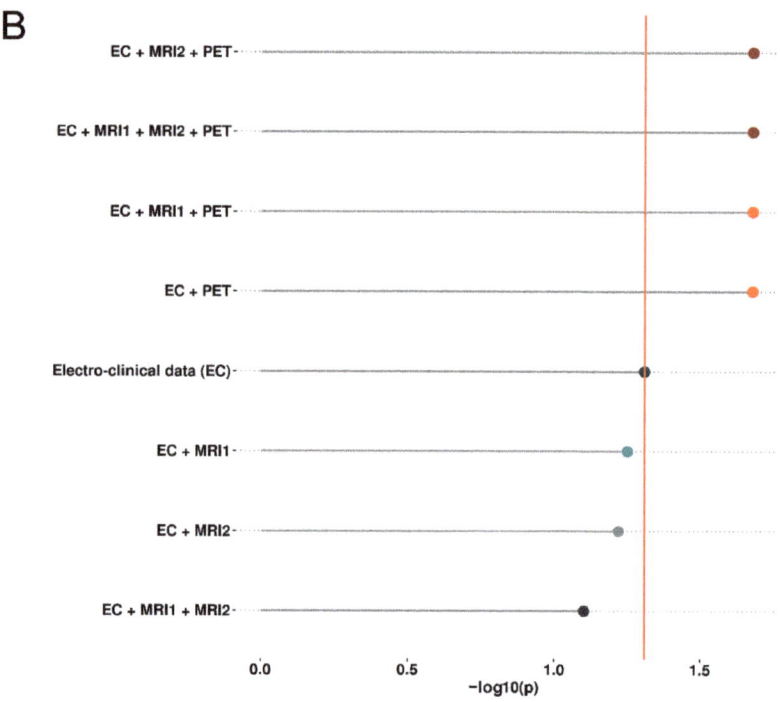

Figure 3. Clinical data concordance (CDC) of "Grouping Method 2." Boxplots of the eight CDC parameters, depending on the two-way classified clinical decisions (CD2). (**A**) When the "operable" and "implantable" groups were integrated into the "invasive" group, only PET-related CDC variants were able to significantly differentiate between "invasive" and "inoperable" categories. (**B**) Analyzed by Mann–Whitney tests with FDR-correction, p-values are shown on the segments in the charts; Negative log10 transformed p values also confirmed the high relevance of PET-based measurements since the vertical line corresponding to $p = 0.05$ separates the non-significant and significant comparisons.

4. Discussion

In our study, the electroclinical data of patients with drug-resistant epilepsy presented a widely discordant pattern. The aim of our prospective study was to test the performance of dual-modality [^{18}F]-FDG PET/MRI in patients with pharmacoresistant epilepsy. Using an objective statistical method, we demonstrated that metabolic hybrid PET/MRI technology may significantly contribute to the clinical decision-making in patients with discordant electroclinical and imaging data. The decisions of the EPI team were based on professional knowledge and skills. However, the decision-making was subjective and carried the potential for diagnostic uncertainty among patients with discordant data, which could be even more challenging in the case of MRI-negative patients [2,14]. For this purpose, we introduced a novel concordance analysis method, which demonstrated that PET matrices are of high importance and well-suited to support clinical decisions, especially the matrices including both PET and 3T MRI.

Numerous previous publications suggested the advantages of simultaneous PET/MRI technology over the diagnostic algorithm, with only MRI and electroclinical data [2,11–13,15,17,26–28,42,43]; however, recent studies have applied a mathematical model to confirm its reliability. Both statistical and concordance analysis highlighted the role of PET imaging for the non-invasive localization of epileptogenic foci, especially in patients with discordant electroclinical data and MRI scans without a definitive epileptogenic lesion or patients with multiple abnormalities.

A concordance analysis demonstrated that PET/MRI examination is able to differentiate between the "invasive" (eligible for invasive treatment) and "inoperable" groups. PET was particularly important in the selection of inoperable patients and confirmed MRI-positive lesions. MRI-assisted PET post-processing techniques (such as the brain atlas-based asymmetry index calculation and SPM analysis) also held additional supportive value for defining clinical decisions. Comparing the visual PET assessment and quantitative PET data, an association between the asymmetry index parameters and visual PET localization proved to be significant, especially for both temporal lobes.

Albeit MR imaging is fundamental in decision-making, it is not sufficient to differentiate between "operable" and "inoperable" patient groups. Additionally, MAP07 measurements did not provide significant conclusions either. The results of our PET/MRI analysis are in line with previously published data in the literature [2,17,19–22,24,25,27,28,38,42].

Moreover, besides its good feasibility and proper applicability, the hybrid PET/MRI was justified by reductions in radiation exposure, time savings, anesthesia, simplification of study-related organizational and design factors, a range of personalized diagnostic tests, and a range of comorbidity and medication data that may arise [18,23,43,44].

Another non-invasive alternative for localizing epileptogenic foci is simultaneous fMRI and EEG recording. In our study, the positive predictive value of interictal epileptiform discharges, associated with BOLD changes within 2 cm of the epileptogenic zone, was 78%, and the negative predictive value was 81% [45]. Additionally, EEG-fMRI can distinguish between ictal onset-, spread-, and preictal-related BOLD changes [46–48]. Besides the single-pass EEG/PET/fMRI [20], the recently reported sub-second analysis method [49] and the topography-related EEG-fMRI [50] may also improve the detection rate of epileptic foci.

In summary, our model confirmed the relevance of simultaneous PET/MRI for epileptic treatment planning. Additionally, the proposed clinical concordance calculation could support the development of a novel artificial intelligence-based decision system in the near future.

5. Conclusions

The fully integrated hybrid [^{18}F]-FDG PET/MRI has demonstrated a significant impact on the presurgical evaluation workflow of patients with pharmacoresistant epilepsy. The diagnostic algorithm of presurgical evaluation should not miss the comprehensive compliance of PET/MRI, mainly for precarious, subtle lesions or uncertain metabolic patterns. The introduction of a concordance analysis may help the EPI team in clinical decision-making in the future.

Author Contributions: K.B.: corresponding author, initiator of the study, study design, concordance model test, PET planning and analysis, and manuscript preparation. M.E. and D.F. (Dániel Fajtai): database handling, mathematical elaboration of the concordance model, image processing, and statistics and figures. I.K.: manuscript revision and figure editing. T.B. and M.W.: manuscript revision. M.T.: patient examination, semiology, and manuscript revision. J.S.: statistical and manuscript revision. P.B. and Z.V.: MRI analysis. E.P.: histopathology. Z.T.: PET analysis and manuscript revision. T.D.: EPI team and initiator of the study. G.B., D.F. (Dániel Fabó), J.J., Z.J., D.F. (Dániel Fajtai), A.K., V.J., F.N., M.M. and D.N.: EPI-team (patient analysis and semiology). J.L.: patients' preparation, conceptual design and test of concordance analysis, and manuscript preparation. I.R.: patients' preparation, study design, and project leader. All authors have read and agreed to the published version of the manuscript.

Funding: Recent work was financially supported by EU Social Fund (EFOP-3.6.2-16-2017-00008 "The role of neuro-inflammation in neurodegeneration: from molecules to clinics"). Supported by the Medical School of Pécs.

Institutional Review Board Statement: The study was conducted in accordance with the Declaration of Helsinki and approved by the Somogy County Moritz Kaposi Teaching Hospital's Scientific Research Ethics Committee of the Medical Research Council (008899/2016/OTIG).

Informed Consent Statement: Informed consent was obtained from all subjects involved in the study.

Data Availability Statement: Database contains personal information. Datasets may be available for special request in anonymized form from Miklós Emri and Imre Repa.

Conflicts of Interest: The authors declare no conflict of interest.

References

1. Collaborators, G.B.D.E. Global, regional, and national burden of epilepsy, 1990–2016: A systematic analysis for the Global Burden of Disease Study 2016. *Lancet Neurol.* **2019**, *18*, 357–375. [CrossRef]
2. Duncan, J.S.; Winston, G.P.; Koepp, M.J.; Ourselin, S. Brain imaging in the assessment for epilepsy surgery. *Lancet Neurol.* **2016**, *15*, 420–433. [CrossRef]
3. Wang, G.-B.; Long, W.; Li, X.-D.; Xu, G.-Y.; Lu, J.-X. Dynamic Contrast-Enhanced Magnetic Resonance Imaging (DCE-MRI) Combined with Positron Emission Tomography-Computed Tomography (PET-CT) and Video-Electroencephalography (VEEG) Have Excellent Diagnostic Value in Preoperative Localization of Epileptic Foci in Children with Epilepsy. *Med. Sci. Monit.* **2017**, *23*, 1–10. [CrossRef] [PubMed]
4. Kogias, E.; Klingler, J.-H.; Urbach, H.; Scheiwe, C.; Schmeiser, B.; Doostkam, S.; Zentner, J.; Altenmüller, D.-M. 3 Tesla MRI-negative focal epilepsies: Presurgical evaluation, postoperative outcome and predictive factors. *Clin. Neurol. Neurosurg.* **2017**, *163*, 116–120. [CrossRef]
5. Ahmed, R.; Rubinger, L.; Go, C.; Drake, J.M.; Rutka, J.T.; Snead, O.C.; Widjaja, E. Utility of additional dedicated high-resolution 3T MRI in children with medically refractory focal epilepsy. *Epilepsy Res.* **2018**, *143*, 113–119. [CrossRef]
6. McGrath, H.; Mandel, M.; Sandhu, M.R.S.; Lamsam, L.; Adenu-Mensah, N.; Farooque, P.; Spencer, D.D.; Damisah, E.C. Optimizing the surgical management of MRI-negative epilepsy in the neuromodulation era. *Epilepsia Open* **2022**, *7*, 151–159. [CrossRef]
7. Engel, J., Jr. Surgery for Seizures. *N. Engl. J. Med.* **1996**, *334*, 647–653. [CrossRef]
8. Wiebe, S.; Blume, W.T.; Girvin, J.P.; Eliasziw, M.; Effectiveness and Efficiency of Surgery for Temporal Lobe Epilepsy Study Group. A Randomized, Controlled Trial of Surgery for Temporal-Lobe Epilepsy. *N. Engl. J. Med.* **2001**, *345*, 311–318. [CrossRef]
9. Téllez-Zenteno, J.F.; Ronquillo, L.H.; Moien-Afshari, F.; Wiebe, S. Surgical outcomes in lesional and non-lesional epilepsy: A systematic review and meta-analysis. *Epilepsy Res.* **2010**, *89*, 310–318. [CrossRef]
10. Taussig, D.; Montavont, A.; Isnard, J. Invasive EEG explorations. *Neurophysiol. Clin.* **2015**, *45*, 113–119. [CrossRef]
11. Desarnaud, S.; Mellerio, C.; Semah, F.; Laurent, A.; Landre, E.; Devaux, B.; Chiron, C.; Lebon, V.; Chassoux, F. 18F-FDG PET in drug-resistant epilepsy due to focal cortical dysplasia type 2: Additional value of electroclinical data and coregistration with MRI. *Eur. J. Nucl. Med. Mol. Imaging* **2018**, *45*, 1449–1460. [CrossRef] [PubMed]
12. Rathore, C.; Dickson, J.C.; Teotónio, R.; Ell, P.; Duncan, J.S. The utility of 18F-fluorodeoxyglucose PET (FDG PET) in epilepsy surgery. *Epilepsy Res.* **2014**, *108*, 1306–1314. [CrossRef] [PubMed]
13. Feng, R.; Hu, J.; Pan, L.; Shi, J.; Qiu, C.; Lang, L.; Gu, X.; Guo, J. Surgical Treatment of MRI-Negative Temporal Lobe Epilepsy Based on PET: A Retrospective Cohort Study. *Ster. Funct. Neurosurg.* **2014**, *92*, 354–359. [CrossRef] [PubMed]
14. Chapman, K.; Wyllie, E.; Najm, I.; Ruggieri, P.; Bingaman, W.; Lüders, J.; Kotagal, P.; Lachhwani, D.; Dinner, D.; O Lüders, H. Seizure outcome after epilepsy surgery in patients with normal preoperative MRI. *J. Neurol. Neurosurg. Psychiatry* **2005**, *76*, 710–713. [CrossRef]
15. Kim, Y.K.; Lee, D.S.; Lee, S.K.; Chung, C.K.; Chung, J.K.; Lee, M.C. (18)F-FDG PET in localization of frontal lobe epilepsy: Comparison of visual and SPM analysis. *J. Nucl. Med.* **2002**, *43*, 1167–1174.
16. Sebastiano, D.R.; Tassi, L.; Duran, D.; Visani, E.; Gozzo, F.; Cardinale, F.; Nobili, L.; Del Sole, A.; Rubino, A.; Dotta, S.; et al. Identifying the epileptogenic zone by four non-invasive imaging techniques versus stereo-EEG in MRI-negative pre-surgery epilepsy patients. *Clin. Neurophysiol.* **2020**, *131*, 1815–1823. [CrossRef]
17. Ding, Y.; Zhu, Y.; Jiang, B.; Zhou, Y.; Jin, B.; Hou, H.; Wu, S.; Zhu, J.; Wang, Z.I.; Wong, C.H.; et al. 18F-FDG PET and high-resolution MRI co-registration for pre-surgical evaluation of patients with conventional MRI-negative refractory extra-temporal lobe epilepsy. *Eur. J. Nucl. Med. Mol. Imaging* **2018**, *45*, 1567–1572. [CrossRef]
18. Fernández, S.; Donaire, A.; Serès, E.; Setoain, X.; Bargalló, N.; Falcón, C.; Sanmartí, F.; Maestro, I.; Rumià, J.; Pintor, L.; et al. PET/MRI and PET/MRI/SISCOM coregistration in the presurgical evaluation of refractory focal epilepsy. *Epilepsy Res.* **2015**, *111*, 1–9. [CrossRef]
19. Paldino, M.J.; Yang, E.; Jones, J.Y.; Mahmood, N.; Sher, A.; Zhang, W.; Hayatghaibi, S.; Krishnamurthy, R.; Seghers, V. Comparison of the diagnostic accuracy of PET/MRI to PET/CT-acquired FDG brain exams for seizure focus detection: A prospective study. *Pediatr. Radiol.* **2017**, *47*, 1500–1507. [CrossRef]
20. Grouiller, F.; Delattre, B.M.A.; Pittau, F.; Heinzer, S.; Lazeyras, F.; Spinelli, L.; Iannotti, G.R.; Seeck, M.; Ratib, O.; Vargas, M.I.; et al. All-in-one interictal presurgical imaging in patients with epilepsy: Single-session EEG/PET/(f)MRI. *Eur. J. Nucl. Med. Mol. Imaging* **2015**, *42*, 1133–1143. [CrossRef]
21. Oldan, J.D.; Shin, H.W.; Khandani, A.H.; Zamora, C.; Benefield, T.; Jewells, V. Subsequent experience in hybrid PET-MRI for evaluation of refractory focal onset epilepsy. *Seizure* **2018**, *61*, 128–134. [CrossRef] [PubMed]
22. Shin, H.W.; Jewells, V.; Sheikh, A.; Zhang, J.; Zhu, H.; An, H.; Gao, W.; Shen, D.; Hadar, E.; Lin, W. Initial experience in hybrid PET-MRI for evaluation of refractory focal onset epilepsy. *Seizure* **2015**, *31*, 1–4. [CrossRef]

23. Shang, K.; Wang, J.; Fan, X.; Cui, B.; Ma, J.; Yang, H.; Zhou, Y.; Zhao, G.; Lu, J. Clinical Value of Hybrid TOF-PET/MR Imaging–Based Multiparametric Imaging in Localizing Seizure Focus in Patients with MRI-Negative Temporal Lobe Epilepsy. *AJNR Am. J. Neuroradiol.* **2018**, *39*, 1791–1798. [CrossRef] [PubMed]
24. Werner, P.; Barthel, H.; Drzezga, A.; Sabri, O. Current status and future role of brain PET/MRI in clinical and research settings. *Eur. J. Pediatr.* **2015**, *42*, 512–526. [CrossRef]
25. Jadvar, H.; Colletti, P.M. Competitive advantage of PET/MRI. *Eur. J. Radiol.* **2014**, *83*, 84–94. [CrossRef]
26. Traub-Weidinger, T.; Muzik, O.; Sundar, L.K.S.; Aull-Watschinger, S.; Beyer, T.; Hacker, M.; Hahn, A.; Kasprian, G.; Klebermass, E.-M.; Lanzenberger, R.; et al. Utility of Absolute Quantification in Non-lesional Extratemporal Lobe Epilepsy Using FDG PET/MR Imaging. *Front. Neurol.* **2020**, *11*, 54. [CrossRef] [PubMed]
27. Zhang, M.; Liu, W.; Huang, P.; Lin, X.; Huang, X.; Meng, H.; Wang, J.; Hu, K.; Li, J.; Lin, M.; et al. Utility of hybrid PET/MRI multiparametric imaging in navigating SEEG placement in refractory epilepsy. *Seizure* **2020**, *81*, 295–303. [CrossRef]
28. Guo, K.; Wang, J.; Cui, B.; Wang, Y.; Hou, Y.; Zhao, G.; Lu, J. [18F]FDG PET/MRI and magnetoencephalography may improve presurgical localization of temporal lobe epilepsy. *Eur. J. Radiol.* **2021**, 1–11. [CrossRef]
29. Varrone, A.; Asenbaum, S.; Borght, T.V.; Booij, J.; Nobili, F.; Någren, K.; Darcourt, J.; Kapucu, Ö.L.; Tatsch, K.; Bartenstein, P.; et al. EANM procedure guidelines for PET brain imaging using [18F]FDG, version 2. *Eur. J. Nucl. Med. Mol. Imaging* **2009**, *36*, 2103–2110. [CrossRef]
30. FreeSurfer Software Suite. Available online: http://surfer.nmr.mgh.harvard.edu (accessed on 21 March 2020).
31. Dale, A.M.; Fischl, B.; Sereno, M.I. Cortical surface-based analysis. I. Segmentation and surface reconstruction. *NeuroImage* **1999**, *9*, 179–194. [CrossRef]
32. Fischl, B.; Sereno, M.I.; Dale, A.M. Cortical Surface-Based Analysis. II: Inflation, Flattening, and a Surface-Based Coordinate System. *NeuroImage* **1999**, *9*, 195–207. [CrossRef] [PubMed]
33. Jenkinson, M.; Beckmann, C.F.; Behrens, T.E.; Woolrich, M.W.; Smith, S.M. FSL. *NeuroImage* **2012**, *62*, 782–790. [CrossRef]
34. Avants, B.B.; Tustison, N.J.; Song, G.; Cook, P.A.; Klein, A.; Gee, J.C. A reproducible evaluation of ANTs similarity metric performance in brain image registration. *NeuroImage* **2011**, *54*, 2033–2044. [CrossRef] [PubMed]
35. Della Rosa, P.A.; Cerami, C.; Gallivanone, F.; Prestia, A.; Caroli, A.; Castiglioni, I.; Gilardi, M.C.; Frisoni, G.; Friston, K.; Ashburner, J.; et al. A Standardized [18F]-FDG-PET Template for Spatial Normalization in Statistical Parametric Mapping of Dementia. *Neuroinformatics* **2014**, *12*, 575–593. [CrossRef] [PubMed]
36. Desikan, R.S.; Ségonne, F.; Fischl, B.; Quinn, B.T.; Dickerson, B.C.; Blacker, D.; Buckner, R.L.; Dale, A.M.; Maguire, R.P.; Hyman, B.T.; et al. An automated labeling system for subdividing the human cerebral cortex on MRI scans into gyral based regions of interest. *NeuroImage* **2006**, *31*, 968–980. [CrossRef]
37. Ashburner, J. SPM: A history. *NeuroImage* **2012**, *62*, 791–800. [CrossRef]
38. House, P.M.; Lanz, M.; Holst, B.; Martens, T.; Stodieck, S.; Huppertz, H.-J. Comparison of morphometric analysis based on T1- and T2-weighted MRI data for visualization of focal cortical dysplasia. *Epilepsy Res.* **2013**, *106*, 403–409. [CrossRef]
39. Benjamini, Y.; Drai, D.; Elmer, G.; Kafkafi, N.; Golani, I. Controlling the false discovery rate in behavior genetics research. *Behav. Brain Res.* **2001**, *125*, 279–284. [CrossRef]
40. Gwet, K.L. Computing inter-rater reliability and its variance in the presence of high agreement. *Br. J. Math. Stat. Psychol.* **2008**, *61*, 29–48. [CrossRef]
41. Wongpakaran, N.; Wongpakaran, T.; Wedding, D.; Gwet, K.L. A comparison of Cohen's Kappa and Gwet's AC1 when calculating inter-rater reliability coefficients: A study conducted with personality disorder samples. *BMC Med. Res. Methodol.* **2013**, *13*, 61. [CrossRef] [PubMed]
42. Salamon, N.; Kung, J.; Shaw, S.J.; Koo, J.; Koh, S.; Wu, J.Y.; Lerner, J.T.; Sankar, R.; Shields, W.D.; Engel, J., Jr.; et al. FDG-PET/MRI coregistration improves detection of cortical dysplasia in patients with epilepsy. *Neurology* **2008**, *71*, 1594–1601. [CrossRef] [PubMed]
43. Sun, K.; Ren, Z.; Yang, D.; Wang, X.; Yu, T.; Ni, D.; Qiao, L.; Xu, C.; Gao, R.; Lin, Y.; et al. Voxel-based morphometric MRI post-processing and PET/MRI co-registration reveal subtle abnormalities in cingulate epilepsy. *Epilepsy Res.* **2021**, *171*, 106568. [CrossRef]
44. Kikuchi, K.; Togao, O.; Yamashita, K.; Momosaka, D.; Nakayama, T.; Kitamura, Y.; Kikuchi, Y.; Baba, S.; Sagiyama, K.; Ishimatsu, K.; et al. Diagnostic accuracy for the epileptogenic zone detection in focal epilepsy could be higher in FDG-PET/MRI than in FDG-PET/CT. *Eur. Radiol.* **2021**, *31*, 2915–2922. [CrossRef] [PubMed]
45. Coan, A.C.; Chaudhary, U.J.; Grouiller, F.; Campos, B.M.; Perani, S.; De Ciantis, A.; Vulliemoz, S.; Diehl, B.; Beltramini, G.C.; Carmichael, D.W.; et al. EEG-fMRI in the presurgical evaluation of temporal lobe epilepsy. *J. Neurol. Neurosurg. Psychiatry* **2016**, *87*, 642–649. [CrossRef]
46. Meletti, S.; Vignoli, A.; Benuzzi, F.; Avanzini, P.; Ruggieri, A.; Pugnaghi, M.; Nichelli, P.; Canevini, M.P. Ictal involvement of the nigrostriatal system in subtle seizures of ring chromosome 20 epilepsy. *Epilepsia* **2012**, *53*, e156–e160. [CrossRef]
47. Chaudhary, U.J.; Carmichael, D.W.; Rodionov, R.; Thornton, R.C.; Bartlett, P.; Vulliemoz, S.; Micallef, C.; McEvoy, A.W.; Diehl, B.; Walker, M.C.; et al. Mapping preictal and ictal haemodynamic networks using video-electroencephalography and functional imaging. *Brain J. Neurol.* **2012**, *135*, 3645–3663. [CrossRef]
48. Vaudano, A.E.; Carmichael, D.W.; Salek-Haddadi, A.; Rampp, S.; Stefan, H.; Lemieux, L.; Koepp, M.J. Networks involved in seizure initiation: A reading epilepsy case studied with EEG-fMRI and MEG. *Neurology* **2012**, *79*, 249–253. [CrossRef] [PubMed]

49. Ito, Y.; Maesawa, S.; Bagarinao, E.; Okai, Y.; Nakatsubo, D.; Yamamoto, H.; Kidokoro, H.; Usui, N.; Natsume, J.; Hoshiyama, M.; et al. Subsecond EEG-fMRI analysis for presurgical evaluation in focal epilepsy. *J. Neurosurg.* **2020**, *134*, 1027–1036. [CrossRef] [PubMed]
50. Chatzistefanidis, D.; Huang, D.; Dümpelmann, M.; Jacobs, J.; Schulze-Bonhage, A.; LeVan, P. Topography-Related EEG-fMRI in Surgically Confirmed Epileptic Foci: A Comparison to Spike-Related EEG-fMRI in Clinical Practice. *Brain Topogr.* **2021**, *34*, 373–383. [CrossRef] [PubMed]

Article

A Single Application of Cerebellar Transcranial Direct Current Stimulation Fails to Enhance Motor Skill Acquisition in Parkinson's Disease: A Pilot Study

Lidio Lima de Albuquerque [1], Milan Pantovic [2], Mitchell Clingo [3], Katherine Fischer [2], Sharon Jalene [2], Merrill Landers [4], Zoltan Mari [5] and Brach Poston [2,*]

1. School of Health and Applied Human Sciences, University of North Carolina Wilmington, Wilmington, NC 28403, USA; limadeal@uncw.edu
2. Department of Kinesiology and Nutrition Sciences, University of Nevada Las Vegas, Las Vegas, NV 89154, USA; milan.pantovic@unlv.edu (M.P.); fische74@unlv.nevada.edu (K.F.); sharon.jalene@unlv.edu (S.J.)
3. School of Medicine, University of Nevada Las Vegas, Las Vegas, NV 89154, USA; clingom@unlv.nevada.edu
4. Department of Physical Therapy, University of Nevada Las Vegas, Las Vegas, NV 89154, USA; merrill.landers@unlv.edu
5. Movement Disorders Program, Cleveland Clinic Lou Ruvo Center for Brain Health, Las Vegas, NV 89106, USA; mariz@ccf.org
* Correspondence: brach.poston@unlv.edu

Abstract: Parkinson's disease (PD) is a progressive neurodegenerative disorder that leads to numerous impairments in motor function that compromise the ability to perform activities of daily living. Practical and effective adjunct therapies are needed to complement current treatment approaches in PD. Transcranial direct current stimulation applied to the cerebellum (c-tDCS) can increase motor skill in young and older adults. Because the cerebellum is involved in PD pathology, c-tDCS application during motor practice could potentially enhance motor skill in PD. The primary purpose was to examine the influence of c-tDCS on motor skill acquisition in a complex, visuomotor isometric precision grip task (PGT) in PD in the OFF-medication state. The secondary purpose was to determine the influence of c-tDCS on transfer of motor skill in PD. The study utilized a double-blind, SHAM-controlled, within-subjects design. A total of 16 participants completed a c-tDCS condition and a SHAM condition in two experimental sessions separated by a 7-day washout period. Each session involved practice of the PGT concurrent with either c-tDCS or SHAM. Additionally, motor transfer tasks were quantified before and after the practice and stimulation period. The force error in the PGT was not significantly different between the c-tDCS and SHAM conditions. Similarly, transfer task performance was not significantly different between the c-tDCS and SHAM conditions. These findings indicate that a single session of c-tDCS does not elicit acute improvements in motor skill acquisition or transfer in hand and arm tasks in PD while participants are off medications.

Keywords: Parkinson's disease; transcranial direct current stimulation; motor skill; cerebellum; cerebellar stimulation; motor learning; manual dexterity; dopamine; basal ganglia; transfer of motor learning

1. Introduction

Parkinson's disease (PD) is the second most common neurodegenerative disorder and affects approximately one million people in the United States with annual costs approaching USD 11 billion [1]. The cardinal pathologic feature of PD is the loss of dopaminergic neurons in the substantia nigra pars compacta, which leads to striatal dopamine depletion. The decrease in dopamine is associated with a variety of motor deficits such as rigidity, bradykinesia, tremor, and postural instability that lead to severe impairments in the ability to perform daily living activities. Current surgical and pharmacological treatments may be affected by many problems including side effects, costs, and limited efficacy [2]. For example, Levodopa combined with other medications represents the standard treatment for PD, but its efficacy diminishes over time and leads to side effects such as dyskinesia [3]. Therefore, the development of practical and effective therapeutic adjuncts to complement current treatments remains an important priority in PD.

Transcranial direct current stimulation (tDCS) is a non-invasive brain stimulation technique that can increase motor skill in healthy adults [4–6] (for review see [7]) and in PD [2,8] when delivered to the primary motor cortex (M1-tDCS). Although M1 has been the brain region most frequently targeted with tDCS, several studies have shown that the tDCS of the cerebellum (c-tDCS) can also enhance motor abilities [9]. For example, c-tDCS improved motor skill [10], motor learning [11], and performance in motor adaptation paradigms in young and older adults [12]. These studies could be relevant to intervention therapy development in PD because the cerebellum contributes to PD pathophysiology [13,14]. Specifically, the approach most often proposed [7] is to utilize the methodology developed from motor skill and learning studies involving tDCS to rehabilitation protocols used in clinical practice. The strategy of simultaneously combining tDCS with existing motor rehabilitation techniques would likely improve motor function to a greater extent than rehabilitation alone [7]. These effects have been shown to occur in a number of M1-tDCS studies and accumulating evidence has begun to demonstrate that c-tDCS could have similar or even greater effects [15] on motor skill compared to M1-tDCS in certain experimental conditions or motor tasks. Thus, c-tDCS could be a valuable and viable intervention for improving motor function in PD if it could enhance motor skill learning to a similar degree as seen in studies involving young and older adults.

Although PD is primarily a basal ganglia disorder, cerebellar involvement in PD pathophysiology provides a basis for targeting it with tDCS [13,14]. While M1 plays the predominant role in skilled execution of hand and arm movements [16], the descending drive of M1 to the spinal motor neuron pools of upper limb muscles depends on input from many motor areas onto intracortical interneurons [17] including crucial cerebellum contributions [17,18]. Furthermore, previously unknown bi-directional pathways have recently been discovered between the cerebellum and basal ganglia [19]. The cerebellar connections to basal ganglia and M1 are important because the effects of tDCS can extend to brain areas not stimulated directly. For example, M1-tDCS has been shown in animal, imaging, and pharmacological studies to induce remote effects in interconnected regions including the basal ganglia [20], thalamus [21], and the spinal cord [22]. Accordingly, M1-tDCS activation of basal ganglia in PD monkeys was associated with enhanced motor function [23]. This provides theoretical support that c-tDCS could indirectly impact M1 and basal ganglia activity. Cerebellar dysfunction in PD could also be a compensatory mechanism to diminish the negative effects of altered basal ganglia activity as people with PD with greater cerebellar activity exhibit better motor function [13]. Thus, c-tDCS could possibly augment motor skill in PD by heightening compensatory processes through increased cerebellar activation [24]. Finally, the increases in motor skill elicited by c-tDCS in older adults [12] are promising because evidence suggests that the cerebellum is the primary brain area responsible for movement impairments in older adults [25]. These factors along with the motor performance improvements elicited by c-tDCS in young adults [10,11,26] provide strong rationale for the investigation of c-tDCS to improve motor function in PD.

Despite these lines of reasoning, only two studies [27,28] have examined the influence of c-tDCS on upper motor limb motor skill acquisition in PD, which is much fewer than the number of M1-tDCS investigations in PD [2,8]. Two additional c-tDCS studies have focused entirely on the lower extremities. One study only involved seven subjects [29] and found that only one of four different c-tDCS electrode montages improved balance performance. The other study found that c-tDCS did not improve dual task gait performance in PD [30]. Additionally, Ferrucci et al. (2016) reported that five days of c-tDCS did not improve any motor or cognitive rating scale measures except dyskinesia scores [31]. In the two aforementioned studies conducted in our laboratory, individuals with PD were only tested in the ON-medication state while c-tDCS was delivered [27,28]. Furthermore, these studies also had the limitation of being between-subjects experimental designs, which introduces numerous interindividual genetic and physiological differences that could potentially impact results [32,33]. Therefore, the primary purpose was to examine the influence of c-tDCS on motor performance in a complex, visuomotor isometric precision grip task (PGT) in PD in the OFF-medication state. The secondary purpose was to determine the influence of c-tDCS on the transfer of motor performance in PD as all but one of the previous c-tDCS studies in PD did not evaluate the transfer of motor skill learning [27,29–31]. It was hypothesized that c-tDCS would increase motor skill acquisition in the PGT compared to the SHAM stimulation. Finally, it was predicted that c-tDCS would increase motor skill in the transfer tasks to a greater extent than SHAM stimulation.

2. Materials and Methods

2.1. Experimental Design

This pilot study utilized a double-blind, SHAM-controlled, within-subjects, counterbalanced design. The study was designed to determine the influence of c-tDCS on both motor skill acquisition and the transfer of motor skill. The assessment of the effect of c-tDCS on motor skill acquisition was accomplished by applying c-tDCS simultaneously with a task that was practiced extensively (PGT). In contrast, the transfer of motor skill measurement was accomplished by measuring performance in motor tasks involving many of the same hand and arm muscles as the PGT when c-tDCS was not applied concurrently and the tasks were not practiced extensively. The transfer tasks (see Section 2.6) included maximum voluntary contractions (MVCs), the Unified Parkinson's Disease Rating Scale Part III (UPDRS-III), the Purdue Pegboard Test (PPT), and the Jebsen Taylor Hand Function Test (JTT). Overall, the rationale was that if c-tDCS could successfully enhance motor skill acquisition when applied during a motor task as well as elicit performance improvements in other hand and arm tasks, it would provide strong evidence that c-tDCS application could be translated to clinical settings and paired with practice and rehabilitation tasks.

2.2. Participants

Sixteen participants diagnosed with idiopathic PD (10 males, 6 females; mean age: 68.4 ± 11.8) participated in the study with 5, 9, and 2 participants being Hoehn and Yahr scale 1, 2, and 3, respectively. Thirteen participants were right-hand dominant and predominantly right-side affected, whereas three participants were left-hand dominant and predominantly left-side affected. The Montreal Cognitive Assessment (MoCA) was used to screen for early identification of cognitive impairment. Participants were required to have a MoCA score of 26 or higher to participate in the study (mean score 28.31 ± 1.70). Participants were free of other neurological disorders and did not meet international exclusion criteria for non-invasive brain stimulation studies [34]. The study was conducted according to the Declaration of Helsinki and approved by the Institutional Review Board at the University of Nevada Las Vegas.

2.3. Experimental Procedures

Two experimental sessions were performed and separated by a 7-day washout period. This within-subject, fully counterbalanced design was chosen for several reasons: (1) The substantial interindividual differences in the responsiveness to tDCS due to physiological, biological, and anatomical factors are mitigated [32,33] with within-subjects designs. For the cerebellum in particular, there are variations in nerve fiber orientation and convolution of the cerebellar cortex beneath where the tDCS electrodes are placed [35]. (2) The within-subjects design allowed for greater statistical power compared with a between-subjects design [36] such as that employed in previous c-tDCS and PD studies performed in our laboratory [27,28]. (3) Many prior M1-tDCS studies in PD [8] and a previous c-tDCS study in PD [29] have had success with within-subject designs using similar motor tasks and washout periods, despite having fewer participants than the current study.

In both experimental sessions, participants reported to the lab in the morning after a 12 h medication withdrawal. This corresponds to the practically defined OFF-medication condition [37], which standardizes clinical responses. All patients kept their medication schedule constant throughout the study period. Participants were tested in the OFF-medication state so that the influence of c-tDCS on motor performance in the basic disease state could be determined and because the aforementioned previous c-tDCS studies in PD from our laboratory were performed in the ON-medication state in a between-subjects design [27,28]. The PGT was performed over a 25 min period concurrent with either c-tDCS or SHAM stimulation with the predominately affected hand. Additionally, the transfer tasks (MVCs, UPDRS-III, PPT, and JTT) were completed before and after stimulation (pre- and post-tests; see below) and were all performed with the predominately affected hand. These tasks were considered transfer tasks because they were not conducted simultaneously with c-tDCS and were not practiced. Accordingly, each experiment was performed in the order prescribed: (1) a familiarization that included acquainting participants with the motor tasks along with visual demonstrations by the investigators; (2) pre-tests were completed; (3) c-tDCS or SHAM stimulation was applied and 10 trials of the PGT were performed during the stimulation period; and (4) post-tests were completed (Figure 1).

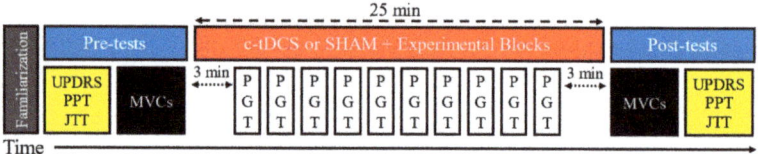

Figure 1. Schematic representation of the experimental protocol that comprised a familiarization, pre-tests (UPDRS-III, PPT, JTT, MVCs), 25 min of either c-tDCS or SHAM stimulation concurrent with 10 trials of the PGT, and post-tests (MVCs, UPDRS, PPT, JTT) in the order depicted.

2.4. Pinch Grip Task (PGT)

The PGT arrangement was similar to previous studies [27,38]. Briefly, participants were seated with the dominant arm abducted to 45°, the elbow flexed to 90°, and the hand semi-supinated while resting on a table. The PGT involved accurately matching a target sine wave (0.5 Hz) on a monitor by producing isometric force using a precision grip (index finger and thumb) against a grip device instrumented with force transducers. The sine wave minimums and maximums were 5% and 25% of the pre-test MVC force for all PGT trials. Thus, the average force produced during each trial was approximately 15% of MVC, but the participants had to modulate this force between 5% and 25% of MVC by accurate force production and force relaxation within this range. Each PGT trial involved matching the template for 30 s and a total of 10 trials were performed concurrent with either c-tDCS or SHAM. The stimulator was turned on for three minutes prior to performing the first PGT trial and was kept on (~1–3 min) after the last trial [10].

The PGT was the motor task chosen to be paired with stimulation for several inter-related reasons: (1) Numerous M1-tDCS studies [7,39,40] and a c-tDCS study in young adults [11] have found that tDCS elicits large, acute performance increases in precision grip tasks. Thus, the PGT had potential for improvement due to c-tDCS. (2) fMRI has revealed that the cerebellum participates in force amplitude and rate modulation in the precision grip [41]. (3) The precision grip is a functional multi-muscle task required in everyday living. (4) There is high cerebellar involvement in muscle activation timing, error detection [42] in voluntary movements, and in visuomotor tracking [43], which are all motor control aspects of the PGT. (5) A series of behavioral and fMRI studies in PD by Vaillancourt and colleagues have shown that the basal ganglia is highly involved in various aspects of pinch grip task performance (e.g., amplitude modulation, rate of force production, force relaxation) and displays differences compared to healthy controls and other disease states [44–51].

2.5. Cerebellar Transcranial Direct Current Stimulation (c-tDCS)

A NeuroConn DC Stimulator delivered anodal tDCS via two rubber electrodes (5 × 5 cm) encased in saline-soaked sponges. c-tDCS was applied over the cerebellum ipsilateral to the predominantly affected hand (anode 3 cm lateral to the inion, cathode over the ipsilateral buccinator muscle, current strength 2 mA, 25 min duration). These c-tDCS parameters have elicited large, immediate motor performance increases in young and older adults [10–12,26]. For SHAM, the current was ramped up and down over 30 s according to standard SHAM procedures. The stimulator was programmed by an investigator who did not participate in data collection and the investigators who conducted the experiments were blind to the experimental conditions as in our previous studies [10,27,28,52].

2.6. Transfer Tasks

Four tasks were employed to quantify transfer of motor performance to tasks that were not performed during stimulation or practiced as extensively as the PGT. The transfer tasks (MVCs, UPDRS, PPT, and JTT) were administered immediately before and after the stimulation and practice period on the predominantly affected hand/arm. Execution of the tasks after stimulation was an important study design aspect because numerous studies have shown that tDCS can elicit performance enhancements for at least 30 min after stimulation. Accordingly, the transfer tasks were able to be completed in this 30 min time period after the application of c-tDCS had ended.

Three MVC trials were completed in the identical experimental arrangement and hand posture as in the PGT. Similar to previous studies, participants exerted maximum force in the shortest time possible and held the maximum for 5 s [53]. The MVC served three purposes: (1) the pre-test MVC force was used as a reference value to calculate the PGT target forces; (2) the difference between the pre- and post-test MVCs was used to rule out the influence of muscle fatigue on the PGT results; and (3) MVC served as a transfer task representing the motor ability of maximum strength as a recent study in young adults found that c-tDCS could acutely enhance maximal isometric force production in a full-body task [54]. The UPDRS-III was administered by an investigator trained by a movement disorder neurologist. The UPDRS-III was chosen as a transfer task because it is the gold standard clinical test to rate motor symptoms in PD. The PPT is a standard test to evaluate arm and hand function and entails picking up and placing pegs in small holes as fast as possible over 30 s. Similarly, the JTT is a manual dexterity assessment used in aging, movement disorder, and tDCS studies. Six tasks are performed that imitate common tasks of daily living as quickly as possible with the hand and arm. The PPT and JTT were each performed for three trials. The PPT and JTT were selected as transfer tasks as they are among the most common manual dexterity tests utilized in movement disorder research and tDCS studies. Collectively, these transfer tasks were chosen because they are well-characterized in the literature, provide information on several aspects of motor function, have varying emphasis on proximal and distal upper limb muscle control, and exhibit varying degrees of overlap of the muscle groups involved in the PGT.

2.7. Data Analysis

The force error in the PGT was the primary dependent variable, whereas MVC, UPDRS-III, PPT, and JTT were secondary dependent variables. Force error in the PGT was calculated as the average error in force relative to the target over each 30 s trial [27]. Specifically, the force error was calculated in the following steps: (1) the difference in the target force displayed on the template and the force produced was quantified at each sampling point for the 30 s trial; (2) the absolute value of each of these differences was calculated; (3) the average of all of these absolute values was quantified for the entire trial; and (4) the final force error value was taken as the average of the 10 PGT trials (grand average). MVC force was quantified as the average force produced during the plateau period for each trial and the highest force among the 3 trials was denoted as the MVC. The UPDRS score was quantified as the sum of the items on the motor examination Part III. The PPT score was calculated as the average number of pegs over 3 trials. For the JTT, the total time to complete the 6 tasks was computed for each trial and averaged over 3 trials.

2.8. Statistical Analysis

Force error in the PGT between the c-tDCS and SHAM conditions was compared with a two-tailed paired *t*-test, whereas MVC, UPDRS, PPT, and JTT were analyzed with two-way (2 *condition* (c-tDCS, SHAM) × 2 *test* (pre, post)) within-subjects ANOVAs. The significance level was α = 0.05 and data are indicated as means ± standard errors in the figures. Similar to our previous study [28], an interim futility analysis was conducted after the completion of 16 participants to estimate the sample size needed for the primary outcome variables (PGT, UPDRS-III, MVC, Pegboard, JTT).

3. Results

3.1. PGT

The force error was not significantly different between the c-tDCS and SHAM conditions (Figure 2; Table 1).

Table 1. Summary of statistical values. The corresponding statistical test, *p* values, and partial eta squared values for each of the dependent variables described in the text and figures above.

Dependent Variable	Statistical Test		*p*	η_p^2
PGT (N)	Paired *t*-test		0.322	
MVC (N)	2 × 2 within-subjects ANOVA	*condition*	0.224	0.158
		test	0.749	0.007
		condition × *test*	0.446	0.036
UPDRS-III (Score)	2 × 2 within-subjects ANOVA	*condition*	0.709	0.010
		test	0.920	0.001
		condition × *test*	0.341	0.061
Purdue Pegboard (pegs)	2 × 2 within-subjects ANOVA	*condition*	0.412	0.045
		test	0.268	0.081
		condition × *test*	0.222	0.098
JTT (sec)	2 × 2 within-subjects ANOVA	*condition*	0.607	0.018
		test	0.004	0.427
		condition × *test*	0.872	0.002

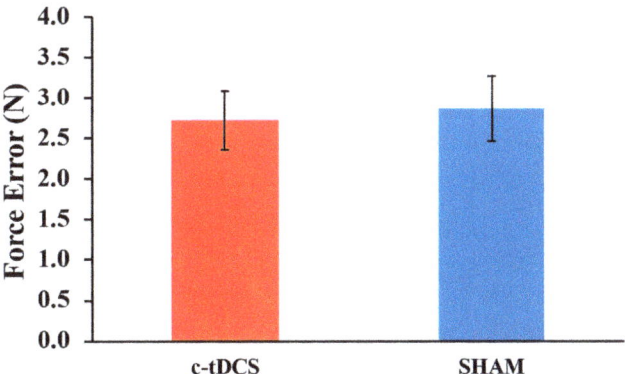

Figure 2. Force error in the PGT for the c-tDCS and SHAM conditions. The force error was not significantly different between the c-tDCS and SHAM conditions ($p = 0.322$).

3.2. Transfer Tasks

For the MVC, the main effect for *condition*, main effect for *test*, and *condition* × *test* interaction were all non-significant (Figure 3A; Table 1). Similarly, the main effect for *condition*, main effect for *test*, and *condition* × *test* interaction were all non-significant for the UPDRS-III (Figure 3B; Table 1). For the PPT, the main effect for *condition*, main effect for *test*, and *condition* × *test* interaction were all non-significant (Figure 4A; Table 1). For the JTT, the main effect for *condition* and *condition* × *test* interaction were non-significant (Figure 4B; Table 1). However, there was a significant main effect for *test*, which indicated that JTT time was shorter in the post-test compared to the pre-test (Figure 4B; Table 1).

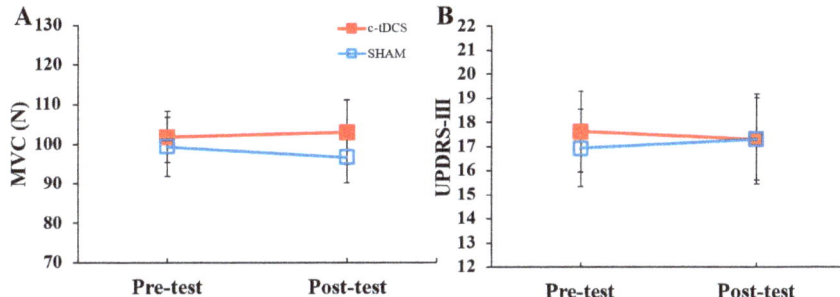

Figure 3. MVC forces and UPDRS-III scores in the pre- and post-tests for the c-tDCS (closed squares) and SHAM conditions (open squares). (**A**) MVC forces were not significantly different for the pre- and post-tests ($p = 0.749$) or between the c-tDCS and SHAM conditions ($p = 0.114$). (**B**) UPDRS scores were not significantly different for the pre- and post-tests ($p = 0.920$) or between the c-tDCS and SHAM conditions ($p = 0.709$).

3.3. Futility Analyses

Interim futility analyses were conducted on all the dependent variables to determine if additional participant recruitment was needed. Using the means, standard deviations, and test statistics from these analyses and the "Conditional Power and Sample Size Reestimation of Paired T-Tests" and the "Conditional Power and Sample Size Reestimation of Tests for Two Means in a 2 × 2 Cross-Over Design" modules on PASS 20.0.10 (NCSS, LLC, Kaysville, UT, USA), it was determined that the following numbers of participants were needed to achieve sufficient power to find statistically significant differences: 115 (PGT), 125 (UPDRS-III), 220 (MVC), 73 (Pegboard), and 4676 (JTT). Based on these estimates and the impracticality of recruiting these numbers, it was decided to terminate recruitment of additional participants for futility because of the lack of meaningful treatment effects.

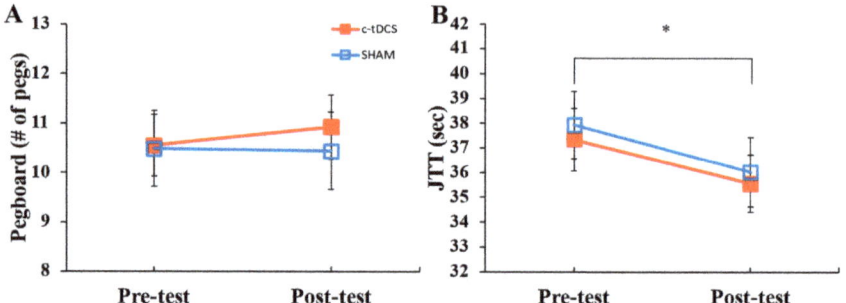

Figure 4. PPT scores and JTT times in the pre- and post-tests for the c-tDCS (closed squares) and SHAM conditions (open squares). (**A**) PPT scores were not significantly different for the pre- and post-tests ($p = 0.268$) or between the c-tDCS and SHAM conditions ($p = 0.412$). (**B**) JTT times were significantly lower in the post-test compared to the pre-test ($p = 0.004$) but not between the c-tDCS and SHAM conditions ($p = 0.607$). * Indicates a significant difference between the pre- and post-tests.

In summary, the statistical results clearly indicated that c-tDCS failed to elicit significant increases in motor skill acquisition or transfer compared to SHAM stimulation. In fact, the mean changes in all of the dependent variables were almost identical between the c-tDCS and SHAM conditions and no trends for any c-tDCS effects emerged. Accordingly, the futility analysis indicated that it was highly unlikely that the lack of significant differences between the c-tDCS and SHAM conditions was due to the sample size of the current study.

4. Discussion

Parkinson's disease (PD) is a progressive neurodegenerative disorder that leads to numerous impairments in motor function that compromise the ability to perform activities of daily living. The current pharmaceutical, surgical, and management strategies for PD are directed towards relieving the symptoms associated with the disease. Levodopa combined with other medications represents the standard treatment for PD, but its efficacy diminishes over time and leads to side effects such as dyskinesia. Accordingly, practical and effective adjunct therapies are needed to complement current treatment approaches in PD. Non-invasive brain stimulation techniques such as M1-tDCS and c-tDCS have emerged as potential valuable adjunct interventions with a realistic potential to be translated into clinical practice to improve motor performance in PD. Based on the available motor skill and rehabilitation studies to date, the most common strategy proposed to realize this goal has been to concurrently apply tDCS with existing motor rehabilitation techniques, which should improve function to a greater degree than rehabilitation alone.

Therefore, the primary purpose was to examine the influence of c-tDCS on motor skill acquisition in a complex, visuomotor isometric precision grip task (PGT) in PD, whereas the secondary purpose was to determine the influence of c-tDCS on the transfer of motor skill in PD. This was accomplished by delivering c-tDCS simultaneously with a motor task (PGT) during practice to measure skill acquisition. The transfer of motor skill measurement was achieved by measuring performance before and after c-tDCS in motor tasks involving the same hand and arm muscles as the PGT. The study produced two main findings. First, c-tDCS did not significantly improve motor performance in the PGT task relative to SHAM. Second, transfer task performance was not enhanced following c-tDCS application relative to SHAM. Taken together, the results indicate that a single session of c-tDCS does not elicit improvements in motor skill acquisition or transfer of motor skill in hand and arm tasks in PD in the OFF-medication state.

The current study sought to extend previous studies that found that c-tDCS applied concurrently with motor task execution could enhance motor skill acquisition and motor learning in young and older adults [9–12]. Based on these observations and the cerebellar involvement in PD, the study investigated the effects of c-tDCS on motor skill acquisition and transfer in PD. It was originally hypothesized that force error in the PGT would be lower during c-tDCS stimulation compared with SHAM stimulation. Contrary to this prediction, force error in the PGT during c-tDCS application was only ~5% lower in the c-tDCS condition, but this small difference did not approach statistical significance ($p = 0.322$). This is in contrast to most previous c-tDCS studies in young and old adults, including a study from our laboratory [10] where c-tDCS increased throwing accuracy in young adults. The results are also not consistent with the motor function improvements observed in the majority of M1-tDCS studies in PD [2,8]. However, a study in young adults reported that c-tDCS failed to improve performance in a whole-body dynamic balance task [55]. Additionally, a single session of c-tDCS did not enhance clinical writing task scores of people with dystonia [56]. This is relevant because, similar to PD, dystonia is primarily a basal ganglia disorder that is also characterized by cerebellar contributions to impaired movement. Accordingly, a previous study from our laboratory involving a between-subjects design by Albuquerque et al. (2020) [27] found that a single application of c-tDCS did not enhance motor skill learning in PD while participants were in the ON-medication state, which confirms and extends the current findings. Overall, it appears that c-tDCS may not be effective, at least in acute conditions for upper limb tasks, at improving motor function in the movement disorders such as dystonia and PD where cerebellar deficits play a partial role.

A critical issue in tDCS studies and the field of motor control is whether performance improvements realized in a given task can be generalized (transferred) to other motor tasks [57]. Any modality will have limited utility if effects are only elicited when given simultaneously with a particular motor task, because it would be impractical for people with PD to train every impaired task of daily living. Surprisingly, the effects of tDCS on motor transfer have only been investigated in a few studies in any population and have yielded conflicting results [58–60]. In the present study, c-tDCS failed to improve performance of any of the transfer tasks as indicated by the lack of change between the pre-tests and the post-tests. These findings are in contrast to an M1-tDCS study in young adults, which demonstrated that tDCS increased transfer in some but not all aspects of arm movement performance [59]. In contrast, the results are consistent with an older adult study where improvements in the trained task conducted simultaneously with M1-tDCS did not generalize to other hand tasks [60]. Furthermore, M1-tDCS-induced improvements in a pinch grip task did not transfer to PPT or JTT performance in people who have had a stroke [58], which is particularly noteworthy as these motor tasks were almost the exact same as the motor tasks employed in the present study. Overall, these findings suggest that M1-tDCS and c-tDCS may have limited ability to induce the transfer of motor performance in several populations including PD.

The dissimilar findings between the present study and the preponderance of M1-tDCS studies in PD and c-tDCS studies in young and older adults imply that it should not be presumed that c-tDCS always enhances motor abilities. Most importantly, the outcomes suggest that results in healthy populations do not always translate directly to PD. Although the current results were unexpected, there are several possible factors responsible for the failure of c-tDCS to improve motor performance.

One possible explanation is that the balance of excitatory and inhibitory pathways from the cerebellum to M1 and basal ganglia are so altered in PD compared to healthy adults that c-tDCS application does not induce the same net motor effects. More specifically, the impairments in motor function in PD are mainly considered to be due to the loss of dopaminergic cells in the substantia nigra pars compacta that project to the striatum [3]. This results in lower levels of dopamine input onto the medium spiny neurons of the striatum that also receive cortical inputs and form part of the direct and indirect pathways which ultimately project back to the cortex. However, the motor dysfunctions in PD do not result solely from striatal dopamine depletion but are also due to impairments in the motor loops between the cerebellum and the cortex [3,13,14]. In healthy adults, transcranial magnetic stimulation (TMS) or tDCS of the cerebellum activates a cerebellar–thalamic–cortical pathway that bifurcates such that one pathway elicits a net inhibition on corticospinal output cells in M1, whereas the second pathway elicits a net facilitation [17]. In addition, two other TMS studies found that two interneuronal networks in M1 differ in how they process cerebellar inputs [61,62]. These studies also demonstrated that these pathways change during motor skill learning, which underscores their functional relevance [18]. Furthermore, similar effects could occur if there are imbalances in the bi-directional pathways between the cerebellum and basal ganglia [19]. Taken together, the widespread network dysfunction in numerous neural circuits between the cerebellum, basal ganglia, and M1 in PD might have led to a lack of positive c-tDCS effects on motor performance.

A second possibility is that one acute c-tDCS application may be insufficient to increase motor function and multi-day stimulation (3–5 sessions) might be necessary. Consistent with this line of reasoning, it was argued in the aforementioned negative c-tDCS study in dystonia that one c-tDCS session is unlikely to be sufficient to override negative motor adaptations that have developed due to the disease over many years [40]. This proposal is supported by the fact that M1-tDCS studies [39,40,58] and a c-tDCS study [11] reported cumulative motor learning effects over 3–5 days of practice performed concurrent with stimulation. Nonetheless, in these studies, the effects of tDCS on performance also reached significance within the first day. Furthermore, the vast majority of M1-tDCS studies in healthy adults and in PD have been single-session studies and have reported significant effects [2,8]. Thus, it is not mandatory that repeated daily application of c-tDCS is necessary to detect enhancements in motor function in PD if they occur. Accordingly, a recent study from our laboratory found that 9 days of c-tDCS application over a 2-week period did not improve motor learning or transfer of motor learning to a greater extent than practice alone (SHAM stimulation) in PD [28]. That study differed from the current study in that testing was performed in both ON- and OFF-medication states. However, the lack of an effect of c-tDCS even though nine stimulation sessions were performed supports the single-session motor performance results of the current study. Specifically, nine stimulation sessions should have been more than enough time for c-tDCS effects to appear if present based on numerous 3–5 day M1-tDCS and c-tDCS studies [11,39,40,58].

It could also be argued that the c-tDCS parameters (montage, current, and duration) were not optimal as other studies in various other populations have had at least some success with slightly different parameters [9]. Although this is possible, it seems highly unlikely as identical parameters were successful in our previous study [6] and in other studies from a different research group [11,12,26,63,64] in young and older adults. These same c-tDCS parameters were selected for the present study and a previous c-tDCS study in PD [27] because they had elicited positive effects in the greatest number of studies and the magnitude of the performance improvements was quite high. Therefore, they were deemed the most likely c-tDCS parameters to initially utilize as no c-tDCS studies existed at the time in PD. However, it cannot be ruled out that other c-tDCS parameters may be more effective in PD. Recently, Workman et al. (2020) [29] compared the ability of four different c-tDCS montage/current strength paradigms (unilateral and bilateral; 2 mA and 4 mA) to improve gait and balance in PD. The findings indicated that only the bilateral electrode montage with a current strength of 4 mA improved balance performance in PD, whereas gait performance was not enhanced in any of the four c-tDCS conditions relative to SHAM. The use of a current strength of 4 mA was especially novel as only a handful of the hundreds of tDCS studies available in any population have employed such a high stimulation intensity. However, this study only involved seven participants and did not report if the testing was conducted in the ON- or OFF-medication state. Despite these issues and the fact that lower extremity function was tested as opposed to fine motor performance in the current study, the results of Workman et al. (2020) [29] demonstrate that many other combinations of c-tDCS parameters are possible and could potentially induce positive effects on motor skill in PD. Similarly, it could be argued that the c-tDCS montages employed have had more overall variability across studies compared with M1-tDCS montage arrangements. Although some M1-tDCS studies have employed bi-hemispheric montages or electrode arrangements where the reference electrode is on the shoulder, the vast majority have used the standard M1-supraorbital montage. In contrast, c-tDCS studies appear to have had more relative variability in montage parameters such as unilateral versus bilateral and the location of the reference electrode (e.g., shoulder versus buccinator muscle). Furthermore, some computational modeling research [65] has indicated that the most common and effective c-tDCS electrode montage, which was also used in the present study, can lead to a dispersion of current so that some current spills over to the contralateral cerebellar hemisphere. This effect was present in all age groups but was greater at ages 75 and above and was due to cerebellar shrinkage with age. Therefore, this phenomenon could have influenced the results of the present study due to the age of the participants. However, this c-tDCS montage has still elicited motor performance improvements in old adults [12], despite these possible effects. Taken together, these issues highlight the need for future research to investigate other promising c-tDCS stimulation protocols other than the one used in the present study and point to the possibility that the stimulation parameters of c-tDCS may need to be individualized for optimal results. Finally, the negative results on motor performance in the present study could be due to some combination of all the aforementioned factors above.

The study was subject to several limitations that should be acknowledged. First, it could be argued that the study had a relatively small sample size that did not allow the identification of performance improvements due to c-tDCS. Accordingly, the low sample sizes that have been used in neuroscience research in general have been recognized and can lead to problems involving reproducibility and incorrect conclusions [66,67]. However, the results of our futility analyses clearly indicated that the effect sizes were very small and there were no apparent treatment effects. Furthermore, the sample size of 16 in the current study was actually larger than the average tDCS motor skill study in healthy adults and in PD. Specifically, a close examination of an extensive tDCS motor skill study review [7] in healthy adults reveals that the average sample size per group was approximately 13 (see their tables 1–3), with 75–80% of these studies showing positive tDCS effects. Similarly, a review article and associated table of upper limb studies in PD [8] appears to show that the average sample size per group was approximately 11. Nonetheless, the current results need to be replicated in larger studies using appropriate sample size estimation to observe clinically relevant effects.

A second limitation is that more than one c-tDCS session would be needed to be able to elicit statistically significant motor skill augmentations. This is a typical argument made in tDCS research in healthy adults and especially in motor disorder studies [56] where it is argued that one session cannot overcome years of disease-induced deficits in motor function. In addition, the fact that a series of M1-tDCS studies in healthy adults [39,40] and a c-tDCS study [11] found large cumulative effects over 3–5 days of stimulation supports this view. However, several lines of evidence argue against the lack of multiple sessions as a major reason for single-session tDCS studies failing to show positive performance effects: (1) all of the aforementioned multiple-day studies also reported significant effects within the first day; (2) the vast majority of acute studies in both healthy adults and in PD have shown positive effects (for reviews, see [2,7,8]); (3) a study in our lab that involved 9 days of c-tDCS in PD found no improvements in motor learning [28]; and (4) a recent meta-analytical review [68] found that tDCS efficacy was not affected by the number of stimulation sessions in healthy older adults or PD. Thus, it appears that while multiple tDCS sessions are highly desirable, they are not obligatory to demonstrate positive tDCS effects if they exist.

A final limitation was that the study did not have an age-matched healthy control group consisting of older adults, which would have allowed a direct comparison between groups in the same experimental and laboratory conditions. If the control group would show improvement, this would be stronger evidence that c-tDCS can be effective in older adults but not in PD due to their widespread basal ganglia, cortical, and cerebellar dysfunction. Thus, the current results can only be compared to prior studies by other research groups that have shown that c-tDCS can improve motor skill in healthy older adults [12,69]. In summary, the results of the present study should be interpreted with caution based on the aforementioned limitations and more work is warranted to address these limitations in future research.

In summary, one session of c-tDCS did not enhance motor skill or transfer of motor skill acquisition in hand and arm tasks in PD in the OFF-medication state. Taken together, this study provides evidence that the c-tDCS applied using the parameters that have enhanced motor skill in young [10,11,63,64] and old adults [12] does not elicit the same motor performance benefits in PD. There are several avenues for future c-tDCS research in PD. For example, some evidence has shown that c-tDCS can modulate some aspects of cognition in PD [70]. Another opportunity for future research is the use of tACS applied to the cerebellum as opposed to tDCS. Accordingly, tACS applied to the cerebellum [71] as well as to M1 and the cerebellum concurrently [72–74] has been shown to enhance motor function in other populations, but no cerebellar tACS studies in PD have been conducted to date. In addition, future c-tDCS studies should examine multiple stimulation sessions and different parameters of stimulation to fully determine the viability of c-tDCS as an intervention to improve motor function in PD. Specifically, individualized placement of tDCS electrodes using anatomical data from MRI and higher current strengths [29] than typically used could overcome the recently described interindividual differences in cerebellar anatomy that influence the amount of current reaching cerebellar neurons [35]. Future research in all of these areas will be needed to determine the viability of c-tDCS as a modality to improve motor function in PD and to utilize it in clinical settings.

Author Contributions: Conceptualization, L.L.d.A., B.P. and M.L; methodology, L.L.d.A., B.P., M.L. and Z.M.; software, M.C. and S.J.; formal analysis, L.L.d.A.; investigation, L.L.d.A., K.F. and M.P.; resources, B.P and L.L.d.A.; data curation, L.L.d.A.; writing—original draft preparation, L.A and B.P.; writing—review and editing L.L.d.A., B.P., M.L. and Z.M.; visualization, L.L.d.A.; supervision, B.P.; project administration, L.L.d.A.; funding acquisition, B.P. All authors have read and agreed to the published version of the manuscript.

Funding: This research was supported by a Mountain West Clinical Translational Research-Infrastructure Network (CTR-IN IDEA), NIGMS, NIH, Grant #U54GM104944.

Institutional Review Board Statement: The study was conducted according to the guidelines of the Declaration of Helsinki and approved by the Institutional Review Board of the University of Nevada Las Vegas (protocol code 724185, initial approval 15 April 2015).

Informed Consent Statement: Informed consent was obtained from all subjects involved in the study.

Data Availability Statement: The data presented in this study are available on request from the corresponding author.

Conflicts of Interest: The authors declare no conflict of interest.

References

1. Chen, J.J. Parkinson's Disease: Health-Related Quality of Life, Economic Cost, and Implications of Early Treatment. *Am. J. Manag. Care* **2010**, *16*, S87–S93. [PubMed]
2. Broeder, S.; Nackaerts, E.; Heremans, E.; Vervoort, G.; Meesen, R.; Verheyden, G.; Nieuwboer, A. Transcranial Direct Current Stimulation in Parkinson's Disease: Neurophysiological Mechanisms and Behavioral Effects. *Neurosci. Biobehav. Rev.* **2015**, *57*, 105–117. [CrossRef] [PubMed]
3. Caligiore, D.; Helmich, R.C.; Hallett, M.; Moustafa, A.A.; Timmermann, L.; Toni, I.; Baldassarre, G. Parkinson's Disease as a System-Level Disorder. *NPJ Park. Dis.* **2016**, *2*, 16025. [CrossRef] [PubMed]
4. Nitsche, M.A.; Schauenburg, A.; Lang, N.; Liebetanz, D.; Exner, C.; Paulus, W.; Tergau, F. Facilitation of Implicit Motor Learning by Weak Transcranial Direct Current Stimulation of the Primary Motor Cortex in the Human. *J. Cogn. Neurosci.* **2003**, *15*, 619–626. [CrossRef] [PubMed]

5. Meek, A.W.; Greenwell, D.; Poston, B.; Riley, Z.A. Anodal Tdcs Accelerates On-Line Learning of Dart Throwing. *Neurosci. Lett.* **2021**, *764*, 136211. [CrossRef]
6. Wilson, M.A.; Greenwell, D.; Meek, A.W.; Poston, B.; Riley, Z.A. Neuroenhancement of a Dexterous Motor Task with Anodal Tdcs. *Brain Res.* **2022**, *1790*, 147993. [CrossRef]
7. Buch, E.R.; Santarnecchi, E.; Antal, A.; Born, J.; Celnik, P.A.; Classen, J.; Gerloff, C.; Hallett, M.; Hummel, F.C.; Nitsche, M.A.; et al. Effects of Tdcs on Motor Learning and Memory Formation: A Consensus and Critical Position Paper. *Clin. Neurophysiol.* **2017**, *128*, 589–603. [CrossRef]
8. Simpson, M.W.; Mak, M. The Effect of Transcranial Direct Current Stimulation on Upper Limb Motor Performance in Parkinson's Disease: A Systematic Review. *J. Neurol.* **2020**, *267*, 3479–3488. [CrossRef]
9. Oldrati, V.; Schutter, D.J.L.G. Targeting the Human Cerebellum with Transcranial Direct Current Stimulation to Modulate Behavior: A Meta-Analysis. *Cerebellum* **2018**, *17*, 228–236. [CrossRef]
10. Jackson, A.K.; de Albuquerque, L.L.; Pantovic, M.; Fischer, K.M.; Guadagnoli, M.A.; Riley, Z.A.; Poston, B. Cerebellar Transcranial Direct Current Stimulation Enhances Motor Learning in a Complex Overhand Throwing Task. *Cerebellum* **2019**, *18*, 813–816. [CrossRef]
11. Cantarero, G.; Spampinato, D.; Reis, J.; Ajagbe, L.; Thompson, T.; Kulkarni, K.; Celnik, P. Cerebellar Direct Current Stimulation Enhances On-Line Motor Skill Acquisition through an Effect on Accuracy. *J. Neurosci.* **2015**, *35*, 3285–3290. [CrossRef] [PubMed]
12. Hardwick, R.M.; Celnik, P.A. Cerebellar Direct Current Stimulation Enhances Motor Learning in Older Adults. *Neurobiol. Aging* **2014**, *35*, 2217–2221. [CrossRef] [PubMed]
13. Wu, T.; Hallett, M. The Cerebellum in Parkinson's Disease. *Brain* **2013**, *136 Pt 3*, 696–709. [CrossRef] [PubMed]
14. Ni, Z.; Pinto, A.D.; Lang, A.E.; Chen, R. Involvement of the Cerebellothalamocortical Pathway in Parkinson Disease. *Ann. Neurol.* **2010**, *68*, 816–824. [CrossRef]
15. Galea, J.M.; Vazquez, A.; Pasricha, N.; de Xivry, J.J.; Celnik, P. Dissociating the Roles of the Cerebellum and Motor Cortex During Adaptive Learning: The Motor Cortex Retains What the Cerebellum Learns. *Cereb. Cortex.* **2011**, *21*, 1761–1770. [CrossRef]
16. Rathelot, J.A.; Strick, P.L. Subdivisions of Primary Motor Cortex Based on Cortico-Motoneuronal Cells. *Proc. Natl. Acad. Sci. USA* **2009**, *106*, 918–923. [CrossRef]
17. Reis, J.; Swayne, O.B.; Vandermeeren, Y.; Camus, M.; Dimyan, M.A.; Harris-Love, M.; Perez, M.A.; Ragert, P.; Rothwell, J.C.; Cohen, L.G. Contribution of Transcranial Magnetic Stimulation to the Understanding of Cortical Mechanisms Involved in Motor Control. *J. Physiol.* **2008**, *586*, 325–351. [CrossRef]
18. Opie, G.M.; Liao, W.Y.; Semmler, J.G. Interactions between Cerebellum and the Intracortical Excitatory Circuits of Motor Cortex: A Mini-Review. *Cerebellum* **2022**, *21*, 159–166. [CrossRef] [PubMed]
19. Bostan, A.C.; Dum, R.P.; Strick, P.L. The Basal Ganglia Communicate with the Cerebellum. *Proc. Natl. Acad. Sci. USA* **2010**, *107*, 8452–8456. [CrossRef]
20. Tanaka, T.; Takano, Y.; Tanaka, S.; Hironaka, N.; Kobayashi, K.; Hanakawa, T.; Watanabe, K.; Honda, M. Transcranial Direct-Current Stimulation Increases Extracellular Dopamine Levels in the Rat Striatum. *Front. Syst. Neurosci.* **2013**, *7*, 6. [CrossRef]
21. Polanía, R.; Paulus, W.; Nitsche, M.A. Modulating Cortico-Striatal and Thalamo-Cortical Functional Connectivity with Transcranial Direct Current Stimulation. *Hum. Brain Mapp.* **2012**, *33*, 2499–2508. [CrossRef] [PubMed]
22. Roche, N.; Lackmy, A.; Achache, V.; Bussel, B.; Katz, R. Effects of Anodal Transcranial Direct Current Stimulation over the Leg Motor Area on Lumbar Spinal Network Excitability in Healthy Subjects. *J. Physiol.* **2011**, *589 Pt 11*, 2813–2826. [CrossRef] [PubMed]
23. Li, H.; Lei, X.; Yan, T.; Li, H.; Huang, B.; Li, L.; Xu, L.; Liu, L.; Chen, N.; Lü, L.; et al. The Temporary and Accumulated Effects of Transcranial Direct Current Stimulation for the Treatment of Advanced Parkinson's Disease Monkeys. *Sci. Rep.* **2015**, *5*, 12178. [CrossRef]
24. Krakauer, J.W.; Mazzoni, P. Human Sensorimotor Learning: Adaptation, Skill, and Beyond. *Curr. Opin. Neurobiol.* **2011**, *21*, 636–644. [CrossRef] [PubMed]
25. Boisgontier, M.P. Motor Aging Results from Cerebellar Neuron Death. *Trends Neurosci.* **2015**, *38*, 127–128. [CrossRef]
26. Block, H.; Celnik, P. Stimulating the Cerebellum Affects Visuomotor Adaptation but not Intermanual Transfer of Learning. *Cerebellum* **2013**, *12*, 781–793. [CrossRef]
27. Lima de Albuquerque, L.; Pantovic, M.; Clingo, M.; Fischer, K.; Jalene, S.; Landers, M.; Mari, Z.; Poston, B. An Acute Application of Cerebellar Transcranial Direct Current Stimulation does not Improve Motor Performance in Parkinson's Disease. *Brain Sci.* **2020**, *10*, 735. [CrossRef]
28. Lima de Albuquerque, L.; Pantovic, M.; Clingo, M.G.; Fischer, K.M.; Jalene, S.; Landers, M.R.; Mari, Z.; Poston, B. Long-Term Application of Cerebellar Transcranial Direct Current Stimulation does not Improve Motor Learning in Parkinson's Disease. *Cerebellum* **2022**, *21*, 333–349. [CrossRef]
29. Workman, C.D.; Fietsam, A.C.; Uc, E.Y.; Rudroff, T. Cerebellar Transcranial Direct Current Stimulation in People with Parkinson's Disease: A Pilot Study. *Brain Sci.* **2020**, *10*, 96. [CrossRef]
30. Wong, P.L.; Yang, Y.R.; Huang, S.F.; Fuh, J.L.; Chiang, H.L.; Wang, R.Y. Transcranial Direct Current Stimulation on Different Targets to Modulate Cortical Activity and Dual-Task Walking in Individuals with Parkinson's Disease: A Double Blinded Randomized Controlled Trial. *Front. Aging Neurosci.* **2022**, *14*, 807151. [CrossRef]

31. Ferrucci, R.; Cortese, F.; Bianchi, M.; Pittera, D.; Turrone, R.; Bocci, T.; Borroni, B.; Vergari, M.; Cogiamanian, F.; Ardolino, G.; et al. Cerebellar and Motor Cortical Transcranial Stimulation Decrease Levodopa-Induced Dyskinesias in Parkinson's Disease. *Cerebellum* **2016**, *15*, 43–47. [CrossRef] [PubMed]
32. Li, L.M.; Uehara, K.; Hanakawa, T. The Contribution of Interindividual Factors to Variability of Response in Transcranial Direct Current Stimulation Studies. *Front. Cell Neurosci.* **2015**, *9*, 181. [CrossRef] [PubMed]
33. Pellegrini, M.; Zoghi, M.; Jaberzadeh, S. Biological and Anatomical Factors Influencing Interindividual Variability to Noninvasive Brain Stimulation of the Primary Motor Cortex: A Systematic Review and Meta-Analysis. *Rev. Neurosci.* **2018**, *29*, 199–222. [CrossRef]
34. Rossi, S.; Hallett, M.; Rossini, P.M.; Pascual-Leone, A. Screening Questionnaire before Tms: An Update. *Clin. Neurophysiol.* **2011**, *122*, 1686. [CrossRef]
35. Miterko, L.N.; Baker, K.B.; Beckinghausen, J.; Bradnam, L.V.; Cheng, M.Y.; Cooperrider, J.; DeLong, M.R.; Gornati, S.V.; Hallett, M.; Heck, D.H.; et al. Consensus Paper: Experimental Neurostimulation of the Cerebellum. *Cerebellum* **2019**, *18*, 1064–1097. [CrossRef] [PubMed]
36. MacInnis, M.J.; McGlory, C.; Gibala, M.J.; Phillips, S.M. Investigating Human Skeletal Muscle Physiology with Unilateral Exercise Models: When One Limb Is More Powerful than Two. *Appl. Physiol. Nutr. Metab.* **2017**, *42*, 563–570. [CrossRef]
37. Defer, G.L.; Widner, H.; Marie, R.M.; Remy, P.; Levivier, M. Core Assessment Program for Surgical Interventional Therapies in Parkinson's Disease (Capsit-Pd). *Mov. Disord.* **1999**, *14*, 572–584. [CrossRef]
38. Lidstone, D.E.; Miah, F.Z.; Poston, B.; Beasley, J.F.; Mostofsky, S.H.; Dufek, J.S. Children with Autism Spectrum Disorder Show Impairments during Dynamic Versus Static Grip-Force Tracking. *Autism. Res.* **2020**, *13*, 2177–2189. [CrossRef]
39. Reis, J.; Fischer, J.T.; Prichard, G.; Weiller, C.; Cohen, L.G.; Fritsch, B. Time- but not Sleep-Dependent Consolidation of Tdcs-Enhanced Visuomotor Skills. *Cereb. Cortex.* **2015**, *25*, 109–117. [CrossRef]
40. Reis, J.; Schambra, H.M.; Cohen, L.G.; Buch, E.R.; Fritsch, B.; Zarahn, E.; Celnik, P.A.; Krakauer, J.W. Noninvasive Cortical Stimulation Enhances Motor Skill Acquisition over Multiple Days through an Effect on Consolidation. *Proc. Natl. Acad. Sci. USA* **2009**, *106*, 1590–1595. [CrossRef]
41. Spraker, M.B.; Corcos, D.M.; Kurani, A.S.; Prodoehl, J.; Swinnen, S.P.; Vaillancourt, D.E. Specific Cerebellar Regions Are Related to Force Amplitude and Rate of Force Development. *Neuroimage* **2012**, *59*, 1647–1656. [CrossRef] [PubMed]
42. Tseng, Y.W.; Diedrichsen, J.; Krakauer, J.W.; Shadmehr, R.; Bastian, A.J. Sensory Prediction Errors Drive Cerebellum-Dependent Adaptation of Reaching. *J. Neurophysiol.* **2007**, *98*, 54–62. [CrossRef]
43. Vaillancourt, D.E.; Thulborn, K.R.; Corcos, D.M. Neural Basis for the Processes That Underlie Visually Guided and Internally Guided Force Control in Humans. *J. Neurophysiol.* **2003**, *90*, 3330–3340. [CrossRef] [PubMed]
44. Burciu, R.G.; Ofori, E.; Shukla, P.; Planetta, P.J.; Snyder, A.F.; Li, H.; Hass, C.J.; Okun, M.S.; McFarland, N.R.; Vaillancourt, D.E. Distinct Patterns of Brain Activity in Progressive Supranuclear Palsy and Parkinson's Disease. *Mov. Disord.* **2015**, *30*, 1248–1258. [CrossRef] [PubMed]
45. Chung, J.W.; Burciu, R.G.; Ofori, E.; Coombes, S.A.; Christou, E.A.; Okun, M.S.; Hess, C.W.; Vaillancourt, D.E. Beta-Band Oscillations in the Supplementary Motor Cortex Are Modulated by Levodopa and Associated with Functional Activity in the Basal Ganglia. *Neuroimage Clin.* **2018**, *19*, 559–571. [CrossRef] [PubMed]
46. Neely, K.A.; Planetta, P.J.; Prodoehl, J.; Corcos, D.M.; Comella, C.L.; Goetz, C.G.; Shannon, K.L.; Vaillancourt, D.E. Vaillancourt. Force Control Deficits in Individuals with Parkinson's Disease, Multiple Systems Atrophy, and Progressive Supranuclear Palsy. *PLoS ONE* **2013**, *8*, e58403. [CrossRef]
47. Planetta, P.J.; McFarland, N.R.; Okun, M.S.; Vaillancourt, D.E. Mri Reveals Brain Abnormalities in Drug-Naive Parkinson's Disease. *Exerc. Sport Sci. Rev.* **2014**, *42*, 12–22. [CrossRef]
48. Prodoehl, J.; Corcos, D.M.; Vaillancourt, D.E. Basal Ganglia Mechanisms Underlying Precision Grip Force Control. *Neurosci. Biobehav. Rev.* **2009**, *33*, 900–908. [CrossRef]
49. Prodoehl, J.; Planetta, P.J.; Kurani, A.S.; Comella, C.L.; Corcos, D.M.; Vaillancourt, D.E. Differences in Brain Activation between Tremor- and Nontremor-Dominant Parkinson Disease. *JAMA Neurol.* **2013**, *70*, 100–106. [CrossRef]
50. Spraker, M.B.; Prodoehl, J.; Corcos, D.M.; Comella, C.L.; Vaillancourt, D.E. Basal Ganglia Hypoactivity During Grip Force in Drug Naive Parkinson's Disease. *Hum. Brain Mapp.* **2010**, *31*, 1928–1941. [CrossRef]
51. Vaillancourt, D.E.; Slifkin, A.B.; Newell, K.M. Intermittency in the Visual Control of Force in Parkinson's Disease. *Exp. Brain Res.* **2001**, *138*, 118–127. [CrossRef] [PubMed]
52. Albuquerque, L.L.; Fischer, K.M.; Pauls, A.L.; Pantovic, M.; Guadagnoli, M.A.; Riley, Z.A.; Poston, B. An Acute Application of Transcranial Random Noise Stimulation does not Enhance Motor Skill Acquisition or Retention in a Golf Putting Task. *Hum. Mov. Sci.* **2019**, *66*, 241–248. [CrossRef] [PubMed]
53. Poston, B.; Christou, E.A.; Enoka, J.A.; Enoka, R.M. Timing Variability and not Force Variability Predicts the Endpoint Accuracy of Fast and Slow Isometric Contractions. *Exp. Brain Res.* **2010**, *202*, 189–202. [CrossRef] [PubMed]
54. Kenville, R.; Maudrich, T.; Maudrich, D.; Villringer, A.; Ragert, P. Cerebellar Transcranial Direct Current Stimulation Improves Maximum Isometric Force Production during Isometric Barbell Squats. *Brain Sci.* **2020**, *10*, 235. [CrossRef]
55. Steiner, K.M.; Enders, A.; Thier, W.; Batsikadze, G.; Ludolph, N.; Ilg, W.; Timmann, D. Cerebellar Tdcs does not Improve Learning in a Complex Whole Body Dynamic Balance Task in Young Healthy Subjects. *PLoS ONE* **2016**, *11*, e0163598. [CrossRef]

56. Sadnicka, A.; Hamada, M.; Bhatia, K.P.; Rothwell, J.C.; Edwards, M.J. Cerebellar Stimulation Fails to Modulate Motor Cortex Plasticity in Writing Dystonia. *Mov. Disord.* **2014**, *29*, 1304–1307. [CrossRef]
57. Krakauer, J.W.; Mazzoni, P.; Ghazizadeh, A.; Ravindran, R.; Shadmehr, R. Generalization of Motor Learning Depends on the History of Prior Action. *PLoS Biol.* **2006**, *4*, e316. [CrossRef]
58. Hamoudi, M.; Schambra, H.M.; Fritsch, B.; Schoechlin-Marx, A.; Weiller, C.; Cohen, L.G.; Reis, J. Transcranial Direct Current Stimulation Enhances Motor Skill Learning but not Generalization in Chronic Stroke. *Neurorehabil. Neural. Repair* **2018**, *32*, 295–308. [CrossRef]
59. Orban de Xivry, J.J.; Marko, M.K.; Pekny, S.E.; Pastor, D.; Izawa, J.; Celnik, P.; Shadmehr, R. Stimulation of the Human Motor Cortex Alters Generalization Patterns of Motor Learning. *J. Neurosc.* **2011**, *31*, 7102–7110. [CrossRef]
60. Parikh, P.J.; Cole, K.J. Effects of Transcranial Direct Current Stimulation in Combination with Motor Practice on Dexterous Grasping and Manipulation in Healthy Older Adults. *Physiol. Rep.* **2014**, *2*, e00255. [CrossRef]
61. Spampinato, D.A.; Celnik, P.A.; Rothwell, J.C. Cerebellar-Motor Cortex Connectivity: One or Two Different Networks? *J. Neurosci.* **2020**, *40*, 4230–4239. [CrossRef]
62. Hamada, M.; Galea, J.M.; Di Lazzaro, V.; Mazzone, P.; Ziemann, U.; Rothwell, J.C. Two Distinct Interneuron Circuits in Human Motor Cortex Are Linked to Different Subsets of Physiological and Behavioral Plasticity. *J. Neurosci.* **2014**, *34*, 12837–12849. [CrossRef] [PubMed]
63. Galea, J.M.; Jayaram, G.; Ajagbe, L.; Celnik, P. Modulation of Cerebellar Excitability by Polarity-Specific Noninvasive Direct Current Stimulation. *J. Neurosci.* **2009**, *29*, 9115–9122. [CrossRef] [PubMed]
64. Jayaram, G.; Tang, B.; Pallegadda, R.; Vasudevan, E.V.; Celnik, P.; Bastian, A. Modulating Locomotor Adaptation with Cerebellar Stimulation. *J. Neurophysiol.* **2012**, *107*, 2950–2957. [CrossRef] [PubMed]
65. Rezaee, Z.; Dutta, A. Lobule-Specific Dosage Considerations for Cerebellar Transcranial Direct Current Stimulation During Healthy Aging: A Computational Modeling Study Using Age-Specific Magnetic Resonance Imaging Templates. *Neuromodulation* **2020**, *23*, 341–365. [CrossRef]
66. Consideration of Sample Size in Neuroscience Studies. *J. Neurosci.* **2020**, *40*, 4076–4077. [CrossRef]
67. Szucs, D.; Ioannidis, J.P. Sample Size Evolution in Neuroimaging Research: An Evaluation of Highly-Cited Studies (1990–2012) and of Latest Practices (2017–2018) in High-Impact Journals. *Neuroimage* **2020**, *221*, 117164. [CrossRef]
68. Siew-Pin Leuk, J.; Yow, K.E.; Zi-Xin Tan, C.; Hendy, A.M.; Kar-Wing Tan, M.; Hock-Beng Ng, T.; Teo, W.P. A Meta-Analytical Review of Transcranial Direct Current Stimulation Parameters on Upper Limb Motor Learning in Healthy Older Adults and People with Parkinson's Disease. *Rev. Neurosci.* **2023**, *34*, 325–348. [CrossRef]
69. Samaei, A.; Ehsani, F.; Zoghi, M.; Yosephi, M.H.; Jaberzadeh, S. Online and Offline Effects of Cerebellar Transcranial Direct Current Stimulation on Motor Learning in Healthy Older Adults: A Randomized Double-Blind Sham-Controlled Study. *Eur. J. Neurosci.* **2017**, *45*, 1177–1185. [CrossRef]
70. Ruggiero, F.; Dini, M.; Cortese, F.; Vergari, M.; Nigro, M.; Poletti, B.; Priori, A.; Ferrucci, R. Anodal Transcranial Direct Current Stimulation over the Cerebellum Enhances Sadness Recognition in Parkinson's Disease Patients: A Pilot Study. *Cerebellum* **2022**, *21*, 234–243. [CrossRef]
71. Naro, A.; Bramanti, A.; Leo, A.; Manuli, A.; Sciarrone, F.; Russo, M.; Bramanti, P.; Calabro, R.S. Effects of Cerebellar Transcranial Alternating Current Stimulation on Motor Cortex Excitability and Motor Function. *Brain Struct. Funct.* **2017**, *222*, 2891–2906. [CrossRef] [PubMed]
72. Miyaguchi, S.; Inukai, Y.; Matsumoto, Y.; Miyashita, M.; Takahashi, R.; Otsuru, N.; Onishi, H. Effects on Motor Learning of Transcranial Alternating Current Stimulation Applied over the Primary Motor Cortex and Cerebellar Hemisphere. *J. Clin. Neurosci.* **2020**, *78*, 296–300. [CrossRef] [PubMed]
73. Miyaguchi, S.; Otsuru, N.; Kojima, S.; Saito, K.; Inukai, Y.; Masaki, M.; Onishi, H. Transcranial Alternating Current Stimulation with Gamma Oscillations over the Primary Motor Cortex and Cerebellar Hemisphere Improved Visuomotor Performance. *Front. Behav. Neurosci.* **2018**, *12*, 132. [CrossRef] [PubMed]
74. Miyaguchi, S.; Otsuru, N.; Kojima, S.; Yokota, H.; Saito, K.; Inukai, Y.; Onishi, H. Gamma Tacs over M1 and Cerebellar Hemisphere Improves Motor Performance in a Phase-Specific Manner. *Neurosci. Lett.* **2019**, *694*, 64–68. [CrossRef]

Disclaimer/Publisher's Note: The statements, opinions and data contained in all publications are solely those of the individual author(s) and contributor(s) and not of MDPI and/or the editor(s). MDPI and/or the editor(s) disclaim responsibility for any injury to people or property resulting from any ideas, methods, instructions or products referred to in the content.

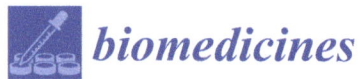

Article

Sedation Therapy in Intensive Care Units: Harnessing the Power of Antioxidants to Combat Oxidative Stress

Gen Inoue [1], Yuhei Ohtaki [2], Kazue Satoh [1], Yuki Odanaka [3], Akihito Katoh [1], Keisuke Suzuki [1], Yoshitake Tomita [1], Manabu Eiraku [1], Kazuki Kikuchi [1], Kouhei Harano [1], Masaharu Yagi [1], Naoki Uchida [4] and Kenji Dohi [1,2,*]

[1] Department of Emergency, Disaster and Critical Care Medicine, School of Medicine, Showa University, 1-5-8 Hatanodai, Shinagawa-ku, Tokyo 142-8555, Japan; gen.musashi83@gmail.com (G.I.)
[2] Department of Emergency Medicine, School of Medicine, The Jikei University, 3-25-8 Nishishinbashi, Minato-ku, Tokyo 105-8461, Japan
[3] Center for Instrumental Analysis, School of Pharmacy, Showa University, 1-5-8 Hatanodai, Shinagawa-ku, Tokyo 142-8555, Japan
[4] Clinical Research Institute for Clinical Pharmacology and Therapeutics, Showa University Karasuyama Hospital, 6-11-11 Kitakarasuyama, Setagaya-ku, Tokyo 157-8577, Japan
* Correspondence: kdop@med.showa-u.ac.jp; Tel.: +81-33784-8744

Abstract: In critically ill patients requiring intensive care, increased oxidative stress plays an important role in pathogenesis. Sedatives are widely used for sedation in many of these patients. Some sedatives are known antioxidants. However, no studies have evaluated the direct scavenging activity of various sedative agents on different free radicals. This study aimed to determine whether common sedatives (propofol, thiopental, and dexmedetomidine (DEX)) have direct free radical scavenging activity against various free radicals using in vitro electron spin resonance. Superoxide, hydroxyl radical, singlet oxygen, and nitric oxide (NO) direct scavenging activities were measured. All sedatives scavenged different types of free radicals. DEX, a new sedative, also scavenged hydroxyl radicals. Thiopental scavenged all types of free radicals, including NO, whereas propofol did not scavenge superoxide radicals. In this retrospective analysis, we observed changes in oxidative antioxidant markers following the administration of thiopental in patients with severe head trauma. We identified the direct radical-scavenging activity of various sedatives used in clinical settings. Furthermore, we reported a representative case of traumatic brain injury wherein thiopental administration dramatically affected oxidative-stress-related biomarkers. This study suggests that, in the future, sedatives containing thiopental may be redeveloped as an antioxidant therapy through further clinical research.

Keywords: oxidative stresses; neuroinflammation; traumatic brain injuries; intensive care; sedatives; antioxidant effects; biologic monitoring; barbiturates; electron spin resonance; translational research

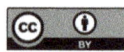

1. Introduction

The extent to which the oxidant–antioxidant balance in the body is disrupted by the generation of excess reactive oxygen species (ROS)/reactive nitrogen species (RNS) is called oxidative stress [1,2]. Oxidative stress plays an important role in the pathogenesis of many acute diseases, including neurological emergencies as well as age-related diseases, such as arthritis, diabetes, dementia, cancer, atherosclerosis, vascular diseases, obesity, osteoporosis, and metabolic syndromes [3–5]. ROS/RNS are produced in vivo via oxygen and regulatory cellular activities like cell survival, stress response, and inflammation [5]. Among ROS, superoxides ($O_2^{\bullet-}$), hydroxyl radicals, and nitric oxide (NO) are free radicals with unpaired electrons. Because of their strong biological reactivity, they are major participants in inflammatory reactions. NO production in vivo is mediated by NO synthase (NOS). Among the three NOS isozymes, overproduced NO via the expression of inducible NOS (iNOS) has a role as an inflammation mediator [6,7]. The reactivity of $ONOO^-$, which is generated via the reaction of $O_2^{\bullet-}$ and NO, is also crucial [8,9]. Oxidative stress also plays an important role during various acute crisis situations, including acute inflammation, surgical stress, ischemia-reperfusion, and trauma [10]. Recently, oxidative stress was reported to play a role in COVID-19 infection [11]. A case series of COVID-19 patients treated with vitamin C reported decreased mortality, significant reductions in inflammatory markers, and a trend toward decreased oxygen demand [12]. Obvious methods to control the critical situation caused by this imbalance are to balance or eliminate the generation of ROS [10]. Numerous animal studies have demonstrated that the administration of free radical scavengers and antioxidants dramatically reduces organ damage [10,13]. Although experimental studies showed positive results, there is very little evidence that antioxidant therapy is clinically beneficial, and few antioxidants have been used in clinical settings. Oxygen consumption in the brain is very high, and neurological emergencies are considered typical conditions in which antioxidant therapy may be useful. Edaravone, a hydroxyl radical scavenger, is the only clinically applicable agent for ischemic stroke [14–18]. Therefore, there is a critical need to develop clinically available antioxidants and new antioxidant therapies.

Sedatives are widely used in acutely critically ill patients, generally to maintain sedation in intensive care units. Sedation therapy in ICUs is performed for sedation and to decrease oxygen consumption and metabolism throughout the body [19]. Some sedatives are known to have beneficial pharmacological effects in addition to simple anesthetic effects [20]. Moreover, sedatives are also used during neurological emergencies for patients with increased intracranial pressure and status epilepticus. In patients with head trauma, barbiturates decrease cerebral oxygen consumption and cerebral blood flow and correspondingly decrease intracranial pressure (ICP). In addition to decreased ICP, increased partial pressure of oxygen in brain tissue ($PbtO_2$) and decreased excitatory amino acids have been reported [21]. Propofol (2,6-diisopropylphenol) is reported to have powerful antioxidant properties, having a chemical structure similar to that of the endogenous antioxidant α-tocopherol (vitamin E) [20].

Free radicals are products of normal cellular metabolism [1–5]. When cells utilize oxygen, redox processes produce free radicals, usually ROS and RNS [22]. Free radicals can be defined as molecular bodies or molecular fragments that can exist independently. Free radicals have one or more unpaired electrons in their outer atomic or molecular orbitals [22]. They are described as "free radical" and occur in different types, such as superoxides ($O_2^{\bullet-}$), hydroxyl radicals ($OH^\bullet$), alkoxyl radicals ($RO^\bullet$), peroxyl radicals ($ROO^\bullet$), nitric oxide (nitrogen monoxide) ($NO^\bullet$), and nitrogen dioxide ($NO_2^\bullet$) [23]. The biological effects of each type are known to differ [24], and the free radicals that can be scavenged or inhibited by each antioxidant are different. For example, edaravone, a free radical scavenger used clinically for cerebral infarction, scavenges hydroxyl radicals and nitric oxide (NO) but not superoxide radicals [14]. Therefore, it is crucial to investigate the scavenging ability of antioxidants for each type of free radical. To the best of our knowledge, to date, no study has evaluated the scavenging ability of antioxidant sedatives, such as propofol, for different types of free radicals.

The purpose of this study was to investigate the potential future clinical applications of sedatives as novel antioxidant therapies. Specifically, we used an in vitro electron spin resonance (ESR) assay to investigate whether common clinical sedatives have direct free-radical-scavenging activity for different types of free radicals. Moreover, we presented clinical cases of patients with head trauma treated with thiopental-based barbiturates and described the changes in in vivo oxidative antioxidant biomarkers.

2. Materials and Methods
2.1. Reagents

Xanthine oxidase (XOD), hypoxanthine (HPX), and diethylene triamine penta-acetic acid (DETAPAC) were obtained from Sigma Chemical (St. Louis, MO, USA). The spin trap 5,5-dimethyl-1-pyrroline-N-oxide (DMPO) was obtained from Labotec (Tokyo, Japan). 1-Hydroxy-2-oxo-3-(N-3-methyl-3-aminopropyl)-3-methyl-1-triazene (NOC-7), 2-(4-carboxyphenyl)-4,4,5,5-

tetramethylimidazoline-1-oxyl-3-oxide, and sodium salt (carboxy-PTIO) were obtained from Dojin Chemical (Kumamoto, Japan). A superoxide dismutase (SOD) standard solution kit was purchased from Labotec. Sumatriptan succinate (GR43175 C) was gifted from Glaxo Wellcome (London, UK).

2.2. In Vitro ESR Method

The ESR analysis of the spin adduct was performed at room temperature using a JES-REIX X-band spectrometer (JEOL, Tokyo, Japan). The following ESR measurement conditions were implemented: magnetic field of 335.6 ± 5.0 mT; microwave power of 8.0 mW; sweep time of 2 min/0.03 s; and modulation amplitude of 0.1 mT. Manganese oxide was used as an external standard because it provided a constant signal against which all peak heights were compared.

To calculate the relative peak height, the sample peak height was divided by the manganese oxide peak height.

The superoxide radical ($O_2^{\bullet-}$) was generated with a hypoxanthine XOD system. For the assay, 50 µL of 2 mM hypoxanthine in phosphate-buffered saline, 20 µL of 0.5 mM DETAPAC, 30 µL of each sedative dissolved in dimethyl sulfoxide, 50 µL of 0.46 M DMPO, and 30 µL of 0.5 U/mL XOD were mixed in a test tube. The solution was placed in a special flat cell in which DMPO–superoxide, the spin adduct, was analyzed using ESR (Figure 1a) [24,25].

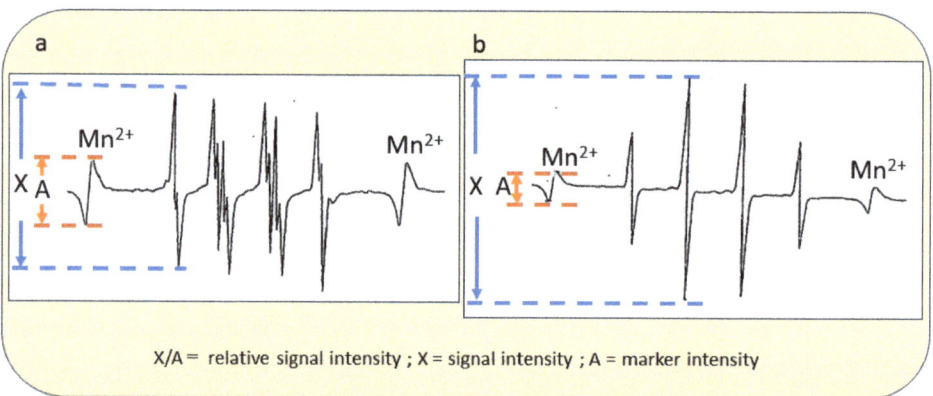

a
Determination of superoxide radical scavenging activity by ESR using the spin trap (DMPO) method.

b
Determination of hydroxyl radical scavenging activity by ESR using the spin trap (DMPO) method.

Figure 1. ESR signals of hydroxyl radicals and superoxide radicals. Determination of hydroxyl radical (**a**) and superoxide radical (**b**) scavenging activities with electron spin resonance using the spin trap method. MnO was used as an external standard. X, signal intensity; A, marker intensity; X/A = 100, relative signal intensity.

A standard curve was constructed with 0.4 to 40 U/mL of superoxide dismutase (SOD) added to the system instead of each sedative.

Hydroxyl radical (OH$^{\bullet}$)-scavenging activity was also measured using the ESR spin trap method (Figure 1b). The reaction mixture comprised 50 µL of 92 mM DMPO, 50 µL of 1 mM FeSO$_4$, 0.02 mM DETAPAC, 50 µL of 1 mM hydrogen peroxide, and 50 µL of each sedative. After rapid stirring, the reaction mixture was placed into an ESR flat cell. Recording of the ESR spectrum was started 60 s after the addition of 1 mM H$_2$O$_2$ [24].

NO-scavenging activity was estimated using carboxy-PTIO. NO was generated from NOC-7. All reagents were dissolved in a 0.1 M phosphate buffer (pH 7.4) except NOC-7, which was diluted to 0.1 mM in a 0.1 N NaOH solution. First, 20 µL of each sedative was added to 140 μL of a 0.1 M potassium buffer followed by 20 μL of 0.1 mM carboxy-PTIO and 20 μL of 0.1 mM NOC-7. Immediately after vortex mixing, the sample solution was transferred into a flat cell (200 μL capacity). ESR measurements were started 1, 3, 5, 7, 10, 12, and 15 min after the addition of NOC-7 (Figure 2) [14].

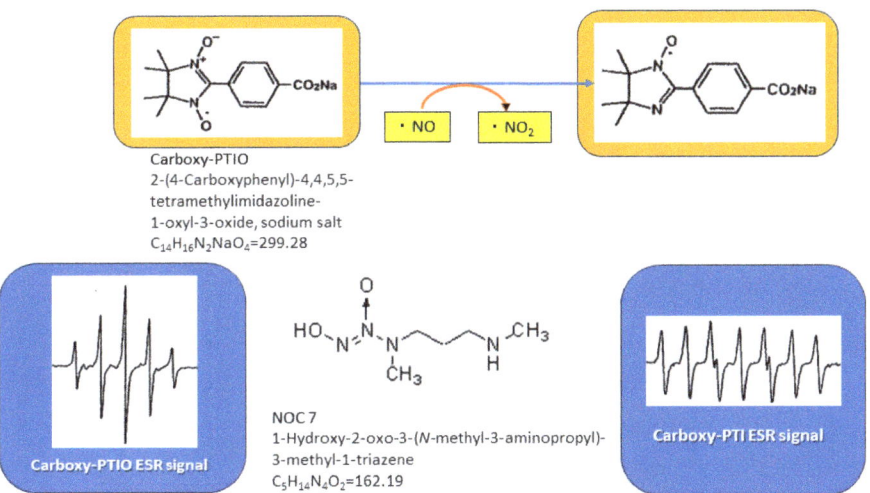

Figure 2. Scheme describing NO reaction using ESR method. Nitric oxide-scavenging activity measured using electron spin resonance spectroscopy. The penta-signal of carboxy-PTIO changed to the hepta-signal of carboxy-PTI.

Singlet oxygen was generated via photosensitization reactions with rose bengal. Singlet oxygen was indirectly estimated as the peak intensity of the 2,2,6,6-tetramethyl-4-4-hydroxy-piperidinyloxy (4-OH TEMPO) radical produced via the oxidation of 2,2,6,6-tetramethyl-4-hydroxy-piperidine (4-OH TEMP) with singlet oxygen (produced via photosensitization with rose bengal) using ESR. Samples were diluted in dimethyl sulfoxide (DMSO) to the required final concentrations. The samples (in 60 μL of DMSO), 10 μL of 1 mM DTPA, 0.1 M phosphate buffer (pH 7.4; 70 μL), 100 mM 4-OH TEMP (40 μL), and 200 μM rose bengal (20 μL) were irradiated for 3 min (1.57 J/cm^2) with a green-light-emitting diode with a λMAX of 540 nm (Simantec Ltd., Tokyo, Japan) [26].

2.3. Statistical Analysis

Data were analyzed using JMP 17 statistical software. Data are presented as means ± standard error. All experiments were performed in triplicate, except for some tests with little or no intensity change. A one-way analysis of variance test was performed to compare. Significance was defined as $p < 0.05$ *.

3. Results

The effects of Propofol and Thiopental on ESR signals of and superoxide radical ($O_2^{\bullet-}$) and hydroxyl radical (OH$^\bullet$) are shown in Figures 3 and 4. Regarding superoxide radical -scavenging activity, ESR showed that the formation of the superoxide radical–DMSO spin adduct was strongly inhibited with 2.06 mM and 20.63 mM thiopental. DEX and propofol did not have direct superoxide-radical-scavenging activity (Figures 3, 5a and 6a).

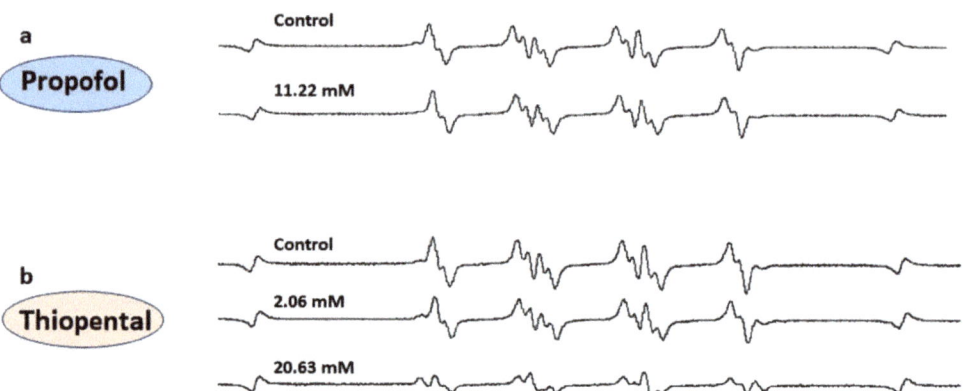

Figure 3. Superoxide-radical-scavenging activity of sedatives. As shown using ESR, the formation of the superoxide radical–DMSO spin adduct was strongly inhibited with thiopental (**b**). Propofol (**a**) did not have direct superoxide-radical-scavenging activity.

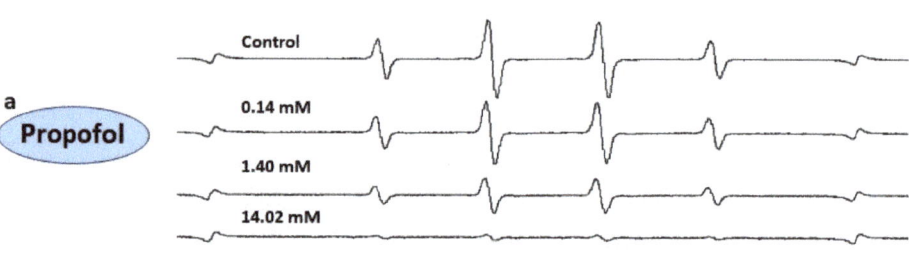

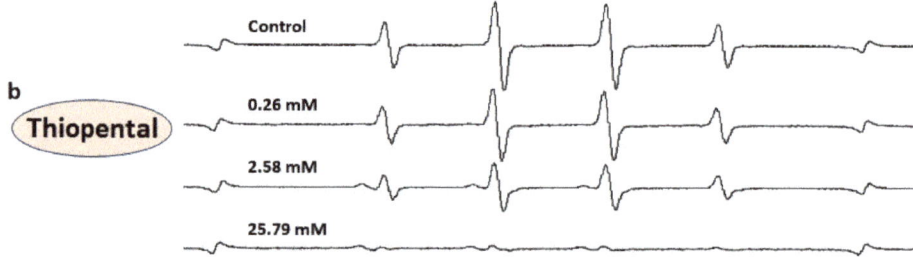

Figure 4. Hydroxy-radical-scavenging activity. As shown using ESR, the formation of the hydroxyl radical–DMSO spin adduct was strongly inhibited with propofol (**a**) and thiopental (**b**).

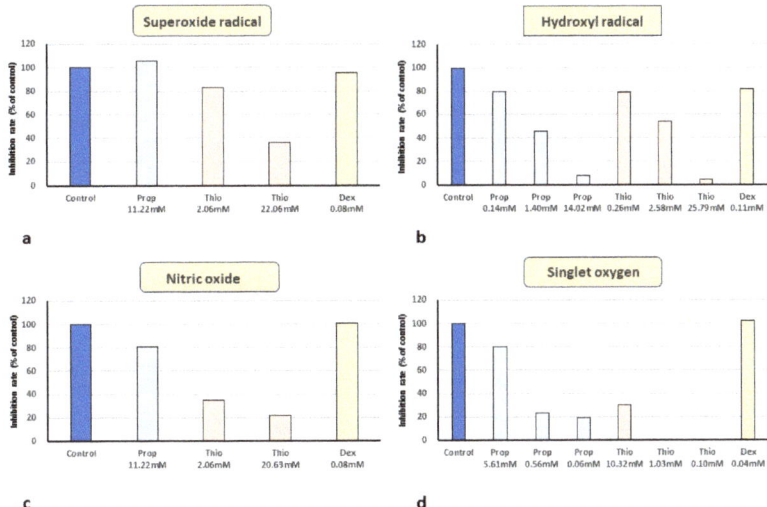

Figure 5. Direct free-radical-scavenging activities of propofol, thiopental, and dexmedetomidine. (**a**) Thiopental has direct superoxide-radical-scavenging activity. (**b**) Hydroxyl-radical-scavenging activity of sedatives. Dexmedetomidine, propofol, and thiopental scavenged hydroxyl radicals. (**c**) Nitric oxide-scavenging activity of sedatives: NO was scavenged by propofol and thiopental. (**d**) Singlet oxygen-scavenging activity of sedatives: propofol and thiopental scavenged singlet oxygen.

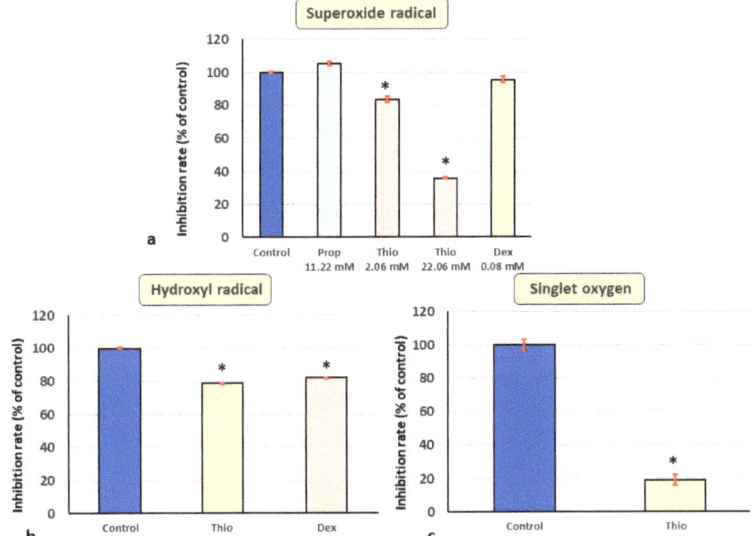

Figure 6. Direct free-radical-scavenging activities of DEX, thiopental, and dexmedetomidine. (**a**) Thiopental significantly scavenged superoxide radicals. * $p < 0.01$. (**b**) Hydroxyl-radical-scavenging activity of thiopental and dexmedetomidine. Thiopental and dexmedetomidine significantly scavenged hydroxyl radicals. * $p < 0.01$. (**c**) Singlet oxygen-scavenging activity of thiopental. Thiopental scavenged singlet oxygen significantly. * $p < 0.01$. Error bar (red) is standard error, SE.

Regarding hydroxyl radical-scavenging activity, ESR showed that the formation of the hydroxyl radical–DMSO spin adduct was inhibited with 0.11 mM DEX strongly inhibited with 1.40 mM and 14.02 mM propofol and with 2.58 mM and 25.79 mM thiopental (Figures 4, 5b and 6b).

Regarding nitric oxide (NO)-scavenging activity, the penta-signal of carboxy-PTIO disappeared and the hepta-signal of carboxy-PTI appeared in the ESR recording after the addition of NOC-7, a NO generator. The appearance of the hepta-signal of carboxy-PTI was inhibited with 11.22 mM propofol and was strongly inhibited with 2.06 mM and 20.63 mM thiopental (Figure 5c).

Regarding singlet oxygen ($^1O_2$)-scavenging activity, propofol and thiopental scavenged singlet oxygen, 10.32 mM thiopental completely inhibited singlet oxygen production, and DEX did not have singlet oxygen-scavenging activity (Figures 5d and 6c).

In summary, propofol, a previously known antioxidant, had direct scavenging activity for hydroxyl radicals, NO, and singlet oxygen. Furthermore, thiopental, a classical sedative, acted as a strong scavenger of all the free radicals examined, including superoxide radicals. Finally, we demonstrated the previously unknown direct hydroxyl-radical-scavenging activity of DEX.

4. Clinical Case

We present a representative case of traumatic brain injury in which thiopental administration dramatically affected oxidative-stress-related biomarkers. A 15-year-old woman was transferred to the emergency department for the trauma inflicted by attempting suicide by jumping onto a train track. Her initial consciousness level was E1V1M4 on the Glasgow Coma Scale (GCS). Dilated pupils were observed, but bilateral contralateral reflections remained slight. Based on these clinical findings, the patient was diagnosed to be in a state of impending cerebral herniation due to severe traumatic brain injury (TBI). Initial brain computed tomography (CT) showed severe diffuse cerebral swelling, acute subdural hemorrhage, and traumatic subarachnoid hemorrhage (Figure 6a). Targeted temperature management therapy to maintain 35 °C and ICP monitoring were immediately started to treat the impending brain herniation associated with increased ICP. At the time of monitor insertion, the ICP exceeded 50 mmHg. After rewarming, the ICP was occasionally elevated above 50 mmHg despite continued normothermia (36 °C). Subsequent CT scans revealed the progressive deterioration of cerebral edema. Consequently, barbiturate coma therapy using thiopental (1 mg/kg/h) was added. Under thiopental administration, ICP was stabilized below 20 mmHg, and the subsequent CT scan on day 10 demonstrated a reduction in cerebral edema. Her consciousness level was improved to E4V5M6/GCS and she was transferred to a psychiatric facility without neurological deficit. With the results of these in vitro ESR experiments, we retrospectively confirmed the in vivo oxidative biomarkers (uric acid (UA), bilirubin (Bil), and carbon-monoxide-binding hemoglobin (COHb)) in this patient. The levels of UA, which is an endogenous antioxidant, were very low before thiopental administration but increased after administration. Moreover, Bil and COHb, metabolites of the stress protein heme oxygenase-1 (HO-1), were decreased after thiopental administration.

5. Discussion

Oxidative stress plays an important role in the pathogenesis of many critical illnesses that require intensive care, such as trauma, severe infections, stroke, and ischemic heart disease [3–5]. For the proper diagnosis and treatment of these diseases and considering their pathologies, it is important to monitor various redox components during disease progression and to regulate the redox balance of the patient with antioxidants. In this study, we evaluated the direct free-radical-scavenging activity of propofol, thiopental, and dexmedetomidine. The present results indicated that the three sedatives had different patterns of free-radical-scavenging activity. Surprisingly, thiopental, a representative sedative, had direct scavenging activity for all four species investigated: superoxide radicals, hydroxyl radicals, NO, and singlet oxygen.

Various drugs and treatments have been developed to maintain the oxidant–antioxidant balance in the body to reduce the damage caused by oxidative stress [2,15,27,28]. Representative drugs and agents include molecular hydrogen (H_2), vitamin C, vitamin E, superoxide dismutase (SOD), and edaravone [29–32]. Meanwhile, with regard to NO, NO donors used as vasodilators and sildenafil used as a treatment for impotence are well known [33–35]. A direct NO scavenger, carboxy-2-phenyl-4,4,5,5,-tetramethylimidazoline-1-oxyl 3-oxide (cyboxy-PTIO), has been applied in various studies but has not yet been applied clinically [36]. The pharmacological effects of vitamin C that could make it a potential option for the prevention and treatment of COVID-19 have recently been reviewed. Clinicians using intravenous vitamin C in severely ill COVID-19 patients have reported positive clinical effects upon administration of 3 g every 6 h, together with steroids and anti-coagulants [11,29,37]. One recent topic is hydrogen's powerful antioxidant properties demonstrated by selectively inhibiting the oxidative effects of the most harmful ROS/RNS, OH and ONOO. H_2 also has a cellular defense function against oxidative stress, eliminating harmful ROS/RNS in the body and suppressing inflammatory responses. Regardless of the method of administration, such as inhalation, intravenous, or oral, H_2 has been reported to be effective in a variety of diseases and conditions due to its high rate of transfer to brain tissue [28].

These drugs are used for the primary purpose of scavenging ROS. Meanwhile, some drugs are known to have antioxidant effects as a secondary action. These drugs are used primarily for their other pharmacological effects but actually possess antioxidant and ROS-scavenging properties. Indomethacin (IND) is a strong cyclooxygenase (COX) inhibitor and has been widely used as a nonsteroidal anti-inflammatory drug (NSAID). Recently, COX inhibitors including IND have been shown to have not only antipyretic and anti-inflammatory effects but also various pharmacological effects (table) including protection against neuronal cell death [24,38]. IND also has direct strong free-radical-scavenging activity [24]. Unlike newly developed drugs, these routinely used drugs are already well experienced in clinical use and have advantages in terms of safety and the occurrence of side effects. Furthermore, the prices of the drugs are also lower, making them more economical than developing a new drug. In addition to these NSAIDs, various sedatives are also routinely used in ICUs and in surgery.

Various sedatives are used for intensive care and surgery. Some sedatives are known to have pharmacological effects other than sedation, with several reported to have antioxidant properties [13]. Propofol is known to have antioxidant properties [13]. The molecular structure of propofol is similar to that of α-tocopherol, one of the strongest endogenous antioxidants [20]. Previous studies have reported that propofol inhibits oxidative stress in preclinical and clinical studies [39].

The present study investigated the direct ROS/RNS-scavenging ability of typical sedatives used in clinical practice, including dexmedetomidine, an α2-adrenoceptor agonist drug for which the antioxidant activity has not yet been investigated using ESR methods. It is also very important to clarify the pharmacological mechanism of action of each drug's antioxidant activity. However, the in vitro ESR method employed in this study can only measure the direct scavenging activity of each ROS and NO radical. The mechanism of the scavenging activity of each drug against each free radical observed in this study requires further investigation.

The results of this study show that propofol scavenges hydroxyl radicals, NO radicals, and singlet oxygen, but not superoxide radicals. Previous in vitro ESR studies have confirmed that propofol inhibits hydroxyl radical generation but not superoxide generation. The present study supports these data and demonstrates the previously unknown ability of propofol to scavenge NO radicals and singlet oxygen.

Dexmedetomidine, a selective and potent alpha 2-adrenergic receptor agonist, was approved by the US Food and Drug Administration for sedation in 1999. In animal studies, dexmedetomidine exerts neuroprotective effects in forebrain ischemia, focal cerebral ischemia, and incomplete forebrain ischemia [40,41]. In this study, DEX had direct scavenging activity for hydroxyl radicals. In recent studies, DEX was found to decrease cerebral ischemia and SCI-induced intracellular ROS production and apoptosis in the brains of rats [42,43]. Akpınar et al. reported that DEX treatment reduces cerebral-ischemia-induced oxidative stress, cell death, and intracellular Ca^{2+} signaling through the inhibition of TRPM2 and TRPV1 [40].

Indeed, barbiturates have been recommended to treat high and refractory ICP since the early 1980s [44,45]. They are still suggested as a second or third line of treatment in US guidelines [46]. Thiopental is a classic sedative with a wide range of uses in serious conditions but is currently less favored in clinical practices. Few studies have examined thiopental and oxidative stress. Barbiturate anesthesia has been reported to inhibit the fatty acid peroxidation of neural tissue after cerebral ischemia and to enhance antioxidant capacity [47,48]. Lee et al. also compared plasma oxidative stress after surgery in dogs sedated with thiopental and propofol [49] and reported lower oxidative stress with propofol than thiopental. The direct ROS/RNS-scavenging potential of thiopental in the present study was found to be dramatic. Thiopental strongly inhibited all the radical species examined in this study. Thiopental scavenged superoxides, hydroxyl radicals, NO, and singlet oxygen in a dose-dependent manner. In addition to its purpose as a sedative, thiopental is sometimes utilized in neurointensive care in patients with decreased ICP and status epilepticus. Thiopental has some serious side effects; for example, pneumonia and hypotension are frequent side effects of barbiturates. The early use of barbiturates was significantly associated with increased ICU mortality [50]. There are few trials that have evaluated barbiturates in severe TBI patients, and none are recent. However, a novel method for the administration of thiopental has been developed to prevent these complications [51,52].

Our data suggest that thiopental has potent superoxide-scavenging activity, which may result in clinically compromised immunity. Within the body, superoxides are a strong bactericidal agent. Additionally, it has been proposed that the thiopental-mediated inhibition of NF-κB induces apoptosis in granulocytes in response to TNF-α stimulation [53]. NF-κB is activated in many cells by a variety of stimulants with redox-regulatory properties, and ROS are involved in activating the NF-κB pathway. ROS were proposed to be involved in the activation of the NF-κB pathway. Clinical reports indicate that following the induction of barbiturate coma for refractory intracranial hypertension, a decrease in white blood cell count is common, occurring in 81% of patients [54]. However, regardless of these complications, superoxide scavenging is an extremely important therapeutic target in neurologic emergencies. Superoxides are considered to be one of the root causes of the production of all types of ROS, oxidative stress activity, and secondary brain damage [27]. Essentially, the cascade of all ROS and lipid peroxidation begins with the generation of superoxide in vivo. Edaravone, which is effective against cerebral infarction, has been applied clinically as a free radical scavenger. However, edaravone only has hydroxyl-radical-scavenging activity, and it does not scavenge superoxides [14,15]. Based on this functionality, further clinical and basic studies on the ROS-scavenging ability of thiopental against various reactive oxygen species, including superoxides, are expected, given that the drug is already used in clinical practice.

Our study reported a case of severe TBI treated with thiopental. The patient received temperature control therapy for an imminent brain herniation due to post-traumatic brain swelling. Initially, the patient was sedated with midazolam. However, because ICP control was very difficult, barbiturate therapy with thiopental was administered. Although the potent ROS-scavenging ability of thiopental was confirmed in this study, endogenous oxidative stress markers such as COHb, Bil, and UA, which were measured with usual blood sampling during the course of this study, were confirmed retrospectively (Figures 7 and 8). Radical-scavenging molecules in vivo include water-soluble ascorbic acid and fat-soluble tocopherols ingested from the diet, and ubiquinone, GSH, Bil, and UA synthesized in vivo [55–58].

UA, a cause of gout, is also known to function as a radical scavenger and endogenous antioxidant [57]. Bil is also known to be an endogenous antioxidant [56]. Bil production is mediated by the induction of HO-1. HO is induced by various stresses and is recognized as a stress-sensitive marker protein [55–58]. Bil elevation was observed after a hemorrhagic stroke, reflecting the intensity of the oxidative stress [56]. Higher Bil was an independent protective factor for arteriosclerotic cardiovascular disease and negatively associated with the prognosis of stroke, acute myocardial infarction, and peripheral arterial disease, but positively associated with in-hospital cardiovascular death and major adverse cardiac events [59]. Plasma Bil concentrations serve as a useful marker of oxidative stress in patients with severe neuronal conditions. Biliverdin, CO, and iron are produced from heme by HO-1. Biliverdin is reduced to bilirubin by reductase. Bil and CO produced via these pathways are also known to possess strong antioxidant properties in vivo. In the present case, ICP was reduced, and intracranial hypertension was improved after the administration of thiopental, which has a strong ROS-scavenging capacity. Bil and COHb concentrations followed a similar time course. Both were decreased with thiopental administration. Thiopental may suppress the stress protein HO-1. The trend in the blood concentration of UA, an antioxidant, was markedly increased by the administration of thiopental. It was suggested that the rapid changes in UA concentration may have been influenced by the administration of thiopental, a potent free radical scavenger. It is known that the oxidative stress level increases in the rewarming phase after targeted temperature management therapy [2]. In this case, the results suggest that thiopental may have had some effect on the oxidant–antioxidant balance in the body. At present, thiopental is used to control intracranial hypertension in neurological emergencies [60]. A patient had markedly elevated ICP; hence, thiopental was administered to prevent cerebral herniation. Thiopental was selected because it can decrease cerebral blood flow, which was observed in CT images showing diffuse cerebral swelling owing to increased cerebral blood flow. Until this observation was noted, its antioxidant effect was not expected. The patient's UA, an endogenous antioxidant, was initially very low, which might have been due to the induction of excessive oxidative stress. In such cases, the administration of thiopental, which has antioxidant properties, may be a better choice than other sedative agents. Alternate clinically relevant methods to assess oxidative stress are required to choose a relevant therapy for a patient.

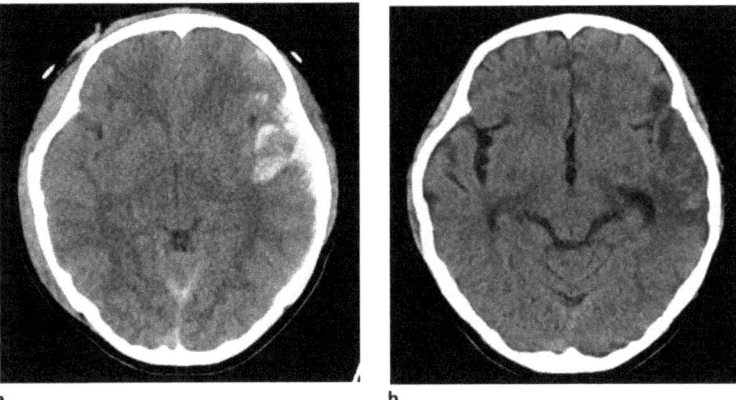

Figure 7. CT images from a case of severe traumatic brain injury. CT on admission (**a**) showing diffuse brain swelling, left acute subdural hematoma, and contusion. The ambient cistern is very narrow, and impending cerebral herniation can be observed. Brain swelling was ameliorated, and hematoma decreased in CT after treatment (**b**).

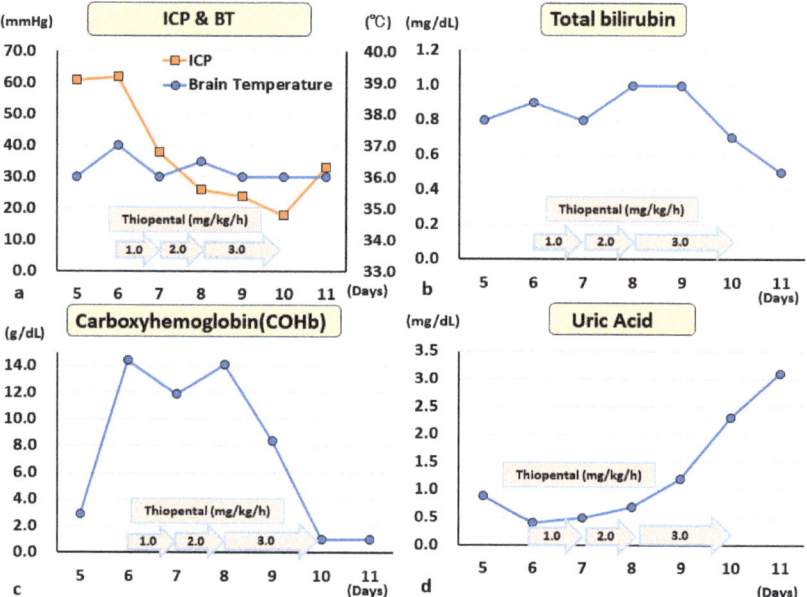

Figure 8. Endogenous oxidant and antioxidant biomarkers in a patient with traumatic brain injury receiving thiopental treatment. Thiopental administration markedly reduced ICP (**a**). The blood bilirubin (**b**) and COHb (**c**) concentrations were similar. Both were decreased with thiopental administration. Thiopental may suppress the stress protein HO-1. The blood concentration of uric acid, an endogenous antioxidant (**d**), markedly increased with thiopental administration. Thus, the rapid changes in uric acid may have been affected by thiopental administration.

This study was only a preliminary case presentation. In clinical practice, data may be influenced by a variety of factors and the condition of the patient prevailing at the time. Therefore, although the changes in UA, CO, and bilirubin data may not be solely due to thiopental administration, no other oxidative-stress-related treatment was being administered to this patient at the time the data were collected. Moreover, there were no pathological changes that would cause such a drastic change.

A major reason for the elementary clinical research on oxidative stress and the development of treatments is that it is very difficult to monitor oxidative stress and the oxidant–antioxidant balance [61]. Basically, the in vivo monitoring of free radicals is extremely difficult to apprehend due to their reaction times. Therefore, most previous studies have discussed clinical results and indirect biomarkers. In a previous study, we used ex vivo ESR to measure alkoxyl radicals in the blood and successfully developed a monitoring method [15]. However, this method could not be implemented at all facilities as the method was complex. In another study, the d-ROMs (diacron reactive oxygen metabolites) method was used to measure hydroperoxide, one of the reactive oxygen metabolites in the blood, to determine the antioxidant effect of hypothermia [2]. Although this monitoring method was simple and practical, it was difficult to determine the origin of these metabolites produced by organs, making it difficult to examine the overall oxidant–antioxidant balance. Tanaka et al. reviewed the use of redox biomarkers in multiple sclerosis (MS), a demyelinating disease of the central nervous system [62]. Reactive chemical species, oxidative enzymes, antioxidants, antioxidant enzymes, degradation products, and end products are potential biomarkers of MS, which can allow early detection and secondary prevention, as well as suggest a possible clinical course, predict MS patients' responses to specific treatments, and provide treatment targets. However, it is very difficult to accurately measure numerous oxidative antioxidant biomarkers, each with different clinical implications, in all patients. The sedative agents evaluated in this study are typical drugs routinely used in ICUs and other settings. These drugs, on top of their well-known pharmacological effects, can potentially influence ROS/RNS, a key factor for many acute diseases. Sedatives may affect a patient's oxidant–antioxidant balance, as observed in the present case. Free-radical-scavenging capacity may have a negative impact on a patient's condition, just as the suppression of superoxide radicals may affect the immune system of a patient with an infectious disease. Therefore, clinicians need to understand the role of oxidative stress in each patient's pathophysiology and the benefits of controlling the oxidant–antioxidant balance when selecting sedatives. To develop novel antioxidant therapies and drugs in the future, a monitoring system is required to solve these issues. Further studies are needed to explore the potential of sedation therapy as an antioxidant as well as its potential use for the control of ICP.

6. Conclusions and Future Perspectives

In this study, we reported that various commonly used sedatives scavenge different collections of radicals. In this study, we found that dexmedetomidine has direct hydroxyl-radical-scavenging activity and thiopental has very potent ROS/RNS-scavenging activity. These results suggest the possibility that this new antioxidant therapy can be developed for clinical application in the future. Each radical plays a different role in various pathologies. Physicians involved in critical care may need to understand the pharmacological properties of each sedative agent as a potential free radical scavenger with respect to other considerations (Figure 9). This report is only an in vitro study and representative case presentation. The free-radical-scavenging activity of sedative agents in vivo studies and in critically ill patients has not yet been studied. Further studies, including in vivo studies and clinical trials involving the effects on oxidative stress and oxidation and antioxidant balance, are needed.

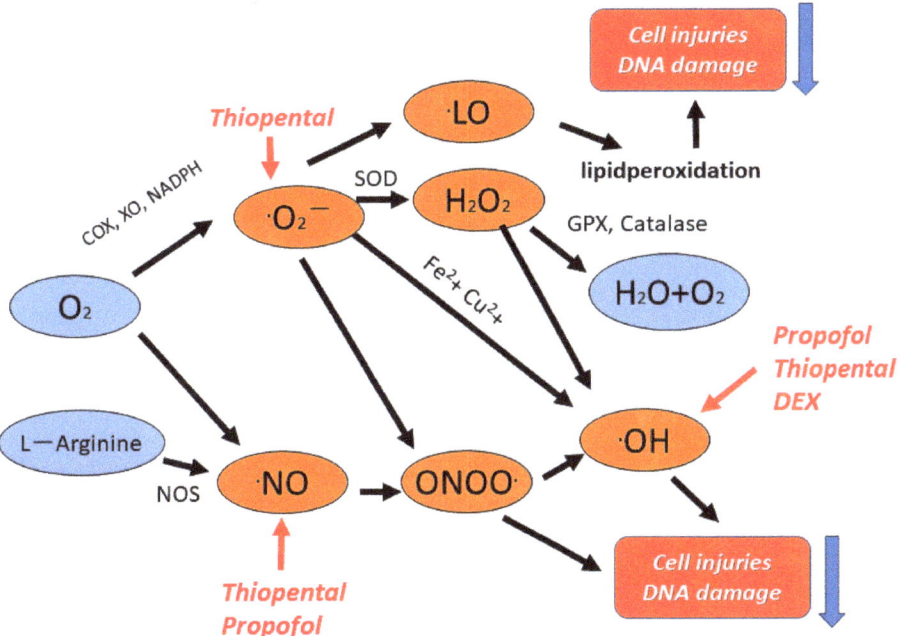

Figure 9. Scheme showing free radical generation under various critical conditions and the role of sedatives. Superoxide radicals contribute to the production of other reactive oxygen species (ROS). Thiopental directly scavenges superoxide radicals, the source of other ROS. Therefore, thiopental may indirectly decrease the production of other ROS.

Author Contributions: Conceptualization, K.D.; methodology, K.S. (Kazue Satoh), K.D. and Y.O. (Yuki Odanaka); investigation, including clinical setting, K.S. (Kazue Satoh), G.I., K.K., M.E., Y.T., K.H., A.K., K.S. (Keisuke Suzuki), M.Y. and Y.O. (Yuki Odanaka); writing—original draft preparation, Y.O. (Yuhei Ohtaki), G.I., N.U. and K.D.; writing—review and editing, K.D.; funding acquisition, K.D. All authors have read and agreed to the published version of the manuscript.

Funding: This work was partially funded by JSPS KAKENHI (grant numbers 21K09082, 19K22779, 21H03036).

Institutional Review Board Statement: Not applicable.

Informed Consent Statement: Not applicable.

Data Availability Statement: Not applicable.

Conflicts of Interest: The authors declare no conflict of interest.

References

1. Jones, D.P. Redefining oxidative stress. *Antioxid. Redox Signal.* **2006**, *8*, 1865–1879. [CrossRef] [PubMed]
2. Dohi, K.; Miyamoto, K.; Fukuda, K.; Nakamura, S.; Hayashi, M.; Ohtaki, H.; Shioda, S.; Aruga, T. Status of systemic oxidative stress during therapeutic hypothermia in patients with post-cardiac arrest syndrome. *Oxidative Med. Cell. Longev.* **2013**, *2013*, 562429. [CrossRef]
3. Tan, B.L.; Norhaizan, M.E.; Huynh, K.; Heshu, S.R.; Yeap, S.K.; Hazilawati, H.; Roselina, K. Water extract of brewers' rice induces apoptosis in human colorectal cancer cells via activation of caspase-3 and caspase-8 and downregulates the Wnt/beta-catenin downstream signaling pathway in brewers' rice-treated rats with azoxymethane-induced colon carcinogenesis. *BMC Complement. Altern. Med.* **2015**, *15*, 205. [CrossRef]
4. Liu, Z.; Zhou, T.; Ziegler, A.C.; Dimitrion, P.; Zuo, L. Oxidative stress in neurodegenerative diseases: From molecular mechanisms to clinical applications. *Oxidative Med. Cell. Longev.* **2017**, *2017*, 2525967. [CrossRef] [PubMed]
5. Tan, B.L.; Norhaizan, M.E.; Liew, W.P.; Sulaiman Rahman, H. Antioxidant and oxidative stress: A mutual interplay in age-related diseases. *Front. Pharmacol.* **2018**, *9*, 1162. [CrossRef] [PubMed]
6. Kröncke, K.D.; Fehsel, K.; Kolb-Bachofen, V. Inducible nitric oxide synthase in human diseases. *Clin. Exp. Immunol.* **1998**, *113*, 147–156. [CrossRef]
7. Geller, D.A.; Billiar, T.R. Molecular biology of nitric oxide synthases. *Cancer Metastasis Rev.* **1998**, *17*, 7–23. [CrossRef]
8. Wink, D.A.; Mitchell, J.B. Chemical biology of nitric oxide: Insights into regulatory, cytotoxic, and cytoprotective mechanisms of nitric oxide. *Free Radic. Biol. Med.* **1998**, *25*, 434–456. [CrossRef]
9. Dohi, K.; Ohtaki, H.; Inn, R.; Ikeda, Y.; Shioda, H.S.; Aruga, T. Peroxynitrite and caspase-3 expression after ischemia/reperfusion in mouse cardiac arrest model. *Acta Neurochir. Suppl.* **2003**, *86*, 87–91. [CrossRef]
10. Biesalski, H.K.; McGregor, G.P. Antioxidant therapy in critical care--is the microcirculation the primary target? *Crit. Care Med.* **2007**, *35*, S577–S583. [CrossRef]
11. Fratta Pasini, A.M.; Stranieri, C.; Cominacini, L.; Mozzini, C. Potential role of antioxidant and anti-inflammatory therapies to prevent severe SARS-Cov-2 complications. *Antioxidants* **2021**, *10*, 272. [CrossRef] [PubMed]
12. Hiedra, R.; Lo, K.B.; Elbashabsheh, M.; Gul, F.; Wright, R.M.; Albano, J.; Azmaiparashvili, Z.; Patarroyo Aponte, G. The use of IV vitamin C for patients with COVID-19: A case series. *Expert Rev. Anti Infect. Ther.* **2020**, *18*, 1259–1261. [CrossRef] [PubMed]
13. Wilson, J.X.; Gelb, A.W. Free radicals, antioxidants, and neurologic injury: Possible relationship to cerebral protection by anesthetics. *J. Neurosurg. Anesthesiol.* **2002**, *14*, 66–79. [CrossRef] [PubMed]
14. Satoh, K.; Ikeda, Y.; Shioda, S.; Tobe, T.; Yoshikawa, T. Edarabone scavenges nitric oxide. *Redox Rep.* **2002**, *7*, 219–222. [CrossRef]
15. Dohi, K.; Satoh, K.; Mihara, Y.; Nakamura, S.; Miyake, Y.; Ohtaki, H.; Nakamachi, T.; Yoshikawa, T.; Shioda, S.; Aruga, T. Alkoxyl radical-scavenging activity of edaravone in patients with traumatic brain injury. *J. Neurotrauma* **2006**, *23*, 1591–1599. [CrossRef]
16. Miyamoto, K.; Ohtaki, H.; Dohi, K.; Tsumuraya, T.; Song, D.; Kiriyama, K.; Satoh, K.; Shimizu, A.; Aruga, T.; Shioda, S. Therapeutic time window for edaravone treatment of traumatic brain injury in mice. *Biomed. Res. Int.* **2013**, *2013*, 379206. [CrossRef]
17. Miyamoto, K.; Ohtaki, H.; Dohi, K.; Tsumuraya, T.; Nakano, H.; Kiriyama, K.; Song, D.; Aruga, T.; Shioda, S. Edaravone increases regional cerebral blood flow after traumatic brain injury in mice. *Acta Neurochir. Suppl.* **2013**, *118*, 103–109. [CrossRef]
18. Dohi, K.; Satoh, K.; Nakamachi, T.; Yofu, S.; Hiratsuka, K.; Nakamura, S.; Ohtaki, H.; Yoshikawa, T.; Shioda, S.; Aruga, T. Does edaravone (MCI-186) act as an antioxidant and a neuroprotector in experimental traumatic brain injury? *Antioxid. Redox Signal.* **2007**, *9*, 281–287. [CrossRef]
19. Hughes, C.G.; McGrane, S.; Pandharipande, P.P. Sedation in the intensive care setting. *Clin. Pharmacol.* **2012**, *4*, 53–63. [CrossRef]
20. Aarts, L.; van der Hee, R.; Dekker, I.; de Jong, J.; Langemeijer, H.; Bast, A. The widely used anesthetic agent propofol can replace alpha-tocopherol as an antioxidant. *FEBS Lett.* **1995**, *357*, 83–85. [CrossRef]
21. Escamilla-Ocañas, C.E.; Albores-Ibarra, N. Current status and outlook for the management of intracranial hypertension after traumatic brain injury: Decompressive craniectomy, therapeutic hypothermia, and barbiturates. *Neurologia* **2023**, *38*, 357–363. [CrossRef] [PubMed]

22. Martemucci, G.; Costagliola, C.; Mariano, M.; D'Andrea, L.; Napolitano, P.; D'Alessandro, A.G. Free radical properties, source and targets, antioxidant consumption and health. *Oxygen* **2022**, *2*, 48–78. [CrossRef]
23. Halliwell, B.; Whiteman, M. Measuring reactive species and oxidative damage in vivo and in cell culture: How should you do it and what do the results mean? *Br. J. Pharmacol.* **2004**, *142*, 231–255. [CrossRef] [PubMed]
24. Ikeda, Y.; Matsumoto, K.; Dohi, K.; Jimbo, H.; Sasaki, K.; Satoh, K. Direct superoxide scavenging activity of nonsteroidal anti-inflammatory drugs: Determination by electron spin resonance using the spin trap method. *Headache* **2001**, *41*, 138–141. [CrossRef] [PubMed]
25. Ikeda, Y.; Jimbo, H.; Shimazu, M.; Satoh, K. Sumatriptan scavenges superoxide, hydroxyl, and nitric oxide radicals: In vitro electron spin resonance study. *Headache* **2002**, *42*, 888–892. [CrossRef]
26. Ao, Y.; Satoh, K.; Shibano, K.; Kawahito, Y.; Shioda, S. Singlet oxygen scavenging activity and cytotoxicity of essential oils from Rutaceae. *J. Clin. Biochem. Nutr.* **2008**, *43*, 6–12. [CrossRef] [PubMed]
27. Dohi, K.; Ohtaki, H.; Nakamachi, T.; Yofu, S.; Satoh, K.; Miyamoto, K.; Song, D.; Tsunawaki, S.; Shioda, S.; Aruga, T. Gp91phox (NOX2) in classically activated microglia exacerbates traumatic brain injury. *J. Neuroinflamm.* **2010**, *7*, 41. [CrossRef]
28. Dohi, K.; Kraemer, B.C.; Erickson, M.A.; McMillan, P.J.; Kovac, A.; Flachbartova, Z.; Hansen, K.M.; Shah, G.N.; Sheibani, N.; Salameh, T.; et al. Molecular hydrogen in drinking water protects against neurodegenerative changes induced by traumatic brain injury. *PLoS ONE* **2014**, *9*, e108034. [CrossRef]
29. Abobaker, A.; Alzwi, A.; Alraied, A.H.A. Overview of the possible role of vitamin C in management of COVID-19. *Pharmacol. Rep.* **2020**, *72*, 1517–1528. [CrossRef] [PubMed]
30. Ikeda, Y.; Mochizuki, Y.; Nakamura, Y.; Dohi, K.; Matsumoto, H.; Jimbo, H.; Hayashi, M.; Matsumoto, K.; Yoshikawa, T.; Murase, H.; et al. Protective effect of a novel vitamin E derivative on experimental traumatic brain edema in rats–preliminary study. *Acta Neurochir. Suppl.* **2000**, *76*, 343–345. [CrossRef]
31. Dohi, K.; Jimbo, H.; Ikeda, Y.; Fujita, S.; Ohtaki, H.; Shioda, S.; Abe, T.; Aruga, T. Pharmacological brain cooling with indomethacin in acute hemorrhagic stroke: Antiinflammatory cytokines and antioxidative effects. *Acta Neurochir. Suppl.* **2006**, *96*, 57–60. [CrossRef] [PubMed]
32. Ikeda, Y.; Matsumoto, K. Hypothermia in neurological diseases. *No Shinkei* **2001**, *53*, 513–524.
33. Kurz, M.A.; Boyer, T.D.; Whalen, R.; Peterson, T.E.; Harrison, D.G. Nitroglycerin metabolism in vascular tissue: Role of glutathione S-transferases and relationship between NO. and NO_2^- formation. *Biochem. J.* **1993**, *292 Pt 2*, 545–550. [CrossRef]
34. Harrison, D.G.; Bates, J.N. The nitrovasodilators. New ideas about old drugs. *Circulation* **1993**, *87*, 1461–1467. [CrossRef] [PubMed]
35. Goldstein, I.; Lue, T.F.; Padma-Nathan, H.; Rosen, R.C.; Steers, W.D.; Wicker, P.A. Oral sildenafil in the treatment of erectile dysfunction. Sildenafil study group. *N. Engl. J. Med.* **1998**, *338*, 1397–1404. [CrossRef]
36. Akaike, T.; Maeda, H. Quantitation of nitric oxide using 2-phenyl-4,4,5,5-tetramethylimidazoline-1-oxyl 3-oxide (PTIO). *Methods Enzymol.* **1996**, *268*, 211–221. [CrossRef]
37. Marik, P.E.; Kory, P.; Varon, J.; Iglesias, J.; Meduri, G.U. MATH+ protocol for the treatment of SARS-CoV-2 infection: The scientific rationale. *Expert Rev. Anti Infect. Ther.* **2021**, *19*, 129–135. [CrossRef]
38. Kondo, F.; Kondo, Y.; Gómez-Vargas, M.; Ogawa, N. Indomethacin inhibits delayed DNA fragmentation of hippocampal CA1 pyramidal neurons after transient forebrain ischemia in gerbils. *Brain Res.* **1998**, *791*, 352–356. [CrossRef]
39. Han, C.; Ding, W.; Jiang, W.; Chen, Y.U.; Hang, D.; Gu, D.; Jiang, G.; Tan, Y.; Ge, Z.; Ma, T. A comparison of the effects of midazolam, propofol and dexmedetomidine on the antioxidant system: A randomized trial. *Exp. Ther. Med.* **2015**, *9*, 2293–2298. [CrossRef]
40. Akpinar, H.; Nazıroğlu, M.; Övey, İ.S.; Çiğ, B.; Akpinar, O. The neuroprotective action of dexmedetomidine on apoptosis, calcium entry and oxidative stress in cerebral ischemia-induced rats: Contribution of TRPM2 and TRPV1 channels. *Sci. Rep.* **2016**, *6*, 37196. [CrossRef] [PubMed]
41. Unchiti, K.; Leurcharusmee, P.; Samerchua, A.; Pipanmekaporn, T.; Chattipakorn, N.; Chattipakorn, S.C. The potential role of dexmedetomidine on neuroprotection and its possible mechanisms: Evidence from in vitro and in vivo studies. *Eur. J. Neurosci.* **2021**, *54*, 7006–7047. [CrossRef] [PubMed]
42. Cai, Y.; Xu, H.; Yan, J.; Zhang, L.; Lu, Y. Molecular targets and mechanism of action of dexmedetomidine in treatment of ischemia/reperfusion injury. *Mol. Med. Rep.* **2014**, *9*, 1542–1550. [CrossRef] [PubMed]
43. Kose, E.A.; Bakar, B.; Kasimcan, O.; Atilla, P.; Kilinc, K.; Muftuoglu, S.; Apan, A. Effects of intracisternal and intravenous dexmedetomidine on ischemia-induced brain injury in rat: A comparative study. *Turk. Neurosurg.* **2013**, *23*, 208–217. [CrossRef] [PubMed]
44. Shapiro, H.M.; Wyte, S.R.; Loeser, J. Barbiturate-augmented hypothermia for reduction of persistent intracranial hypertension. *J. Neurosurg.* **1974**, *40*, 90–100. [CrossRef]
45. Bricolo, A.P.; Glick, R.P. Barbiturate effects on acute experimental intracranial hypertension. *J. Neurosurg.* **1981**, *55*, 397–406. [CrossRef] [PubMed]
46. Carney, N.; Totten, A.M.; O'Reilly, C.; Ullman, J.S.; Hawryluk, G.W.; Bell, M.J.; Bratton, S.L.; Chesnut, R.; Harris, O.A.; Kissoon, N.; et al. Guidelines for the management of severe traumatic brain injury, fourth edition. *Neurosurgery* **2017**, *80*, 6–15. [CrossRef]

47. Smith, D.S.; Rehncrona, S.; Siesjö, B.K. Inhibitory effects of different barbiturates on lipid peroxidation in brain tissue in vitro: Comparison with the effects of promethazine and chlorpromazine. *Anesthesiology* **1980**, *53*, 186–194. [CrossRef] [PubMed]
48. Murphy, P.G.; Davies, M.J.; Columb, M.O.; Stratford, N. Effect of propofol and thiopentone on free radical mediated oxidative stress of the erythrocyte. *Br. J. Anaesth.* **1996**, *76*, 536–543. [CrossRef]
49. Lee, J.Y. Oxidative stress due to anesthesia and surgical trauma and comparison of the effects of propofol and thiopental in dogs. *J. Vet. Med. Sci.* **2012**, *74*, 663–665. [CrossRef]
50. Léger, M.; Frasca, D.; Roquilly, A.; Seguin, P.; Cinotti, R.; Dahyot-Fizelier, C.; Asehnoune, K.; Le Borgne, F.; Gaillard, T.; Foucher, Y.; et al. Early use of barbiturates is associated with increased mortality in traumatic brain injury patients from a propensity score-based analysis of a prospective cohort. *PLoS ONE* **2022**, *17*, e0268013. [CrossRef]
51. Kajiwara, S.; Hasegawa, Y.; Negoto, T.; Orito, K.; Kawano, T.; Yoshitomi, M.; Sakata, K.; Takeshige, N.; Yamakawa, Y.; Jono, H.; et al. Efficacy of a novel prophylactic barbiturate therapy for severe traumatic brain injuries: Step-down infusion of a barbiturate with normothermia. *Neurol. Med. Chir.* **2021**, *61*, 528–535. [CrossRef]
52. Yamakawa, Y.; Morioka, M.; Negoto, T.; Orito, K.; Yoshitomi, M.; Nakamura, Y.; Takeshige, N.; Yamamoto, M.; Takeuchi, Y.; Oda, K.; et al. A novel step-down infusion method of barbiturate therapy: Its safety and effectiveness for intracranial pressure control. *Pharmacol. Res. Perspect.* **2021**, *9*, e00719. [CrossRef] [PubMed]
53. Loop, T.; Humar, M.; Pischke, S.; Hoetzel, A.; Schmidt, R.; Pahl, H.L.; Geiger, K.K.; Pannen, B.H. Thiopental inhibits tumor necrosis factor alpha-induced activation of nuclear factor kappaB through suppression of kappaB kinase activity. *Anesthesiology* **2003**, *99*, 360–367. [CrossRef] [PubMed]
54. Stover, J.F.; Stocker, R. Barbiturate coma may promote reversible bone marrow suppression in patients with severe isolated traumatic brain injury. *Eur. J. Clin. Pharmacol.* **1998**, *54*, 529–534. [CrossRef]
55. Barbagallo, I.; Galvano, F.; Frigiola, A.; Cappello, F.; Riccioni, G.; Murabito, P.; D'Orazio, N.; Torella, M.; Gazzolo, D.; Li Volti, G. Potential therapeutic effects of natural heme oxygenase-1 inducers in cardiovascular diseases. *Antioxid. Redox Signal.* **2013**, *18*, 507–521. [CrossRef]
56. Dohi, K.; Mochizuki, Y.; Satoh, K.; Jimbo, H.; Hayashi, M.; Toyoda, I.; Ikeda, Y.; Abe, T.; Aruga, T. Transient elevation of serum bilirubin (a heme oxygenase-1 metabolite) level in hemorrhagic stroke: Bilirubin is a marker of oxidant stress. *Acta Neurochir. Suppl.* **2003**, *86*, 247–249. [CrossRef] [PubMed]
57. Yisireyili, M.; Hayashi, M.; Wu, H.; Uchida, Y.; Yamamoto, K.; Kikuchi, R.; Shoaib Hamrah, M.; Nakayama, T.; Wu Cheng, X.; Matsushita, T.; et al. Xanthine oxidase inhibition by febuxostat attenuates stress-induced hyperuricemia, glucose dysmetabolism, and prothrombotic state in mice. *Sci. Rep.* **2017**, *7*, 1266. [CrossRef] [PubMed]
58. Drummond, G.S.; Baum, J.; Greenberg, M.; Lewis, D.; Abraham, N.G. HO-1 overexpression and underexpression: Clinical implications. *Arch. Biochem. Biophys.* **2019**, *673*, 108073. [CrossRef] [PubMed]
59. Lan, Y.; Liu, H.; Liu, J.; Zhao, H.; Wang, H. Is serum total bilirubin a predictor of prognosis in arteriosclerotic cardiovascular disease? A meta-analysis. *Medicine* **2019**, *98*, e17544. [CrossRef]
60. Schizodimos, T.; Soulountsi, V.; Iasonidou, C.; Kapravelos, N. An overview of management of intracranial hypertension in the intensive care unit. *J. Anesth.* **2020**, *34*, 741–757. [CrossRef]
61. Vassalle, C.; Maltinti, M.; Sabatino, L. Targeting oxidative stress for disease prevention and therapy: Where do we stand, and where do we go from here. *Molecules* **2020**, *25*, 2653. [CrossRef]
62. Tanaka, M.; Vecsei, L. Monitoring the redox status in multiple sclerosis. *Biomedicines* **2020**, *8*, 406. [CrossRef]

Disclaimer/Publisher's Note: The statements, opinions and data contained in all publications are solely those of the individual author(s) and contributor(s) and not of MDPI and/or the editor(s). MDPI and/or the editor(s) disclaim responsibility for any injury to people or property resulting from any ideas, methods, instructions or products referred to in the content.

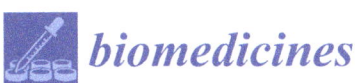

Article

TRPM4 Blocking Antibody Protects Cerebral Vasculature in Delayed Stroke Reperfusion

Bo Chen [1], Shunhui Wei [1], See Wee Low [1], Charlene Priscilla Poore [1], Andy Thiam-Huat Lee [2], Bernd Nilius [3] and Ping Liao [1,2,4,*]

[1] Calcium Signalling Laboratory, Department of Research, National Neuroscience Institute, Singapore 308433, Singapore; bo_chen@nni.com.sg (B.C.)
[2] Health and Social Sciences, Singapore Institute of Technology, Singapore 138683, Singapore
[3] Department of Cellular and Molecular Medicine, KU Leuven, 3000 Leuven, Belgium
[4] Neuroscience Academic Clinical Programme, Duke-NUS Medical School, Singapore 169857, Singapore
* Correspondence: ping_liao@nni.com.sg; Tel.: +65-6357-7611

Abstract: Reperfusion therapy for acute ischemic stroke aims to restore the blood flow of occluded blood vessels. However, successful recanalization is often associated with disruption of the blood-brain barrier, leading to reperfusion injury. Delayed recanalization increases the risk of severe reperfusion injury, including severe cerebral edema and hemorrhagic transformation. The TRPM4-blocking antibody M4P has been shown to alleviate reperfusion injury and improve functional outcomes in animal models of early stroke reperfusion. In this study, we examined the role of M4P in a clinically relevant rat model of delayed stroke reperfusion in which the left middle cerebral artery was occluded for 7 h. To mimic the clinical scenario, M4P or control IgG was administered 1 h before recanalization. Immunostaining showed that M4P treatment improved vascular morphology after stroke. Evans blue extravasation demonstrated attenuated vascular leakage following M4P treatment. With better vascular integrity, cerebral perfusion was improved, leading to a reduction of infarct volume and animal mortality rate. Functional outcome was evaluated by the Rotarod test. As more animals with severe injuries died during the test in the control IgG group, we observed no difference in functional outcomes in the surviving animals. In conclusion, we identified the potential of TRPM4 blocking antibody M4P to ameliorate vascular injury during delayed stroke reperfusion. If combined with reperfusion therapy, M4P has the potential to improve current stroke management.

Keywords: transient receptor potential channels; antibody; reperfusion injury; middle cerebral artery occlusion; model; vascular; protection; hypoxia; stroke; therapy

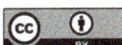

1. Introduction

An ischemic stroke occurs when the blood supply to part of the brain is interrupted or reduced. Insufficient blood supply to the brain results in a limited supply of oxygen and other nutrients to meet tissue metabolic demands, leading to brain damage [1]. Current management for acute ischemic stroke is mainly focused on reperfusion therapy by restoring blood flow to the affected brain tissues. Reperfusion therapies for acute ischemic stroke include pharmacological thrombolysis via the application of tissue plasminogen activator (tPA) and mechanical thrombectomy [2]. The oxygen and nutrients following successful reperfusion thus salvage the brain tissues within the penumbra region that are dysfunctional but not yet dead. Paradoxically, restoring blood supply may injure the brain tissue, which is known as reperfusion injury [3]. Clinical outcomes following reperfusion therapy are often confounded by reperfusion injury. The key pathophysiological change during reperfusion injury is the damage to the blood-brain barrier (BBB) [4]. Disruption of the BBB sometimes results in severe consequences such as vasogenic edema and hemorrhagic transformation. Importantly, the severity of reperfusion injury increases over time, which determines the time window for therapy. The gold-standard treatment of tPA is recommended to be administered to eligible patients given up to 4.5 h after symptom onset [5]. Mechanical thrombectomy is best for patients suffering from a major stroke with a large vessel occlusion. The guidelines recommend thrombectomy to be given 6 to 16 h from the last seen well. Beyond these time windows, the risks of side effects from recanalization outweigh the benefits, causing more morbidity and mortality [6]. Due to the limitation of these time windows, many stroke patients are unable to receive the potent reperfusion treatment because they do no not reach the hospital soon enough [7]. It is thus critical to extend the therapeutic time window to improve reperfusion therapy. How to protect BBB beyond the current time window has become a major challenge for stroke research.

Recently, the transient receptor potential (TRP) channels have emerged to play an important role in stroke pathophysiology [8]. The TRP channels constitute a superfamily that includes at least nine subfamilies: TRPP (polycystin or polycystic kidney disease), TRPML (mucolipin), TRPA (ankyrin), TRPV (vanilloid), TRPVL (vanilloid-like), TRPC (canonical), TRPN (nompC, or no mechanoreceptor potential C), TRPM (melastatin) and TRPS (soromelastatin) [9]. Among the TRP superfamily, the transient receptor potential melastatin-like subfamily member 4 (TRPM4) has recently emerged as an important drug target for stroke therapy [10–17] and many other diseases [18–20]. TRPM4 is a nonselective cation channel, conducting monovalent ions such as sodium [21]. Importantly, TRPM4 is activated by ATP depletion and an increase of intracellular Ca^{2+}, which are important pathological features associated with hypoxia. Under hypoxic conditions such as stroke, TRPM4 activity is greatly enhanced [11,15,16,22]. Furthermore, TRPM4 expression is upregulated in surviving neurons and vascular endothelial cells close to the infarct core [11,22]. As a result of TRPM4 activation, sodium influx induces cell swelling and leads to oncotic cell death in neurons and vascular endothelial cells. Accordingly, blocking TRPM4 attenuates oncotic cell death [15]. The effect of TRPM4 on reperfusion injury is prominent. In an animal model of stroke reperfusion, MRI and PET scans show that TRPM4 inhibition by siRNA resulted in a drastic reduction of cerebral edema and infarction [11]. In a chronic hypoxia model, the application of TRPM4 siRNA was shown to improve spatial memory impairment and hippocampal long-term potentiation deficit [23].

As siRNA acts at the transcriptional level, it must be administered prior to protein upregulation. In an animal stroke model, we found that TRPM4 expression is upregulated as early as 2 h after middle cerebral artery occlusion [11]. Therefore, the application of TRPM4 siRNA beyond 2 h following stroke onset is unlikely to achieve optimal outcomes. It is best to use an antagonist to block the channel directly. However, current available TRPM4 blockers have various limitations, such as lack of specificity, requiring associated subunits, or toxicity [10]. TRPM4 has been reported to interact with sulfonylurea receptor-1 (Sur1) to form a SUR1-TRPM4 channel complex. SUR1 blockers sulfonylureas were shown to inhibit SUR1-TRPM4 function [24]. SUR1 is an auxiliary subunit of the K_{ATP} channel, which senses ATP levels in pancreatic β cells [25]. Sulfonylureas such as glibenclamide are widely used to control blood glucose levels in diabetic patients by regulating insulin secretion. As sulfonylureas are available in clinical practice, multiple trials of glibenclamide were carried out in stroke patients with or without diabetes mellitus. In some studies, the application of sulfonylureas before or after stroke onset reduced hemorrhagic transformation and attenuated cerebral edema with improved neurological outcomes [26–30]. Other retrospective studies on diabetic patients who later developed stroke revealed that sulfonylureas treatment achieved a similar outcome as other antidiabetic therapies [31–35]. Such controversies may arise from differences in patient inclusion criteria, dose of sulfonylureas, or the severity of diabetes mellitus. For example, the dose of glibenclamide was low in the study on stroke as higher doses could induce hypoglycemia in patients [36]. Another study showed that application of sulfonylurea glimepiride achieved neuroprotection against stroke only in normal mice but not in type 2 diabetic mice [37]. This result suggests that the presence of diabetes may be a confounding factor when sulfonylureas are used to manage stroke.

In view of the challenges among current TRPM4 blockers, we have developed a TRPM4-specific blocking antibody M4P [10]. M4P could bind to the TRPM4 channel from the extracellular space and inhibit channel function. In an early 3-h stroke reperfusion animal model, the application of M4P successfully ameliorates reperfusion injury [10]. In this study, we aim to examine the therapeutic effect of M4P during delayed stroke reperfusion. We hypothesize that TRPM4 blocking antibody could reduce delayed stroke reperfusion injury and possibly extend the time window of current reperfusion therapy.

2. Materials and Methods

2.1. Rat Middle Cerebral Artery Occlusion (MCAO) Model and Experimental Protocol

This study was approved by the Institutional Animal Care and Use Committee of Lee Kong Chian School of Medicine from Nanyang Technological University and National Neuroscience Institute. All experiments were performed following the ARRIVE guidelines (Animal Research: Reporting In Vivo Experiments) and in compliance with the NACLAR guidelines (National Advisory Committee for Laboratory Animal Research) of Singapore. A total of 300 adult male Sprague–Dawley rats, weighing 250–300 g, were divided into 4 groups: sham (n = 24), permanent MCAO (n = 20), 3 h transient MCAO (n = 57), and 7-h transient MCAO (n = 199). The animals were housed with a temperature maintained at around 23 °C, and a 12/12-h light/dark cycle was set. Pelleted food and water were available for the animals. The animals were monitored on a daily basis. Allocation of animal treatment was randomized by rolling a dice. All researchers involved in the study were blinded to the intervention. MCAO was induced as previously described [38]. Briefly, rats were anesthetized with ketamine (75 mg/kg) and xylazine (10 mg/kg) intraperitoneally. The rats were placed supine, a midline incision was made in the neck, and the left external carotid artery (ECA), internal carotid artery (ICA), and common carotid artery (CCA) were dissected. A silicon-coated filament (0.37 mm, Cat #403756PK10, Doccol Corp, Redlands, CA, USA) was inserted into the left ICA through ECA. A Laser-Doppler flowmetry (moorVMS-LDF2, Moor Instruments Inc., Wilmington, DE, USA) was used to measure cerebral blood flow. Animals with less than 70% cerebral blood flow reduction were excluded from the study. At 3 h or 7 h after occlusion, the suture and CCA vessel clip were removed, and the ECA was closed. One hour before recanalization, a single dose of 100 μg of antibody (M4P or control rabbit IgG) was injected intravenously via the tail vein. The production of GST-tagged antigens and the generation of M4P have been described previously [10,39]. For permanent MCAO, the filament was left inside ICA. For sham-operated animals, the same anesthetic procedure was applied, but no filament was inserted into the ICA. During the operation in all animals, heart rate, blood pressure, and rectal temperature were monitored using a data acquisition system PowerLab 4/35 from AD Instruments (AD Instruments, Dunedin, New Zealand). The body temperature was maintained at 37 °C $\pm$ 0.5 °C with a warm pad throughout the operation. The mortality rate for permanent MCAO was 10% (2/20); for sham-operated animals, it was 8.3% (2/24); for 3-h stroke reperfusion was 15.7% (9/57), and for 7-h stroke reperfusion (including animals used for immunostaining, TTC staining, and functional analysis) was 49.7% (99/199).

2.2. Cerebral Blood Flow Measurement

The midline scalp was incised to reach the cranial fascia. A subsequent left paramedian incision was made to the cranial fascia for the left MCAO. The skull bone was exposed by blunt dissection, and the bone area was prepared for applying a probe holder. After applying a 3% hydrogen peroxide solution to disinfect and dry the skull surface, the probe holder and the probe were placed on the skull surface at -1 mm from bregma, 5 mm lateral to the midline [40]. The Laser Doppler probe was purchased from Moor Instruments. The cerebral blood flow during the operation was monitored using the moorVMS-LDF laser Doppler monitor (Moor Instruments Inc., Wilmington, DE, USA).

2.3. 2,3,5-Triphenyltetrazolium Chloride (TTC) Staining and Evans Blue Extravasation

TTC staining was performed 24 h after the operation to quantify infarct volume. Brains were collected after the animals were euthanized, and the cerebellum and overlying membranes were removed. Using a brain-sectioning block, the brains were sectioned into 2-mm-thick coronal slices. The brain sections were stained with 0.1% TTC (Sigma, St. Louis, MO, USA) solution at 37 °C for 30 min and then preserved in 4% formalin solution. The sections were scanned, and the infarct was captured with an image analyzer system (Scion image, Microsoft windows, Scion Corporation, Frederick, MA, USA). Calculation of edema-corrected lesion was performed as described previously [41].

Blood-brain barrier permeability was assessed by measuring Evans blue extravasations. Evans blue (E2129; Sigma-Aldrich) was prepared at a concentration of 2%. Half an hour before filament withdrawal, Evans blue was injected into the jugular vein at a dose of 4 mL/kg body weight. Three hours after reperfusion, rats were perfused transcardially with phosphate-buffered saline (PBS). After taking a picture, the ipsilateral and contralateral hemispheres were dissected, weighted, and homogenized in 1:3 weight (mg): volume (µL) ratios of 50% trichloroacetic acid (TCA) (T9159; Sigma-Aldrich, St. Louis, MO, USA) in saline. Following centrifugation at $12,000 \times g$ for 20 min, the supernatant was collected and thoroughly mixed with 95% ethanol (1:3) by repeated pipetting for fluorescence spectroscopy (620 nm/680 nm) using a Tecan infinite plate reader. Results were quantified according to a standard curve and presented as a µg of Evans Blue per gram of brain tissue.

2.4. Immunofluorescent Staining

The rat brains collected at different time points after MCAO were harvested and sectioned at 10 µm in thickness. Following fixation with 4% paraformaldehyde, the brain slice was incubated in 100 µL blocking serum (10% fetal bovine serum in 0.2% PBST) for 1 h. Cerebral vasculature was stained with primary antibody anti-vWF (AB7356, 1:200, Milipore, Burlington, MA, USA), followed by Alexa Fluor 594 conjugated secondary antibody. Images were visualized by a confocal microscope (Fluoview BX61, Olympus, Tokyo, Japan). ImageJ was used to capture the change in vascular morphology. The total vascular area per image was quantified by ImageJ, and the average vascular diameter was determined using the shortest Feret diameter (Feret Min) as described previously [42].

2.5. Rotarod Test

Rotarod (Ugo Basile, Gemonio, Italy) was used to evaluate motor functions post-stroke. Before the operation, the rats received 3 training trials at 15-min intervals for 5 consecutive days. The rotarod was set to accelerate from 4 to 80 rpm within 10 min. The mean duration of time that the animals remained on the device 1 day before MCAO was recorded as internal baseline control. At different time points following surgery, the mean duration of latency was recorded and compared.

2.6. Electrophysiology

Whole-cell patch clamp was used to measure TRPM4 currents in HEK293 cells transfected with pIRES-EGFP-TRPM4 encoding mouse TRPM4 channel using Lipofectamine 2000. TRPM4 currents were recorded 24–48 h after transfection at room temperature (22–23 °C). Patch electrodes were pulled using a Flaming/Brown micropipette puller (Sutter Instrument) and polished with a microforge. Whole-cell currents were recorded using a patch clamp amplifier (Multiclamp 700B equipped with Digidata 1440A, Molecular Devices, San Jose, CA, USA). The bath solution contained (in mmol/L): NaCl 140, $CaCl_2$ 2, KCl 2, $MgCl_2$ 1, glucose 20, and HEPES 20 at pH 7.4. The internal solution contained (in mmol/lL): CsCl 156, $MgCl_2$ 1, EGTA 10, and HEPES 10 at pH 7.2 adjusted with CsOH [20]. Additional Ca^{2+} was added to get 7.4 µM free Ca^{2+} in the pipette solution, calculated using the program WEBMAXC v2.10. Rabbit IgG or M4P was added into the bath solution at a concentration of 20 µg/mL half an hour before recording. ATP depletion was induced by applying a bath solution containing 5 mM NaN_3 and 10 mM 2-deoxyglucose (2-DG) continuously through a MicroFil (34 Gauge, WPI Inc., Sarasota, FL, USA) around 10 µm away from the recording cells. The flow rate was 200 µL/min. The current–voltage relations were measured by applying voltage ramps for 250 ms from −100 to +100 mV from a holding potential of 0 mV.

The sampling rate was 20 kHz, and the filter setting was 1 KHz. Data were analyzed using pClamp10, version 10.2 (Molecular Devices, San Jose, CA, USA).

2.7. Statistical Analysis

Data are expressed as the mean ± s.e.m. Statistical analyses were performed using GraphPad Prism version 6.0. Two-tailed unpaired student's *t*-test was used to compare two means. One-way ANOVA with Bonferroni's multiple comparison tests was used to compare ≥3 means. Two-way ANOVA with Bonferroni's multiple comparison tests was used to analyze motor functions.

3. Results

3.1. Time-Dependent Vascular Injury Post MCAO

To understand the status of vascular health after stroke, MCAO was created in Sprague–Dawley rats. The brains were collected at different time points after occlusion: 3, 6, 9, 12, and 24 h. Immunostaining using an anti-vWF antibody on the ipsilateral hemispheres demonstrated time-dependent morphological changes in the cerebral vasculature (Figure 1A). Quantification of vascular staining revealed that the area of vascular staining decreases gradually after MCAO induction (Figure 1B). Loss of vascular staining indicates the degradation of vascular structure. At 6 h MCAO, the area of vasculature is lower than 3 h MCAO but still higher than those after 9 h MCAO. After 9 h MCAO, there was no change in the vascular areas, indicating that the vasculature loss had reached a maximal level. Vascular health is closely related to the reperfusion injury after stroke. Figure 1C compares two sample brains after 3 h MCAO reperfusion and 10 h MCAO reperfusion. The 10 h transient MCAO brain demonstrated a larger infarct area and a diffused hemorrhage at multiple sections within the infarct area.

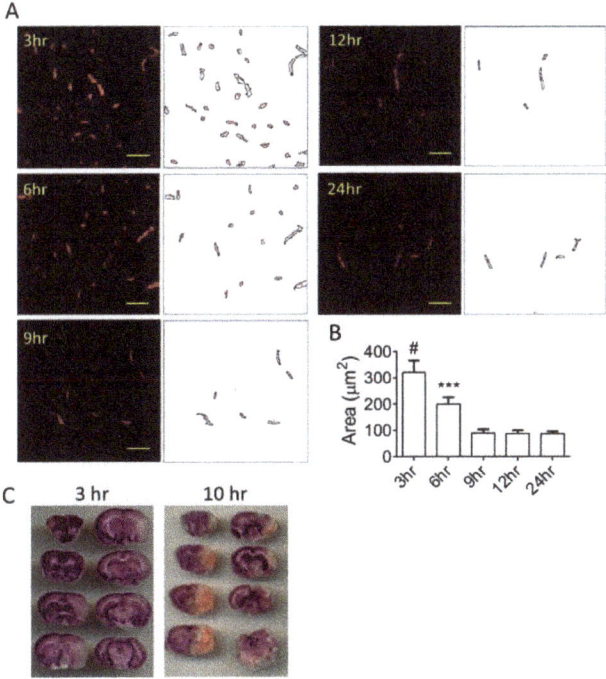

Figure 1. Time-dependent changes in the vasculature during stroke. (**A**) Representative images of cerebral vasculature within the ipsilateral hemispheres were captured at different time points

after stroke induction. Corresponding ImageJ-processed vascular images were shown next to the immunofluorescent staining images. Scale bars: 50 μm. (**B**) Summary of vascular areas. n = 6–9 images from 3 rats. (**C**) Representative images of TTC staining obtained from a 3-h reperfusion rat brain and a 10-h reperfusion rat brain. Statistical analysis was performed by one-way ANOVA with Bonferroni's post hoc analysis. *** $p < 0.001$, # $p < 0.0001$. The numerical data supporting the graphs can be found in Supplementary Table S1.

3.2. M4P Inhibits TRPM4 Current

We have developed a TRPM4-blocking antibody, M4P, which inhibits rodent TRPM4 [10]. TRPM4 currents exhibit a typical outward rectifying property in HEK 293 cells transiently expressing mouse TRPM4 (Figure 2A). Compared to control rabbit IgG, the application of M4P significantly inhibited TRPM4 current (Figure 2B). TRPM4 is known to be activated by ATP depletion and increased intracellular calcium levels [43]. When ATP was depleted, a prominent higher TRPM4 current was observed in cells treated with control IgG (Figure 2C). Again, incubation with M4P significantly reduced TRPM4 current (Figure 2D). These results suggest that M4P suppresses TRPM4 current under both normoxic and hypoxic conditions.

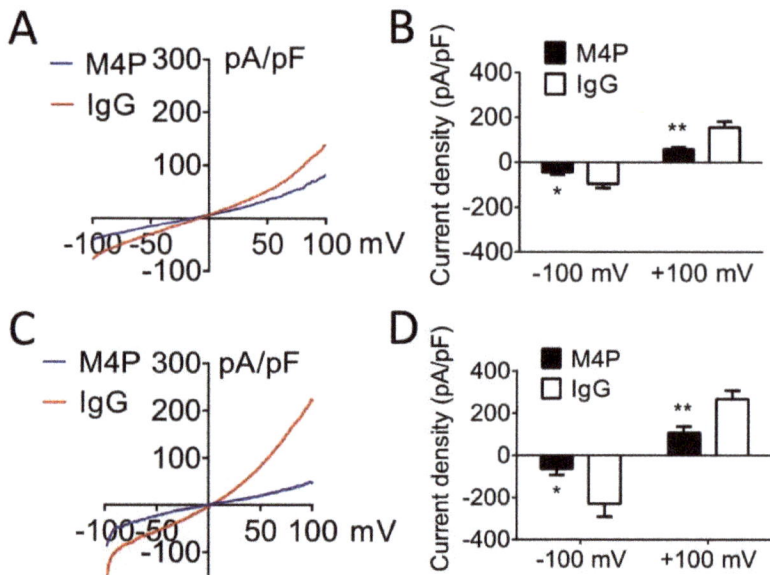

Figure 2. Inhibitory effect of TRPM4 blocking antibody M4P. (**A**) Exemplary current-voltage relationships of TRPM4 channel under the treatment of 20 μg/mL control IgG or 20 μg/mL M4P. Ramp protocols were applied from − 100 to + 100 mV with a holding potential at 0 mV. (**B**) Summary of current density at −100 and +100 mV. M4P: n = 12 cells; control IgG: n = 15 cells. (**C**) Exemplary current–voltage relationships of TRPM4 channel after 7-min ATP depletion. (**D**) Summary of current density under 7-min ATP depletion at −100 and +100 mV. M4P: n = 9 cells; control IgG: n = 12 cells. Statistical analysis was performed by student's t-test. * $p < 0.05$, ** $p < 0.01$. The numerical data supporting the graphs can be found in Supplementary Table S2.

3.3. M4P Reduces Mortality Rate and Infarct Volume in 7-h Stroke Reperfusion

We had reported that the application of M4P at 2 h post-MCAO could reduce reperfusion injury and improve functional recovery when recanalization was achieved at 3 h post-MCAO [10]. To examine the effect of M4P on delayed stroke reperfusion, we performed a 7-h transient MCAO model on rats (Figure 3A). M4P, control IgG, or vehicle was administered intravenously at 6 h post-MCAO. Reperfusion was achieved at 7-h MCAO by removing the filament. As a prolonged operation was performed, we evaluated first how this procedure affects animal mortality. In the permanent MCAO group, the animals received normal MCAO procedures without reperfusion; the mortality rate was 10% (2/20). The remaining animals all survived beyond 24 h. In a sham surgery group, animals received a similar 7-h operation procedure but without exposing carotid arteries. The mortality rate is 8.3% (2/24). In the 7-h transient MCAO group, the mortality rate is 15.6% (31/199) (Figure 3B). This result indicates that prolonged operational procedure with anesthesia increases mortality.

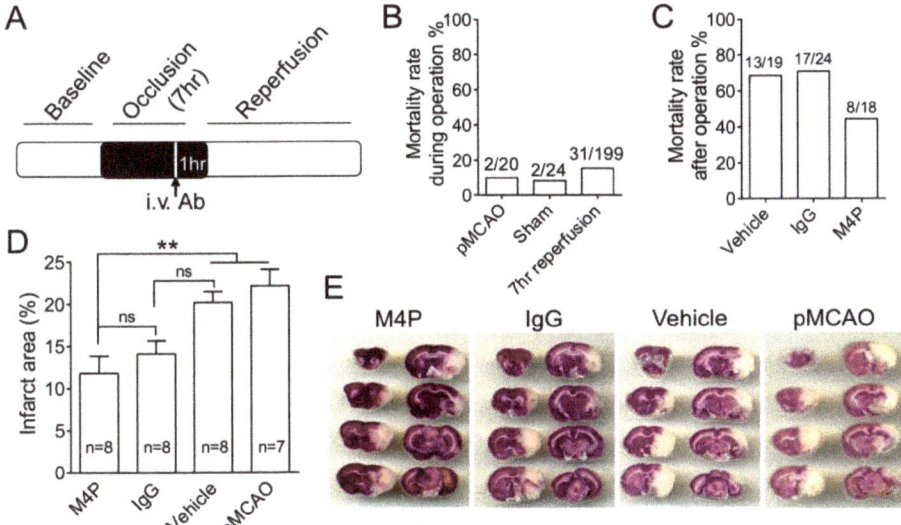

Figure 3. Evaluation of blocking TPRM4 in 7-h stroke reperfusion. (**A**) Diagram showing the experimental protocol for 7-h transient MCAO. M4P (100 μg) or control IgG (100 μg) was injected intravenously 1 h before recanalization. (**B**) Mortality rates during operation. Sham-operated animals received the same operation procedure as the 7-h transient MCAO except for the dissection of arteries and insertion of filaments. (**C**) Mortality rates after recovery from the operation. All 3 groups of animals underwent 7-h transient MCAO and were observed for 14 days post-operation. Vehicle group received i.v. injection of IgG elution buffer. (**D**) Summary of infarct area 24 h after operation. (**E**) Images of TTC-stained rat brains receiving permanent MCAO or 7-h transient MCAO with the treatments of M4P, control IgG, and vehicle. Statistical analysis was performed by one-way ANOVA with Bonferroni's post hoc analysis. ** $p < 0.01$. The numerical data supporting the graphs can be found in Supplementary Table S3.

Next, we calculated the mortality rates in animals that recovered from 7-h operation of transient MCAO and observed for 14 days. In the vehicle treatment group and control IgG treatment group, the mortalities are similar at around 68–70%. In the M4P treatment group, the mortality rate decreases to 44.4% (8/18) (Figure 3C). Further analysis revealed that within the dead animals from the control IgG group, 76.5% (13/17) animals died within 24 h after occlusion, and the remaining 23.5% (4/17) animals died after 24 h post-operation. In M4P-treated animals, the proportion of animals that died after 24 h is 12.5% (1/8), lower than the control IgG group.

To evaluate the tissue damage, infarct volume was quantified in rat brains collected 24 h after occlusion (Figure 3D,E). The infarct volume of the M4P group was significantly lower than the vehicle and permanent MCAO groups. The control IgG group shows no difference from the vehicle and permanent MCAO groups. There is also no difference between the M4P and control IgG groups.

3.4. M4P Improves Vascular Integrity after 7-h Stroke Reperfusion

To understand whether blocking TRPM4 improves vascular integrity, we performed immunostaining on cerebral vasculature one day after occlusion in permanent MCAO animals and in 7-h MCAO reperfusion animals treated with M4P or control IgG (Figure 4A). The vascular diameter was quantified accordingly (Figure 4B). Both control IgG and M4P groups demonstrated a larger vascular diameter than the permanent MCAO. Between the control IgG and M4P groups, animals in the M4P group showed a larger diameter. This result indicates that M4P achieved better reperfusion than IgG.

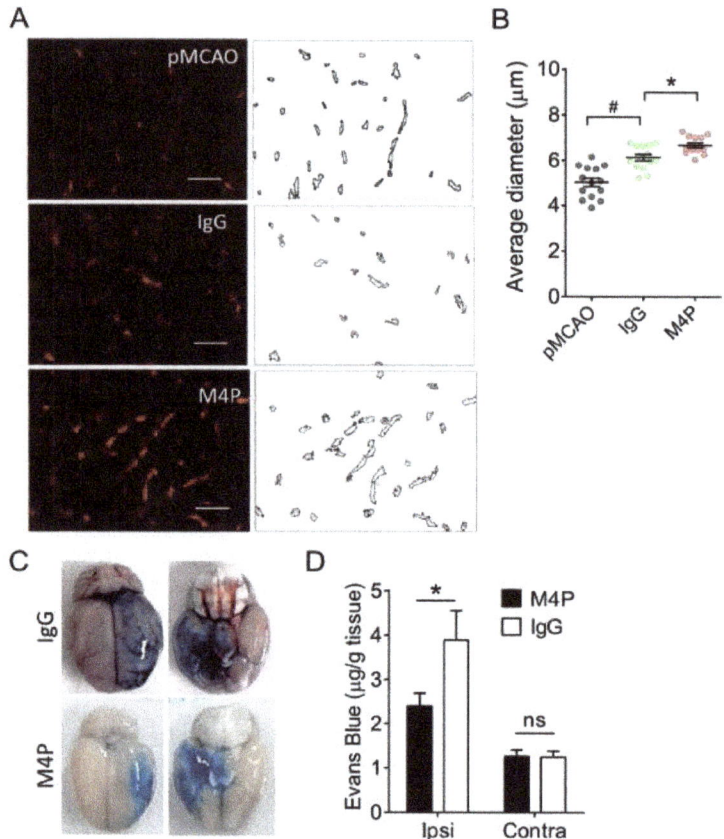

Figure 4. M4P improves vascular integrity during 7-h stroke reperfusion. (**A**) Representative images of immunofluorescent staining and corresponding ImageJ-processed images. 7-h transient MCAO rats receiving 100 µg control IgG or 100 µg M4P compared with permanent MCAO (pMCAO) without treatment. Scale bars: 50 µm. (**B**) Summary of the vascular diameter calculated by the shortest Feret diameter. In each group, $n = 14$ images were taken from 3 rats. (**C**) Dorsal and ventral views of sample rat brains with Evens blue staining. The rat brains were collected 24 h after the operation. (**D**) Summary of Evans blue quantification from ipsilateral and contralateral hemispheres. For M4P, $n = 10$ rats; for IgG, $n = 8$ rats. Statistical analysis was performed by one-way ANOVA with Bonferroni's post hoc analysis for (**B**) and student's t-test for (**D**). * $p < 0.05$, # $p < 0.0001$. The numerical data supporting the graphs can be found in Supplementary Tables S4 and S5.

Next, we compared the vascular integrity between the control IgG and M4P treatments post reperfusion by injecting Evans Blue dye. Extravasation of the dye stained the ipsilateral hemispheres in blue color (Figure 4C). Bleeding was also identified in the control IgG-treated rat brain, suggesting that 7-h stroke reperfusion-induced hemorrhage transformation in this rat. Quantification of Evans Blue dye showed that the leakage of dye was significantly reduced in the ipsilateral hemispheres of M4P-treated animals compared to the control IgG group (Figure 4D). In the contralateral hemispheres, there is no difference between the two treatments.

3.5. M4P on Cerebral Blood Flow and Functional Recovery

To examine whether reperfusion results in improved blood flow, we used a Laser-Doppler flowmetry to monitor the blood flow to the ipsilateral hemispheres at baseline, after MCAO, and after reperfusion (Figure 5A,B). The reperfusion was achieved by removing the filament from the middle cerebral artery at 7 h after occlusion. As illustrated by Figure 5A–C, the blood flow following filament withdrawal does not resume to the baseline level. The blood flow in the M4P group (43%) is significantly higher than the control IgG group (30.2%). We also quantified the blood flow in an early stroke reperfusion model in which the MCAO time was maintained for 3 h, and the antibodies were administered at 2 h post occlusion (Figure 5D). Compared to the 7-h transient MCAO, 3-h stroke reperfusion achieved a much higher blood flow resumption. In the M4P group, the blood flow to the ipsilateral hemisphere was elevated to 89.4% of baseline after recanalization, and from the control IgG group, the blood flow was resumed to 64.3%. Again, the blood flow of the M4P group was significantly higher than the control IgG group.

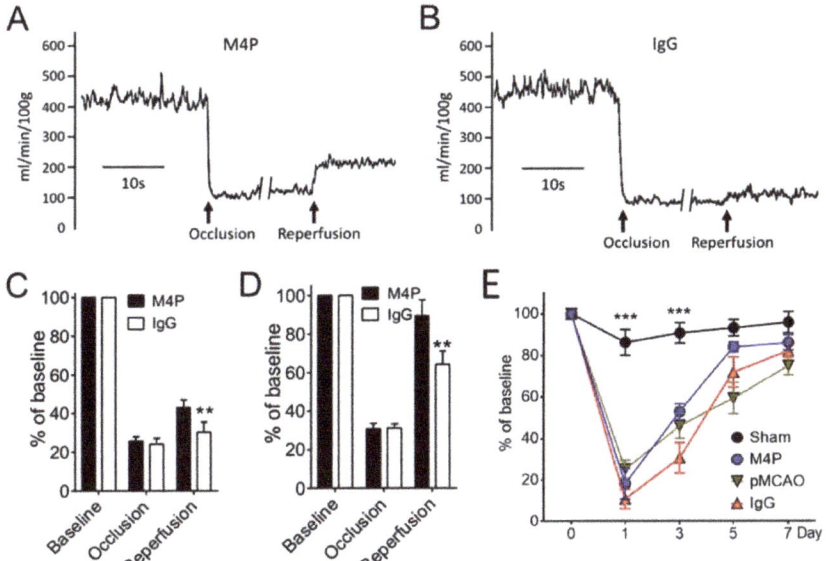

Figure 5. Functional analysis of M4P in 7-h stroke reperfusion. (**A**) Exemplary cerebral blood flow from a rat receiving 7-h MCAO. M4P of 100 μg was injected intravenously 1 h prior to recanalization. The blood flow was recorded using a Laser-Doppler flowmetry. (**B**) Exemplary cerebral blood flow from a rat treated with 100 μg control IgG. (**C**) Summary of cerebral blood flow from M4P and IgG-treated animals. The blood flow was normalized to baseline. For M4P, n = 9 rats; for IgG, n = 6 rats. (**D**) Cerebral blood flow from animals receiving 3-h stroke reperfusion. M4P (100 μg) and IgG (100 μg) were injected 1 h prior to recanalization. For M4P, n = 6 rats; for IgG, n = 10 rats. (**E**) Assessment of motor functions using the Rotarod test (n = 7 rats/group). Statistical analysis was performed by two-way ANOVA with Bonferroni's post hoc analysis. ** $p < 0.01$, *** $p < 0.001$. The numerical data supporting the graphs can be found in Supplementary Tables S6–S8.

Next, we used the Rotarod test to assess the motor functions of animals after 7-h stroke reperfusion (Figure 5E). In sham-operated animals, the motor functions slightly dropped on day 1 post-operation. In the permanent MCAO group and 7-h stroke reperfusion groups treated with M4P or control IgG, motor functions dropped significantly on day 1 post-operation. The motor functions gradually recovered in the following days. However, we did not observe any difference among the three groups of animals receiving MCAO.

4. Discussion

Antibodies have been proposed for stroke therapy [44]. To our knowledge, TRPM4 blocking antibody M4P is the first antibody developed to target an ion channel for stroke therapy. M4P was shown to inhibit the TRPM4 channel function [10]. By binding to an extracellular domain close to the channel pore, M4P inhibits sodium influx and attenuates oncotic cell death in neurons and vascular endothelial cells under hypoxia [15]. In a 3-h transient MCAO animal model, M4P was revealed to ameliorate reperfusion injury and improve functional outcomes [10]. Here, we examined the role of M4P in a delayed 7-h stroke reperfusion animal model. In this model, M4P was given 1 h before filament removal at 7 h post occlusion. We have shown previously that antibodies could reach the occluded blood vessels, possibly via collateral circulation, when injected 1 h prior to recanalization [10]. This 1-h interval was selected based on the clinical observations from stroke patients receiving tPA, most of whom achieved recanalization within 60 min of tPA treatment [45]. This experimental design is to mimic the clinical scenario in which the antibody is proposed to be delivered together with the reperfusion drug tPA. Our study contrasts with other reports using putative neuroprotective agents administered either pre-ischemia, intra-ischemia, or shortly after reperfusion which are irrelevant to clinical situations [46]. Using this clinically relevant animal stroke model, we hypothesized that M4P has the potential to extend the time window of reperfusion therapy when applied together with tPA. Such a hypothesis was supported by the observation that, albeit with a structural loss, vasculature at 6 h post occlusion has a better morphology than the 9 h MCAO brain (Figure 1). Therefore, it is possible to achieve vascular protection at 6 h before the damage reaches a maximum at 9 h. The key question is whether the reperfusion injury induced by delayed reperfusion exceeds the beneficial effect obtained from reperfusion.

Compared to IgG, M4P treatment at 6 h post occlusion improved vascular integrity manifested by a larger vascular diameter after recanalization and a less severe leakage of Evans blue dye. Vascular endothelial swelling often occurs after ischemic onset, further narrowing the occluded blood vessels [4]. M4P has been found to attenuate endothelial swelling [15], which may facilitate perfusion when recanalization is successful. The overall result of vascular protection by M4P leads to a reduction of infarct volume and mortality rate during the delayed reperfusion. However, we did not observe a difference in functional recovery assessed by the Rotarod test. A possible reason is that the infarct volume was quantified 24 h after operation. In contrast, the functional test was performed throughout the whole process of stroke recovery. It should be noted that in the control IgG group, 23.5% of mortality occurred after 24 h. This figure reduces to 12.5% in the M4P group. Animals that died after 24 h may present with a larger infarct volume not captured by the TTC staining. Whereas in the functional study, only animals that completed the full course of tests were included for analysis. The delayed animal death may be caused by the expansion of lesions after recanalization, which has been reported in patients having received reperfusion therapy [47]. Most expansions of infarction were found largely within the reperfusion region. However, in a small portion of patients, the lesion can reach outside the reperfusion area. The possible causes of lesion expansion include newly formed microvascular dysfunction or cortical spreading depression, which warrants further study [47]. Such infarct growth has also been identified in animal models of permanent MCAO [48].

Reopening the occluded blood vessels sometimes does not achieve complete tissue reperfusion, referred to as reperfusion failure. Although the underlying mechanisms are not fully understood, some have been proposed, including capillary constricting and stalling with neutrophils and pericytes, large vessel constriction, microvascular occlusion with microclots, among others. [49]. In this study when the filament was removed at 7 h post-MCAO, we observed a moderately higher blood flow in both M4P and control IgG groups. However, blood reflow upon recanalization is much higher in the 3-h transient MC than in the 7-h transient MCAO. Since the surgical procedures are similar in both models, injury to the vascular wall during operation alone is unlikely to cause the difference. In contrast, the prolonged time of obstruction might be the determining factor. After 7 h occlusion, the vascular structure affected by hypoxia is more severely injured than the 3-h MCAO model. Thus, fewer blood vessels remained intact following filament withdrawal to be reperfused completely and successfully. A second possible reason is that a blood clot may form in the distal part of the blood vessel after prolonged occlusion. Once reperfusion is achieved, this blood clot may travel downstream and occlude distal branches.

5. Limitations and Future Directions

The major limitation or challenge of this study is the prolonged 7-h operational procedure and anesthesia. Although ketamine/xylazine was selected for its safety, ease of administration, and low mortality [50,51], we encountered a high mortality rate even in the sham-operated group. The 8.3% mortality rate (2/24) is close to the 10% permanent MCAO model (2/20), suggesting that prolonged anesthesia is harmful to the animals. Furthermore, repeated operational procedures to the carotid arteries and branches cause additional injuries. The potential for clot formation after 7 h of occlusion also confounded the efficiency of recanalization. We have tried to use tPA in the experiment to dissolve blood clots. However, our attempts failed due to the bleeding disorder during/after the operation. To overcome the limitations of MCAO, less invasive animal models of stroke, such as transcranial occlusion and photothrombosis models [52], can be considered to test the effect of M4P on functional outcomes.

As M4P is a polyclonal antibody against rodent TRPM4, it cannot be used in humans. We are now in the process of developing a humanized antibody against human TRPM4. In addition to reducing reperfusion injury, TRPM4-blocking antibodies can be examined in conjunction with other treatments such as antiplatelets [53], none invasive transcranial stimulation [54,55], and other neuroprotectants [56,57]. Better neuroprotection may be achieved with multiple therapies being used together.

6. Conclusions

We provide evidence showing that TRPM4 blocking antibody M4P can be an effective vascular protective agent in delayed stroke reperfusion. Although it has been reported that reperfusion at 4 h and 12 h does not change infarct volume formation [58], our results suggest that with proper vascular protection, reperfusion injury at a time point longer than 4 h can be alleviated. Although an improvement in vascular integrity and reduced mortality are evidenced, the functional outcomes following M4P treatment require further studies with a lesser invasive animal model. The translation of animal study to clinical practice needs to consider the anatomical and functional differences between human and animal brains [59]. Despite all the challenges, our study provides a novel approach to vascular protection that has the potential to extend the current reperfusion time window of tPA. Furthermore, TRPM4 blocking antibody could benefit patients receiving mechanical thrombectomy, which is performed at a later point than tPA [2]. As a co-therapy, TRPM4 blocking antibody certainly could improve the outcome of thrombectomy [60].

Supplementary Materials: The following supporting information can be downloaded at: https://www.mdpi.com/article/10.3390/biomedicines11051480/s1, Table S1. Summary of vascular areas (Figure 1B). Table S2. TRPM4 current density in control (Figure 2B) and ATP depletion (Figure 2D) condition. Table S3. Summary of infarct area 24 hrs after operation (Figure 3D). Table S4. Summary of the vascular diameter (Figure 4B). Table S5. Summary of Evens blue quantification (Figure 4D). Table S6. Summary of cerebral blood flow (Figure 5C). Table S7. Summary of cerebral blood flow (Figure 5D). Table S8. Assessment of motor functions by Rotarod test (Figure 5E).

Author Contributions: P.L. conceived and directed the project; B.C., S.W., A.T.-H.L., B.N. and P.L. conceived, analyzed data, and wrote the paper; S.W., B.C., S.W.L. and C.P.P. performed experiments and analyzed data. All authors have read and agreed to the published version of the manuscript.

Funding: This work was supported by grants NMRC/CIRG/1469/2017, NMRC/OFIRG/0070/2018, and MOH-000522-00 from the Singapore Ministry of Health's National Medical Research Council.

Institutional Review Board Statement: All rats were housed in the Animal Research Facility, Lee Kong Chian School of Medicine, Nanyang Technological University. All experiments were conducted in accordance with the guidelines of the Institutional Animal Care and Use Committee of the National Neuroscience Institute for the care and use of animals in research. Furthermore, all protocols were approved by the institutional animal care and use committee.

Informed Consent Statement: Not applicable.

Data Availability Statement: All data generated and analyzed for this study are included in this published article.

Conflicts of Interest: The authors declare no conflict of interest.

References

1. Ahad, M.A.; Kumaran, K.R.; Ning, T.; Mansor, N.I.; Effendy, M.A.; Damodaran, T.; Lingam, K.; Wahab, H.A.; Nordin, N.; Liao, P.; et al. Insights into the neuropathology of cerebral ischemia and its mechanisms. *Rev. Neurosci.* **2020**, *31*, 521–538. [CrossRef]
2. Powers, W.J.; Rabinstein, A.A.; Ackerson, T.; Adeoye, O.M.; Bambakidis, N.C.; Becker, K.; Biller, J.; Brown, M.; Demaerschalk, B.M.; Hoh, B.; et al. 2018 Guidelines for the Early Management of Patients with Acute Ischemic Stroke: A Guideline for Healthcare Professionals from the American Heart Association/American Stroke Association. *Stroke* **2018**, *49*, e46–e110. [CrossRef] [PubMed]
3. Nour, M.; Scalzo, F.; Liebeskind, D.S. Ischemia-reperfusion injury in stroke. *Interv. Neurol.* **2013**, *1*, 185–199. [CrossRef]
4. Khatri, R.; McKinney, A.M.; Swenson, B.; Janardhan, V. Blood-brain barrier, reperfusion injury, and hemorrhagic transformation in acute ischemic stroke. *Neurology* **2012**, *79*, S52–S57. [CrossRef] [PubMed]
5. Powers, W.J.; Rabinstein, A.A.; Ackerson, T.; Adeoye, O.M.; Bambakidis, N.C.; Becker, K.; Biller, J.; Brown, M.; Demaerschalk, B.M.; Hoh, B.; et al. Guidelines for the Early Management of Patients with Acute Ischemic Stroke: 2019 Update to the 2018 Guidelines for the Early Management of Acute Ischemic Stroke: A Guideline for Healthcare Professionals from the American Heart Association/American Stroke Association. *Stroke* **2019**, *50*, e344–e418. [CrossRef]
6. The NINDS t-PA Stroke Study Group. Intracerebral hemorrhage after intravenous t-PA therapy for ischemic stroke. *Stroke* **1997**, *28*, 2109–2118. [CrossRef]
7. Henninger, N.; Fisher, M. Extending the Time Window for Endovascular and Pharmacological Reperfusion. *Transl. Stroke Res.* **2016**, *7*, 284–293. [CrossRef] [PubMed]
8. Zhang, E.; Liao, P. Brain transient receptor potential channels and stroke. *J. Neurosci. Res.* **2015**, *93*, 1165–1183. [CrossRef] [PubMed]
9. Himmel, N.J.; Cox, D.N. Transient receptor potential channels: Current perspectives on evolution, structure, function and nomenclature. *Proc. Biol. Sci.* **2020**, *287*, 20201309. [CrossRef]
10. Chen, B.; Gao, Y.; Wei, S.; Low, S.W.; Ng, G.; Yu, D.; Tu, T.M.; Soong, T.W.; Nilius, B.; Liao, P. TRPM4-specific blocking antibody attenuates reperfusion injury in a rat model of stroke. *Pflugers Arch.* **2019**, *471*, 1455–1466. [CrossRef]
11. Chen, B.; Ng, G.; Gao, Y.; Low, S.W.; Sandanaraj, E.; Ramasamy, B.; Sekar, S.; Bhakoo, K.; Soong, T.W.; Nilius, B.; et al. Non-Invasive Multimodality Imaging Directly Shows TRPM4 Inhibition Ameliorates Stroke Reperfusion Injury. *Transl. Stroke Res.* **2019**, *10*, 91–103. [CrossRef] [PubMed]
12. Loh, K.Y.; Wang, Z.; Liao, P. Oncotic Cell Death in Stroke. *Rev. Physiol. Biochem. Pharmacol.* **2019**, *176*, 37–64. [CrossRef]
13. Simard, J.M.; Kahle, K.T.; Gerzanich, V. Molecular mechanisms of microvascular failure in central nervous system injury-synergistic roles of NKCC1 and SUR1/TRPM4. *J. Neurosurg.* **2010**, *113*, 622–629. [CrossRef] [PubMed]
14. Simard, J.M.; Tarasov, K.V.; Gerzanich, V. Non-selective cation channels, transient receptor potential channels and ischemic stroke. *Biochim. Biophys. Acta* **2007**, *1772*, 947–957. [CrossRef]
15. Wei, S.; Low, S.W.; Poore, C.P.; Chen, B.; Gao, Y.; Nilius, B.; Liao, P. Comparison of Anti-oncotic Effect of TRPM4 Blocking Antibody in Neuron, Astrocyte and Vascular Endothelial Cell Under Hypoxia. *Front. Cell Dev. Biol.* **2020**, *8*, 562584. [CrossRef]
16. Low, S.W.; Gao, Y.; Wei, S.; Chen, B.; Nilius, B.; Liao, P. Development and characterization of a monoclonal antibody blocking human TRPM4 channel. *Sci. Rep.* **2021**, *11*, 10411. [CrossRef] [PubMed]
17. Simard, J.M.; Chen, M.; Tarasov, K.V.; Bhatta, S.; Ivanova, S.; Melnitchenko, L.; Tsymbalyuk, N.; West, G.A.; Gerzanich, V. Newly expressed SUR1-regulated NC(Ca-ATP) channel mediates cerebral edema after ischemic stroke. *Nat. Med.* **2006**, *12*, 433–440. [CrossRef] [PubMed]
18. Gao, Y.; Liao, P. TRPM4 channel and cancer. *Cancer Lett.* **2019**, *454*, 66–69. [CrossRef]

19. Gerzanich, V.; Woo, S.K.; Vennekens, R.; Tsymbalyuk, O.; Ivanova, S.; Ivanov, A.; Geng, Z.; Chen, Z.; Nilius, B.; Flockerzi, V.; et al. De novo expression of Trpm4 initiates secondary hemorrhage in spinal cord injury. *Nat. Med.* **2009**, *15*, 185–191. [CrossRef]
20. Schattling, B.; Steinbach, K.; Thies, E.; Kruse, M.; Menigoz, A.; Ufer, F.; Flockerzi, V.; Bruck, W.; Pongs, O.; Vennekens, R.; et al. TRPM4 cation channel mediates axonal and neuronal degeneration in experimental autoimmune encephalomyelitis and multiple sclerosis. *Nat. Med.* **2012**, *18*, 1805–1811. [CrossRef]
21. Vennekens, R.; Nilius, B. Insights into TRPM4 function, regulation and physiological role. In *Transient Receptor Potential (TRP) Channels*; Flockerzi, V., Nilius, B., Eds.; Springer: Berlin/Heidelberg, Germany, 2007; pp. 269–285. [CrossRef]
22. Loh, K.P.; Ng, G.; Yu, C.Y.; Fhu, C.K.; Yu, D.; Vennekens, R.; Nilius, B.; Soong, T.W.; Liao, P. TRPM4 inhibition promotes angiogenesis after ischemic stroke. *Pflugers Arch.* **2014**, *466*, 563–576. [CrossRef]
23. Hazalin, N.; Liao, P.; Hassan, Z. TRPM4 inhibition improves spatial memory impairment and hippocampal long-term potentiation deficit in chronic cerebral hypoperfused rats. *Behav. Brain Res.* **2020**, *393*, 112781. [CrossRef]
24. Woo, S.K.; Kwon, M.S.; Ivanov, A.; Gerzanich, V.; Simard, J.M. The sulfonylurea receptor 1 (Sur1)-transient receptor potential melastatin 4 (Trpm4) channel. *J. Biol. Chem.* **2013**, *288*, 3655–3667. [CrossRef] [PubMed]
25. Nichols, C.G. KATP channels as molecular sensors of cellular metabolism. *Nature* **2006**, *440*, 470–476. [CrossRef] [PubMed]
26. Kunte, H.; Busch, M.A.; Trostdorf, K.; Vollnberg, B.; Harms, L.; Mehta, R.I.; Castellani, R.J.; Mandava, P.; Kent, T.A.; Simard, J.M. Hemorrhagic transformation of ischemic stroke in diabetics on sulfonylureas. *Ann. Neurol.* **2012**, *72*, 799–806. [CrossRef] [PubMed]
27. Kimberly, W.T.; Battey, T.W.; Pham, L.; Wu, O.; Yoo, A.J.; Furie, K.L.; Singhal, A.B.; Elm, J.J.; Stern, B.J.; Sheth, K.N. Glyburide is associated with attenuated vasogenic edema in stroke patients. *Neurocrit. Care* **2014**, *20*, 193–201. [CrossRef]
28. Sheth, K.N.; Simard, J.M.; Elm, J.; Kronenberg, G.; Kunte, H.; Kimberly, W.T. Human Data Supporting Glyburide in Ischemic Stroke. *Acta Neurochir. Suppl.* **2016**, *121*, 13–18. [CrossRef]
29. Sheth, K.N.; Kimberly, W.T.; Elm, J.J.; Kent, T.A.; Yoo, A.J.; Thomalla, G.; Campbell, B.; Donnan, G.A.; Davis, S.M.; Albers, G.W.; et al. Exploratory analysis of glyburide as a novel therapy for preventing brain swelling. *Neurocrit. Care* **2014**, *21*, 43–51. [CrossRef]
30. Sheth, K.N.; Kimberly, W.T.; Elm, J.J.; Kent, T.A.; Mandava, P.; Yoo, A.J.; Thomalla, G.; Campbell, B.; Donnan, G.A.; Davis, S.M.; et al. Pilot study of intravenous glyburide in patients with a large ischemic stroke. *Stroke* **2014**, *45*, 281–283. [CrossRef]
31. Horsdal, H.T.; Mehnert, F.; Rungby, J.; Johnsen, S.P. Type of preadmission antidiabetic treatment and outcome among patients with ischemic stroke: A nationwide follow-up study. *J. Stroke Cerebrovasc. Dis.* **2012**, *21*, 717–725. [CrossRef]
32. Weih, M.; Amberger, N.; Wegener, S.; Dirnagl, U.; Reuter, T.; Einhaupl, K. Sulfonylurea drugs do not influence initial stroke severity and in-hospital outcome in stroke patients with diabetes. *Stroke* **2001**, *32*, 2029–2032. [CrossRef] [PubMed]
33. Tziomalos, K.; Bouziana, S.D.; Spanou, M.; Kostaki, S.; Papadopoulou, M.; Giampatzis, V.; Dourliou, V.; Kostourou, D.T.; Savopoulos, C.; Hatzitolios, A.I. Prior treatment with dipeptidyl peptidase 4 inhibitors is associated with better functional outcome and lower in-hospital mortality in patients with type 2 diabetes mellitus admitted with acute ischaemic stroke. *Diab. Vasc. Dis. Res.* **2015**, *12*, 463–466. [CrossRef]
34. Favilla, C.G.; Mullen, M.T.; Ali, M.; Higgins, P.; Kasner, S.E. Sulfonylurea use before stroke does not influence outcome. *Stroke* **2011**, *42*, 710–715. [CrossRef]
35. Liu, R.; Wang, H.; Xu, B.; Chen, W.; Turlova, E.; Dong, N.; Sun, C.L.; Lu, Y.; Fu, H.; Shi, R.; et al. Cerebrovascular safety of sulfonylureas: The role of KATP channels in neuroprotection and the risk of stroke in patients with type 2 diabetes. *Diabetes* **2016**, *65*, 2795–2809. [CrossRef]
36. King, Z.A.; Sheth, K.N.; Kimberly, W.T.; Simard, J.M. Profile of intravenous glyburide for the prevention of cerebral edema following large hemispheric infarction: Evidence to date. *Drug Des. Dev. Ther.* **2018**, *12*, 2539–2552. [CrossRef]
37. Darsalia, V.; Ortsater, H.; Olverling, A.; Darlof, E.; Wolbert, P.; Nystrom, T.; Klein, T.; Sjoholm, A.; Patrone, C. The DPP-4 inhibitor linagliptin counteracts stroke in the normal and diabetic mouse brain: A comparison with glimepiride. *Diabetes* **2013**, *62*, 1289–1296. [CrossRef] [PubMed]
38. Wei, S.; Behn, J.; Poore, C.P.; Low, S.W.; Nilius, B.; Fan, H.; Liao, P. Binding epitope for recognition of human TRPM4 channel by monoclonal antibody M4M. *Sci. Rep.* **2022**, *12*, 19562. [CrossRef]
39. Liao, P.; Yu, D.; Hu, Z.; Liang, M.C.; Wang, J.J.; Yu, C.Y.; Ng, G.; Yong, T.F.; Soon, J.L.; Chua, Y.L.; et al. Alternative splicing generates a novel truncated Cav1.2 channel in neonatal rat heart. *J. Biol. Chem.* **2015**, *290*, 9262–9272. [CrossRef]
40. Yeo, C.; Kim, H.; Song, C. Cerebral Blood Flow Monitoring by Diffuse Speckle Contrast Analysis during MCAO Surgery in the Rat. *Curr. Opt. Photonics* **2017**, *1*, 433–439. [CrossRef]
41. Walberer, M.; Stolz, E.; Muller, C.; Friedrich, C.; Rottger, C.; Blaes, F.; Kaps, M.; Fisher, M.; Bachmann, G.; Gerriets, T. Experimental stroke: Ischaemic lesion volume and oedema formation differ among rat strains (a comparison between Wistar and Sprague-Dawley rats using MRI). *Lab Anim.* **2006**, *40*, 1–8. [CrossRef] [PubMed]
42. Adapala, R.K.; Thoppil, R.J.; Ghosh, K.; Cappelli, H.C.; Dudley, A.C.; Paruchuri, S.; Keshamouni, V.; Klagsbrun, M.; Meszaros, J.G.; Chilian, W.M.; et al. Activation of mechanosensitive ion channel TRPV4 normalizes tumor vasculature and improves cancer therapy. *Oncogene* **2016**, *35*, 314–322. [CrossRef] [PubMed]
43. Mathar, I.; Jacobs, G.; Kecskes, M.; Menigoz, A.; Philippaert, K.; Vennekens, R. Trpm4. *Handb. Exp. Pharmacol.* **2014**, *222*, 461–487. [CrossRef] [PubMed]
44. Yu, C.Y.; Ng, G.; Liao, P. Therapeutic Antibodies in Stroke. *Transl. Stroke Res.* **2013**, *4*, 477–483. [CrossRef] [PubMed]

45. Christou, I.; Alexandrov, A.V.; Burgin, W.S.; Wojner, A.W.; Felberg, R.A.; Malkoff, M.; Grotta, J.C. Timing of recanalization after tissue plasminogen activator therapy determined by transcranial doppler correlates with clinical recovery from ischemic stroke. *Stroke* **2000**, *31*, 1812–1816. [CrossRef] [PubMed]
46. Liu, F.; McCullough, L.D. Middle cerebral artery occlusion model in rodents: Methods and potential pitfalls. *J. Biomed. Biotechnol.* **2011**, *2011*, 464701. [CrossRef]
47. Zhou, Y.; He, Y.; Yan, S.; Chen, L.; Zhang, R.; Xu, J.; Hu, H.; Liebeskind, D.S.; Lou, M. Reperfusion Injury Is Associated with Poor Outcome in Patients With Recanalization After Thrombectomy. *Stroke* **2023**, *54*, 96–104. [CrossRef]
48. Hossmann, K.A. Pathophysiological basis of translational stroke research. *Folia Neuropathol.* **2009**, *47*, 213–227.
49. El Amki, M.; Gluck, C.; Binder, N.; Middleham, W.; Wyss, M.T.; Weiss, T.; Meister, H.; Luft, A.; Weller, M.; Weber, B.; et al. Neutrophils Obstructing Brain Capillaries Are a Major Cause of No-Reflow in Ischemic Stroke. *Cell Rep.* **2020**, *33*, 108260. [CrossRef]
50. Mousavi, S.M.; Karimi-Haghighi, S.; Chavoshinezhad, S.; Pandamooz, S.; Belem-Filho, I.J.A.; Keshavarz, S.; Bayat, M.; Hooshmandi, E.; Rahimi Jaberi, A.; Salehi, M.S.; et al. The impacts of anesthetic regimens on the middle cerebral artery occlusion outcomes in male rats. *Neuroreport* **2022**, *33*, 561–568. [CrossRef]
51. Hoffmann, U.; Sheng, H.; Ayata, C.; Warner, D.S. Anesthesia in Experimental Stroke Research. *Transl. Stroke Res.* **2016**, *7*, 358–367. [CrossRef]
52. Li, Y.; Zhang, J. Animal models of stroke. *Anim. Model. Exp. Med.* **2021**, *4*, 204–219. [CrossRef] [PubMed]
53. Tornyos, D.; Komocsi, A.; Balint, A.; Kupo, P.; El Abdallaoui, O.E.A.; Szapary, L.; Szapary, L.B. Antithrombotic therapy for secondary prevention in patients with stroke or transient ischemic attack: A multiple treatment network meta-analysis of randomized controlled trials. *PLoS ONE* **2022**, *17*, e0273103. [CrossRef] [PubMed]
54. Wang, W.J.; Zhong, Y.B.; Zhao, J.J.; Ren, M.; Zhang, S.C.; Xu, M.S.; Xu, S.T.; Zhang, Y.J.; Shan, C.L. Transcranial pulse current stimulation improves the locomotor function in a rat model of stroke. *Neural Regen. Res.* **2021**, *16*, 1229–1234. [CrossRef] [PubMed]
55. Wu, Z.; Sun, F.; Li, Z.; Liu, M.; Tian, X.; Guo, D.; Wei, P.; Shan, Y.; Liu, T.; Guo, M.; et al. Electrical stimulation of the lateral cerebellar nucleus promotes neurogenesis in rats after motor cortical ischemia. *Sci. Rep.* **2020**, *10*, 16563. [CrossRef]
56. Battaglia, S.; Di Fazio, C.; Vicario, C.M.; Avenanti, A. Neuropharmacological Modulation of N-methyl-D-aspartate, Noradrenaline and Endocannabinoid Receptors in Fear Extinction Learning: Synaptic Transmission and Plasticity. *Int. J. Mol. Sci.* **2023**, *24*, 5926. [CrossRef]
57. Damodaran, T.; Tan, B.W.L.; Liao, P.; Ramanathan, S.; Lim, G.K.; Hassan, Z. Clitoria ternatea L. root extract ameliorated the cognitive and hippocampal long-term potentiation deficits induced by chronic cerebral hypoperfusion in the rat. *J. Ethnopharmacol.* **2018**, *224*, 381–390. [CrossRef]
58. Engelhorn, T.; von Kummer, R.; Reith, W.; Forsting, M.; Doerfler, A. What is effective in malignant middle cerebral artery infarction: Reperfusion, craniectomy, or both? An experimental study in rats. *Stroke* **2002**, *33*, 617–622. [CrossRef]
59. Ruan, J.; Yao, Y. Behavioral tests in rodent models of stroke. *Brain Hemorrhages* **2020**, *1*, 171–184. [CrossRef]
60. Rajendram, P.; Ikram, A.; Fisher, M. Combined Therapeutics: Future Opportunities for Co-therapy with Thrombectomy. *Neurotherapeutics* **2023**. [CrossRef]

Disclaimer/Publisher's Note: The statements, opinions and data contained in all publications are solely those of the individual author(s) and contributor(s) and not of MDPI and/or the editor(s). MDPI and/or the editor(s) disclaim responsibility for any injury to people or property resulting from any ideas, methods, instructions or products referred to in the content.

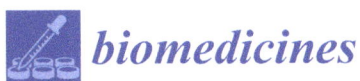

Article

Estradiol Treatment Enhances Behavioral and Molecular Changes Induced by Repetitive Trigeminal Activation in a Rat Model of Migraine

Eleonóra Spekker [1], Zsuzsanna Bohár [1], Annamária Fejes-Szabó [1], Mónika Szűcs [2], László Vécsei [1,3,*] and Árpád Párdutz [3]

[1] ELKH-SZTE Neuroscience Research Group, University of Szeged, Semmelweis u. 6, H-6725 Szeged, Hungary
[2] Department of Medical Physics and Informatics, University of Szeged, Korányi Fasor 9, H-6720 Szeged, Hungary
[3] Department of Neurology, Interdisciplinary Excellence Centre, Albert Szent-Györgyi Medical School, University of Szeged, H-6725 Szeged, Hungary
* Correspondence: vecsei.laszlo@med.u-szeged.hu; Tel.: +36-62-545-351; Fax: +36-62-545-597

Abstract: A migraine is a neurological condition that can cause multiple symptoms. It is up to three times more common in women than men, thus, estrogen may play an important role in the appearance attacks. Its exact pathomechanism is still unknown; however, the activation and sensitization of the trigeminal system play an essential role. We aimed to use an animal model, which would better illustrate the process of repeated episodic migraine attacks to reveal possible new mechanisms of trigeminal pain chronification. Twenty male (M) and forty ovariectomized (OVX) female adult rats were used for our experiment. Male rats were divided into two groups (M + SIF, M + IS), while female rats were divided into four groups (OVX + SIF, OVX + IS, OVX + E2 + SIF, OVX + E2 + IS); half of the female rats received capsules filled with cholesterol (OVX + SIF, OVX + IS), while the other half received a 1:1 mixture of cholesterol and 17β-estradiol (OVX + E2 + SIF, OVX + E2 + IS). The animals received synthetic interstitial fluid (SIF) (M + SIF, OVX + SIF, OVX + E2 + SIF) or inflammatory soup (IS) (M + IS, OVX + IS, OVX + E2 + IS) treatment on the dural surface through a cannula for three consecutive days each week (12 times in total). Behavior tests and immunostainings were performed. After IS application, a significant decrease was observed in the pain threshold in the M + IS ($0.001 < p < 0.5$), OVX + IS ($0.01 < p < 0.05$), and OVX + E2 + IS ($0.001 < p < 0.05$) groups compared to the control groups (M + SIF; OVX + SIF, OVX + E2 + SIF). The locomotor activity of the rats was lower in the IS treated groups (M + IS, $0.01 < p < 0.05$; OVX + IS, $p < 0.05$; OVX + E2 + IS, $0.001 < p < 0.05$), and these animals spent more time in the dark room (M + IS, $p < 0.05$; OVX + IS, $0.01 < p < 0.05$; OVX + E2 + IS, $0.001 < p < 0.01$). We found a significant difference between M + IS and OVX + E2 + IS groups ($p < 0.05$) in the behavior tests. Furthermore, IS increased the area covered by calcitonin gene-related peptide (CGRP) immunoreactive (IR) fibers (M + IS, $p < 0.01$; OVX + IS, $p < 0.01$; OVX + E2 + IS, $p < 0.001$) and the number of neuronal nitric oxide synthase (nNOS) IR cells (M + IS, $0.001 < p < 0.05$; OVX + IS, $0.01 < p < 0.05$; OVX + E2 + IS, $0.001 < p < 0.05$) in the caudal trigeminal nucleus (TNC). There was no difference between M + IS and OVX + IS groups; however, the area was covered by CGRP IR fibers ($0.01 < p < 0.05$) and the number of nNOS IR cells was significantly higher in the OVX + E2 + IS ($p < 0.05$) group than the other two IS- (M + IS, OVX + IS) treated animals. Overall, repeated administration of IS triggers activation and sensitization processes and develops nociceptive behavior changes. CGRP and nNOS levels increased significantly in the TNC after IS treatments, and moreover, pain thresholds and locomotor activity decreased with the development of photophobia. In our model, stable high estradiol levels proved to be pronociceptive. Thus, repeated trigeminal activation causes marked behavioral changes, which is more prominent in rats treated with estradiol, also reflected by the expression of the sensitization markers of the trigeminal system.

Citation: Spekker, E.; Bohár, Z.; Fejes-Szabó, A.; Szűcs, M.; Vécsei, L.; Párdutz, Á. Estradiol Treatment Enhances Behavioral and Molecular Changes Induced by Repetitive Trigeminal Activation in a Rat Model of Migraine. *Biomedicines* **2022**, *10*, 3175. https://doi.org/10.3390/biomedicines10123175

Academic Editor: Marc Ekker

Received: 18 October 2022
Accepted: 6 December 2022
Published: 8 December 2022

Publisher's Note: MDPI stays neutral with regard to jurisdictional claims in published maps and institutional affiliations.

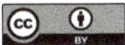

Copyright: © 2022 by the authors. Licensee MDPI, Basel, Switzerland. This article is an open access article distributed under the terms and conditions of the Creative Commons Attribution (CC BY) license (https://creativecommons.org/licenses/by/4.0/).

Keywords: primary headache; migraine; trigeminal system; CGRP; nNOS; neurogenic inflammation; animal model; inflammatory soup; dura mater; estrogen; behavior

1. Introduction

Migraine is a primary headache causing throbbing pain and neurological symptoms such as photophobia, phonophobia, cutaneous allodynia, and decreased physical activity [1]. The disease is three times more common in women than men [2], therefore, the gonadal hormones may play a role in nociceptive processing and the development of migraine attacks. In addition, the increase in the frequency of migraine attacks is one important risk factor contributing to migraine becomes chronic [3].

A widely-used rodent model of migraine is the use of inflammatory soup (IS) [4–7], which reproduces the characteristic features of clinical migraine—both the structural [8] and functional [9] changes. The administration of IS onto the dura mater of the rat can activate the trigeminal system and induces a sterile inflammation [9,10]. Furthermore, it leads to cutaneous mechanical and thermal allodynia [11,12]. Based on these the IS model can be a valuable platform for preclinical studies. However, the current migraine models mostly use single stimulation [12,13], which does not take into account the prolonged and recurrent nature of attacks, which occur usually more than once within a month. With an exception to one study [7], repeated IS application in other models are usually continuous, which does not reflect the characteristics of repeated attacks [14,15]. Therefore, using an animal model in which discontinuous multiple stimulations are carried out on the dura mater would be more in line with recurrent episodic migraine attacks and helps to understand the mechanism of trigeminal pain becoming chronic.

In addition to studying molecular variances, it is crucial to examine behavioral changes as well in this context. The symptoms of migraine, e.g., the headache, the sensitivity to light and sound, and the allodynia are aggravated by physical activity [1,16]. Some experiments suggest that the application of inflammatory mediators directly onto the dura mater elicited tactile allodynia [17,18]. Moreover, in animal models of migraine, the locomotor activity of the animals was decreased [16,19], and photo- and phono-phobia were observed [20,21].

In animals, upon activation of the trigeminal system, neuropeptides are released, such as calcitonin gene-related peptide (CGRP), which has a vital role in migraine [22]. Repetitive electrical stimulation of the dura mater can increase CGRP expression in the trigeminal system [23]. Its release from trigeminal nerve endings may mediate the inflammation, contributing to the associated pain [24]. It has been also shown that CGRP may play an important role in the development of mechanical allodynia, hyperalgesia [25], and photophobia [26].

Some studies suggest that nitric oxide (NO) has a role in the transmission of inflammation [27,28] and can implicate the development of chronic pain [29]. The production of NO is catalyzed by nitric oxide synthase (NOS), and the neuronal isoform is expressed all along the migraine pain pathway, including the dura and pia mater [30]. An association has been demonstrated between the activation of the trigeminovascular system with the production or upregulation of nNOS. of the activation of the trigeminovascular system with the production or upregulation of nNOS [30], and the inhibition of NOS attenuates inflammatory pain [31,32]. Handy and colleagues described that after intraplantar injection of carrageenan, NOS inhibitors could prevent the hyperalgesia in response to a thermal or mechanical stimulus [33].

In our experiment, we used multiple IS stimulations onto the dura mater, based on the appearance of repeated episodic migraine attacks which is defined as less than 15 headache days per month with an attack duration of 4 to 72 h [1]. For mimicking multiple attacks, the rats received twelve IS treatments on three consecutive days for four weeks.

Among the gonadal steroids, mainly estradiol can modify the clinical appearance of migraine. After puberty, migraine occurs two to three times more often in women than in men, and the underlying processes behind the gender dimorphism are not yet known. Estrogen can elicit a pronociceptive effect by activating trigeminal afferents, enhancing glutamatergic tone, and increasing the levels of brain-derived neurotrophic factor (BDNF) or nerve growth factor (NGF) [34]. Based on these, it can be assumed that estrogen plays an important role in migraine attacks, therefore, we examined the effect of chronic, stable high-serum 17β-estradiol levels on trigeminal pain and activation.

Behavioral tests were also performed to examine the pain threshold, locomotor activity, and photophobia of the animals in these models. Furthermore, CGRP and nNOS immunohistochemical stainings were carried out and evaluated based on the somatotopic organization of the trigeminal nerve, which helped to examine the effect of the chemical stimulation of dura in a more specific way.

Our aim was to investigate how repeated IS treatment on the dura mater affects the behavior of the animals and the expression of activation and sensitization markers in TNC. Moreover, we wanted test the effect of a constant high estradiol level in this context, comparing ovariectomized females treated with estradiol to untreated male rats.

2. Materials and Methods

2.1. Animals

The procedures used in our study were approved by the Committee of the Animal Research of the University of Szeged (I-74-6/2020) and the Scientific Ethics Committee for Animal Research of the Protection of Animals Advisory Board (XI./1995/2020). They followed the guidelines the Use of Animals in Research of the International Association for the Study of Pain and the directive of the European Parliament (2010/63/EU).

Twenty male and forty female Sprague-Dawley rats weighing 280–350 g were used. The animals were raised and maintained under standard laboratory conditions with tap water and regular rat chow available ad libitum on a 12-h dark,12 h-light cycle.

2.2. Brief Summary of the Experiment

At week 0, female animals were ovariectomized and capsules were placed subcutaneously. In week 1, behavioral tests were performed with the animals to obtain baseline values. The following day, a craniotomy was carried out and a cannula was inserted into the animals' skulls. The next week, before the treatments, we repeated the behavioral tests, meaning we checked whether the surgery caused any changes in the animals' behavior. The next day we started the treatments. The animals were treated with SIF or IS for 3 consecutive days a week for 4 weeks, and various behavioral tests were performed one h after the treatment. At the end of the week 5 the animals were perfused, and samples were collected. A detailed description of the solutions and methodologies can be found below.

2.3. Experimental Groups

M + SIF: male rats with SIF treatment
M + IS: male rats with IS treatment
OVX + SIF: ovariectomized female + cholesterol capsules + SIF treatment
OVX + IS: ovariectomized female + cholesterol capsules + IS treatment
OVX + E2 + SIF: ovariectomized female + a 1:1 mixture of cholesterol and 17β-estradiol capsules + SIF treatment
OVX + E2 + IS: ovariectomized female + a 1:1 mixture of cholesterol and 17β-estradiol capsules + IS treatment

2.4. Ovariectomy

Forty female Sprague Dawley rats were used. The animals were ovariectomized under isoflurane anesthesia (Tec3 Selectatec Vaporizers, Harvard Apparatus, Holliston, MA, USA). Rats were put in a plastic box as an induction chamber that received a continuous flow of anesthetic gas. During induction, the rats were monitored by observing their respiratory movements and the pink color of their skin. After 10 min in the induction chamber (using induction doses of 5% isoflurane) the rat was quickly removed, and an inhalation mask was applied to it for the maintenance of anesthesia (using 3% isoflurane) during the surgical procedure.

Before surgery, the backs of the rats were shaved with an electric clipper to remove the fur, and Cutasept was used to disinfect the skin. First, a midline dorsal skin incision was made, which was 3 cm long and located approximately halfway between the middle of the back and the base of the tail, and then 1.5 cm-long peritoneal incisions were made on both sides. After access into the peritoneal cavity, the ovarian fat pad was carefully pulled out of the incision. With the help of hemostatic tweezers, the part below the ovary was tightly fixed. Thereafter, two knots were tied under the area to be removed using sterile thread, and then the connection between the fallopian tube and the uterine horn was cut and the ovaries were removed. Afterward, the peritoneal incisions were sutured together with sterile thread. Then, the animals were randomly divided into two groups. (1) In the OVX group, the rats had two 15 mm long silastic capsules (3.18 mm outer diameter and 1.57 mm inner diameter, catalog ID: 508–008; Dow Corning, Midland, MI, USA) filled with cholesterol (15 mg, catalog ID:C8667; Sigma-Aldrich, Darmstadt, Germany) as the control. (2) In the OVX + E2 group, the animals received two 15 mm-long silastic capsules filled with a 1:1 mixture of 17β-estradiol (7.5 mg, catalog ID: 75262; Fluka, Sigma-Aldrich) and cholesterol (7.5 mg), which provide a constant elevated serum estradiol level.

The capsules were placed subcutaneously in the interscapular region, and then the peritoneal cavity and skin were closed with absorbable sutures. All the surgical instruments were sterilized in 70% ethanol. A high degree of aseptic procedure was followed during the procedure with all equipment being sterilized before. To prevent hypothermia, the animals were placed on a warmed pad (30–35 °C) and covered with paper. To relieve pain and avoid inflammation, the animals were injected subcutaneously with carprofen (5 mg/kg body weight) before surgery and 24 and 48 h after surgery. All animals had a six-day recovery period before the craniotomy (Figure 1).

2.5. Implantation of the Cannula

Both male and female animals were deeply anesthetized with an intraperitoneal injection of 4% chloral hydrate (0.4 g/kg body weight, Sigma-Aldrich). The head of the animal was fixed in a stereotaxic frame and lidocaine infiltration (4.5 mg/kg; subcutaneously) on the skull was used before the interventions. An incision was performed to expose the surface of the skull. The bone surface was then treated with 10% hydrogen peroxide to clean the wound and decrease the bleeding. The craniotomy (1 mm in diameter) was performed with an electric drill. The hole, located on the right side of the midline, 1 mm to the junction of the coronal suture and midline was drilled to expose the dura mater. To avoid burning and damage to the dura, a standard saline solution was used to decrease the temperature. After this, stainless steel cannula was made from a 21 G needle [35] and was affixed to the bone around the opening in the skull using small screws and two types of dental cements (Duracryl Plus, Adhesor Zinc Phosphate Cement, Spofa Dental, CZK, Jičín). The cannula's end opened onto the dura and was sealed with an obturator that extends just beyond the end of the cannula over the dura. This prevented scar tissue from growing over the hole. At the end of the craniotomy, the animals received subcutaneous injections of carprofen (5 mg/mL, 0.1 mL/100 g, Pfizer, New York, NY, USA) and gentamicin (0.2 mL/100 g, Pfizer), which were repeated on the next two days after surgery (24 and 48 h). All animals had a six-day recovery period before the actual dural stimulation (Figure 1).

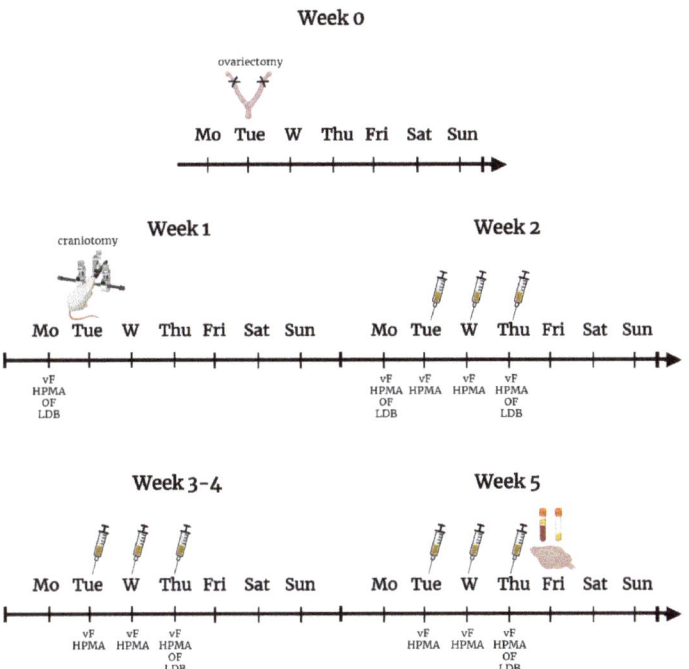

Figure 1. Schematic timeline of the experimental settings. One week before craniotomy, the female rats were overiectomized. After craniotomy, animals received twelve times SIF or IS treatment (needles). Behavioral tests were performed one day before and six days after the craniotomy and on the days when animals received treatment. After the twelfth SIF or IS treatment, the animals were transcardially perfused, and the trigemino-cervical complex was removed for immunohistochemistry. vF—von Frey test, HPMA—hind paw mechanical allodynia test, OF—open field test, LDB—light-dark box test. Created with BioRender.com.

2.6. Application of the Inflammatory Soup or Synthetic Interstitial Fluid

The animals were randomly divided into two groups. Rats were placed in a transparent plastic box, where the treatment was administered to them. The animals in the first group, called the control group, received synthetic interstitial fluid (SIF, 135 mM NaCl, 5 mM KCl, 1 mM $MgCl_2$, 5 mM $CaCl_2$, 10 mM glucose, in 10 mM HEPES buffer, pH 7.3) as treatment. In the second group, we applied inflammatory soup (IS, 1 mM bradykinin, 1 mM serotonin, 1 mM histamine, 0.1 mM prostaglandin in 10 mM HEPES buffer) on the dural surface. The solutions (10 μL) were delivered to the surface of the dura mater through a cannula made of polyethylene tube (PE10) and a 30 G needle manually, using a Hamilton syringe, over 5 min while the rat was freely moving (Figure 1). During the experiment, the animals received a total of 12 treatments (three consecutive days for 4 weeks).

Time points for repeated inflammatory soup treatment were chosen based on the headache criteria. In episodic migraine, the frequency of headache days is less than 15 days per month, and the attacks usually last from 4 to 72 h. Based on these, rats were infused with IS or SIF for three consecutive days per a week to better model the symptoms of migraine patients. With the repeated IS treatment, we mimicked multiple attacks.

2.7. Behavioral Tests

The behavioral tests were performed the day before the craniotomy and the first treatment, as well as on the treatment days one h after SIF or IS administration (Figure 1).

2.7.1. von Frey Test (vF)

The testing procedures were performed during the light phase (between 8 a.m. and 2 p.m.) in a quiet room. Three weeks before the experiment, the rats were habituated to the von Frey filament to get used to touching the area between the eyes with the fibers. The rodents were placed in a transparent plastic box, which prevented the rat from walking away from the sensory testing, but it was large enough for the animals to turn around with some difficulty. During the test, von Frey filaments, identified by manufacturer-assigned force values (Bio-VF-M von Frey Filaments, Bioseb, USA, Florida), were used to touch the area between the two eyes and observe the reaction of the animals. We touched the rats five times in a row with a filament. There was a small 2-min break between the five touches. If the animal jerked its head at least three times out of five touches, the test was positive and over for the animal. If it did not respond to that filament, we used another filament with higher strength (Figure 1).

2.7.2. Hind Paw Mechanical Allodynia Test (HPMA)

Ten minutes after the von Frey test, a hind paw mechanical allodynia test was performed. We used a dynamic plantar aesthesiometer (37450; Ugo Basile, Gemonio, Italy) to measure the touch sensitivity threshold in both hind paws. The device presses the paws of the animals with a maximum force of 50 g, rising continuously from 0 and reaches a maximum of 50 g in 8 s from touching the sole. When the animal showed a paw-withdrawal response, the value of g printed by the machine was recorded. We pressed both feet three times, and then the test was over. During the statistical analysis, we used the mean of these three measurements (Figure 1).

2.7.3. Open Field Test (OF)

An open field test can be used to measure spontaneous locomotor activity. The animals were placed in an open box from above (48 × 48 × 40 cm); then, during the 5 min of the experiment, the time spent moving or grooming and the time spent in the center of the box were detected with a video camera (Basler GigE acA1300-60 gm Ahrensburg, Germany, Ethovision XT 14 software. Noldus Information Technology, Wageningen, The Netherlands) (Figure 1).

2.7.4. Light Dark Box Test (LDB)

This test can be used to determine the anxiety response in rodents and is also suitable for studying photophobia. The animals were placed in a special box (Experimetria Ltd. Hungary, Budapest), which has a dark and a light side. The light compartment is 2/3 of the box and is brightly lit and open. The dark compartment is 1/3 of the total box and is covered and dark. A door of 7 cm connects the two compartments. At the beginning of the test, the animals were placed in the light area. After 5 s, the door opened, then they could go through the dark side. After ten minutes, the test ended, and the animals were removed from the box. The test examined anxiety and photophobia based on how much time the animals spent in the light and dark areas (Figure 1).

During IS treatments, we monitored the animals on a daily basis. We kept track of the changes by scoring the weight change, appearance, posture, ability to move, and respiration. If any given animal reached a critical score, we excluded it from the experiment.

2.8. Measurement of Estradiol Concentration

The serum 17β-estradiol concentration was measured in both groups (n = 5). At the end of the experiment, blood samples were taken from the female rats. The serum was cleared from cellular components of the blood by centrifugation at 12,000 rpm for 10 min at 4 °C and stored at −80 °C until use. An Estradiol EIA Kit (catalog ID: 582251; Cayman Chemical Company, Ann Arbor, MI, USA) was used to assay concentrations according to the guidelines of the manufacturer.

2.9. Immunohistochemistry

At the end of the experiment, the anesthetized animals (4% chloral hydrate) were trancardially perfused (50 mL PBS, 0.1 M, pH 7.4), then fixed with 200 mL 4% paraformaldehyde in phosphate buffer. Afterward, the trigemino-cervical complex was removed, post-fixed overnight in the same fixative., and then processed for CGRP and nNOS immunohistochemical staining. After cryoprotection (10% sucrose for 2 h, 20% sucrose until it sank, and 30% sucrose for 1 night) 30 μm sections were made using a cryostat and serially collected in 12 wells containing cold PBS.

Thirty serials of sections were collected into 10 wells starting from one millimeter rostrally to the obex. Every tenth section was used for staining. The free-floating sections were rinsed in PBS and immersed in 0.3% H_2O_2 in methanol or PBS for 30 min. After several rinses in PBS containing 1% Triton X-100, sections were kept overnight at room temperature in the anti-CGRP antibody (Sigma-Aldrich, Darmstadt, Germany, C8198) at a dilution of 1:20,000, or for two nights at 4 °C in the anti-nNOS antibody (EuroProxima, 2263B220-1, Arnhem, Netherlands) at a dilution of 1:5000. The immunohistochemical reaction was visualized by the avidin-biotin kit (Vectastain, Vector Laboratories, Newark, CA, USA, PK6101) and 3,3′-diaminobenzidine enhanced with nickel ammonium sulfate. The specificity of the immune reaction was controlled by omitting the primary antiserum.

2.10. Data Evaluation

All evaluations were performed by an observer blind to the procedure. The photomicrographs of the CGRP and nNOS stained sections were taken using a Zeiss AxioImager M2 microscope supplied with an AxioCam MRc Rev. 3 camera (Carl Zeiss Microscopy, New York, NY, USA) with a 10_x and 40_x objective with Zeiss Zen Pro 2.6 software. The area covered by CGRP-IR fibers was determined by Image Pro Plus 6.2® image analysis software (Media Cybernetics, USA, MD, Rockville). After image acquisition, the laminae I–II in the dorsal horn were defined manually as areas of interest, and a threshold gray level was validated with the image analysis software. The program calculated the area innervated by the IR fibers as the number of pixels with densities above the threshold; the data were expressed as area fractions (%) of the corresponding immunolabelled structures. The nNOS-IR cells were counted in laminae I-II of the dorsal horn using Nikon Optiphot-2 light microscope (Nikon, Tokyo, Japan) under 10× objective. We measured the covered area by the CGRP-IR fibers and counted the nNOS-IR cells according to the somatotopic representation of the ophthalmic (V/1) branch (Strassman and Vos, 1993).

2.11. Statistical Analysis

Prior to our experiments, we employed the PS Power and Sample Size program to determine the number of animals required. The Shapiro–Wilk test was used to determine the distribution of data. In addition, we used a Q-Q plot to find out if two sets of data come from the same distribution. Our data followed a normal distribution. For CGRP and nNOS immunohistochemistry the differences among the groups and sides were examined with a mixed ANOVA model. The effects of treatments on nNOS cell numbers and the area covered by CGRP-IR fibers at various distances from the obex between the treated and untreated sides were examined with distance, treatment, and side as repeated measures (within-subject factor) and the group as between-subject factors. RM ANOVA test was used to evaluate the results of the behavior tests followed by the Tamhane post hoc test. For the 17β-estradiol concentration of serum paired and independent samples *t*-tests performed the pairwise comparisons with Sidak corrections. All statistical analyses was carried out using SPSS version 24.0 (IBM Corporation, New York, NY, USA). Values $p < 0.05$ were considered statistically significant. Our data are reported as means + SEM for all parameters and groups.

3. Results
3.1. Estradiol Concentration

The ovariectomy kept an approximate steady-state status in serum concentration of 17β-estradiol was maintained for 6 weeks with an average value of 20.96 pg/mL in the OVX and OVX + IS group, and 54.05 pg/mL in the OVX + E2 and OVX + E2 + IS group (Figure 2A).

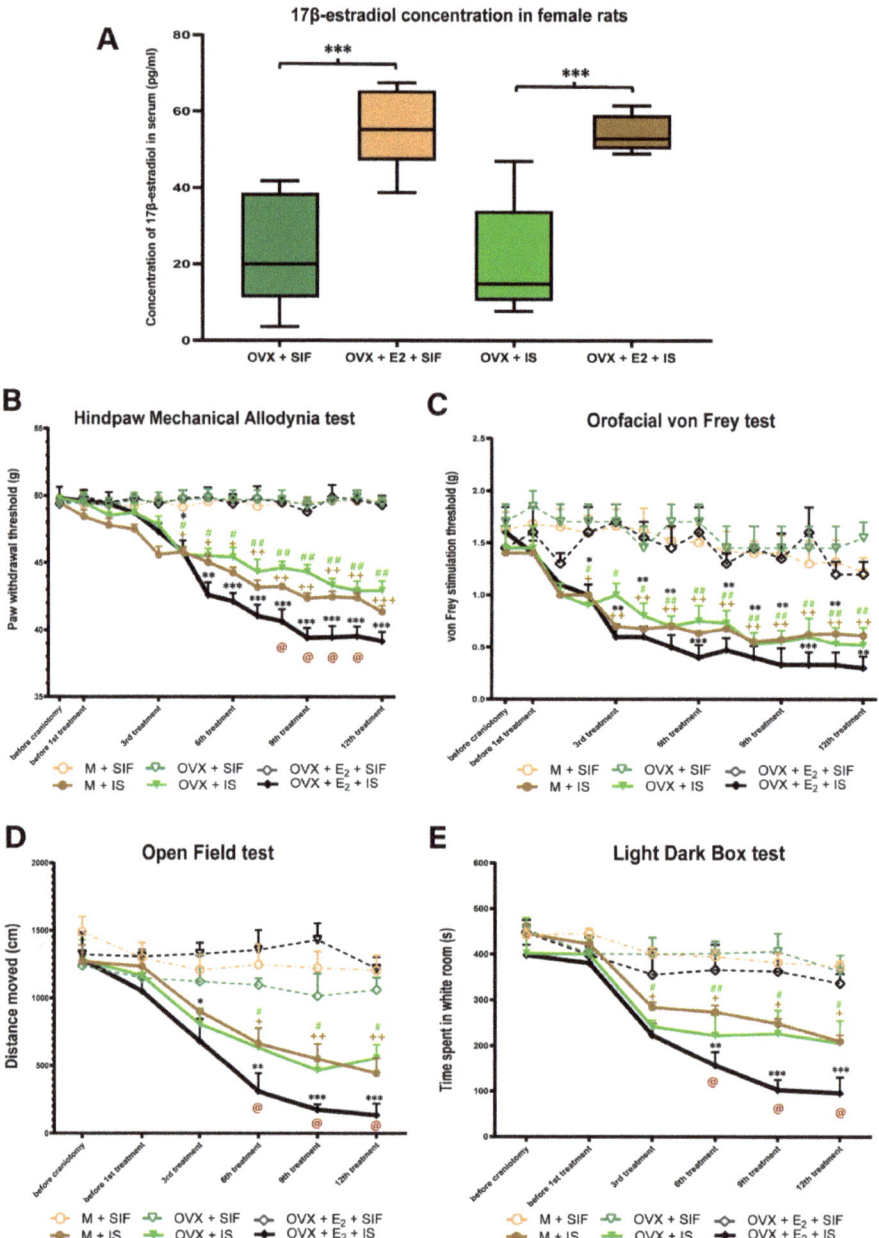

Figure 2. Statistical analysis of the serum concentration of 17-estradiol and behavior tests. (**A**) The concentration of 17β-estradiol in serum (pg/mL) in the female rats. The chronic 17β-estradiol treatment

significantly increases the serum concentration compared with the cholesterol (*** $p < 0.001$). (**B**) Hind Paw Mechanical Allodynia test. The IS treatment significantly decreased the paw withdrawal threshold. In the OVX + E2 + IS group this change was even more significant. (**C**) Orofacial von Frey test. After the second IS administration, the pain threshold was significantly lower in OVX + IS, OVX + E2 + IS and M + IS treated groups compared to the control groups. There was no difference between male and female animals. (**D**) Open Field test. The distance moved by rats was significantly less from the third treatment in the IS treated groups compared to the control groups and 17β-estradiol treatment further reduced this. (**E**) Light Dark box test. The animals in the IS treated groups spent more time in the dark room compared to the control groups. Chronic estrogen treatment reduced the time spent in the light compared to the male rats. + means M + SIF and M + IS, # means OVX + SIF and OVX + IS, and * means OVX + E2 + SIF and OVX + E2 + IS difference. @ means M + IS and OVX + E2 + IS difference. (* p in the range from 0.05 to 0.01; ** p in the range of 0.01 to 0.001; *** $p < 0.0001$).

3.2. Inflammatory Soup and Behavioral Changes

There was no difference in the paw withdrawal threshold between the groups before and after the craniotomy, but a significant decrease was detected in the pain threshold after the fourth IS treatment in the hind paw mechanical allodynia test. Chronic estrogen treatment further reduced the pain threshold compared to the male rats. There was a significant difference between the OVX + E2 + IS and M + IS groups. The OVX + IS group was similar to the M + IS group (Figure 2B).

Similar to the previous behavior tests, before IS treatment, there was no relevant difference between the control and the treated groups in the orofacial von Frey test, but after the second IS infusion, the pain threshold was significantly lower in OVX + IS, OVX + E2 + IS and M + IS treated groups compared to the control groups. There was no significant difference in male and female rats (Figure 2C).

Prior to the cannulation, no noticeable difference in locomotor activities was observed between the control and the treated groups, but the distance moved by rats was significantly decreased from the third treatment in the IS-treated groups compared to the control groups. Similar to HPMA test, in female animals given IS in addition to chronic estradiol treatment, an even greater decrease is observed in the distance traveled compared to male animals (Figure 2D).

In the light-dark box test, the animals of the IS-treated groups spent more time in the dark room compared to the control groups, but in the number of passes there was no difference between the two groups. Chronic estrogen treatment reduced the time spent in the light compared to the male rats. There was a significant difference between the OVX + E2 + IS and M + IS groups. The OVX + IS group was similar to the M + IS group (Figure 2E).

3.3. Inflammatory Soup and Calcitonin Gene-Related Peptide

After CGRP staining of the caudal trigeminal nucleus, CGRP-IR axon fibers were distributed in the laminae I and II in the dorsal horn. In the IS treated groups, the CGRP staining was stronger than in the control groups (Figure 3A). There was a significant increase in the area covered by CGRP IR fibers in the IS-treated groups in the ophthalmic nerve area. In the case of the maxillary nerve and mandibular nerve, the difference is negligible. Higher CGRP immunoreactivity was observed in female animals receiving chronic estrogen treatment and IS compared to the male IS-treated rats. No difference was observed between the OVX + IS and M + IS groups (Figure 3B).

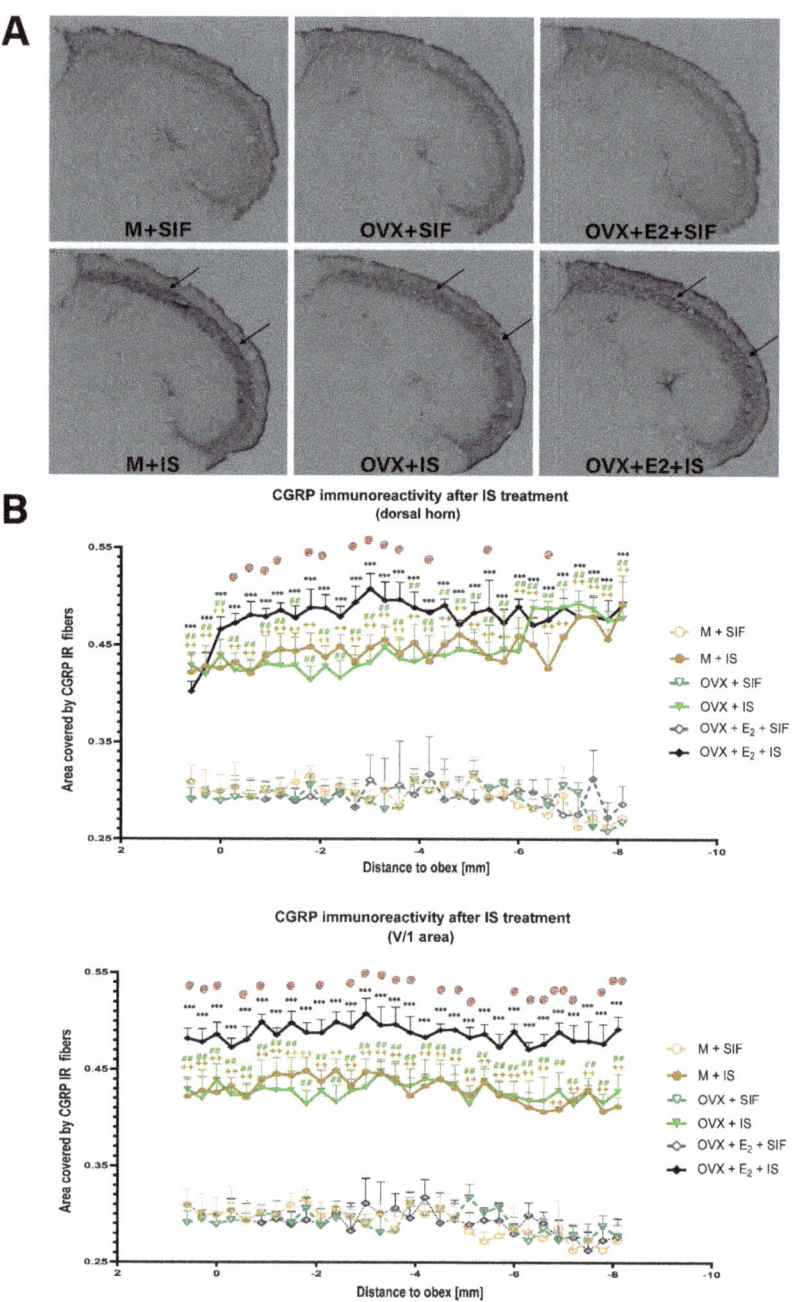

Figure 3. CGRP immunostaining. (**A**) Representative photomicrographs of the CGRP expression in the trigemino-cervical segments. In the IS treated groups, the CGRP staining was stronger compared to the control groups. (**B**) Statistical analysis of CGRP staining. In the IS-treated groups, the area covered by CGRP-IR fibers is significantly higher than in the control groups in the whole dorsal horn and in the ophthalmic nerve area. + means M + SIF and M + IS, # means OVX + SIF and OVX + IS, and * means OVX + E2 + SIF and OVX + E2 + IS difference. @ means M + IS and OVX + E2 + IS difference. (* p in the range from 0.05 to 0.01; ** p in the range of 0.01 to 0.001; *** $p < 0.0001$).

3.4. Inflammatory Soup and Neuronal Nitric Oxide Synthase

Following the nNOS immunohistochemical staining of the TNC, more nNOS-positive cells were observed in the IS-treated groups than the control groups (Figure 4A). After the statistical analysis, the repeated administration of IS was able to increase the number of nNOS IR cells in the whole dorsal horn and the somatotopic representation of the ophthalmic nerve area. This difference is not seen for the maxillary and mandibular nerves. More nNOS-positive cells were found in female animals treated with chronic estrogen and inflammatory soup than in male IS-treated animals. There was no significant difference between the OVX + IS and M + IS groups (Figure 4B).

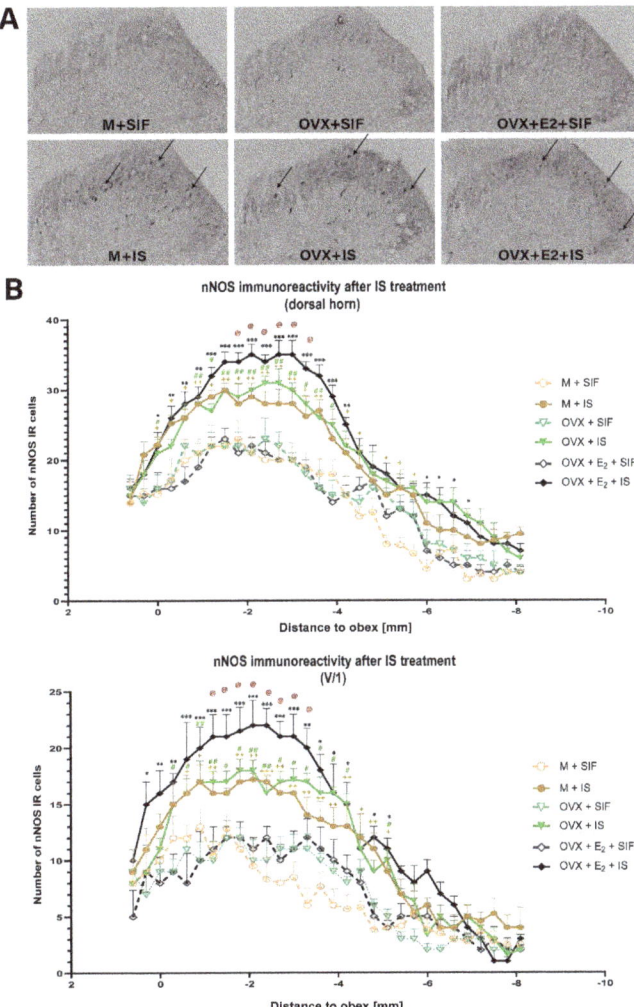

Figure 4. nNOS immunostaining. (**A**) Representative photomicrographs of the nNOS expression in the trigemino-cervical segments In the IS-treated groups, the nNOS staining was more robust than in the control groups. (**B**) Statistical analysis of nNOS staining. The quantitative analysis shows that in the IS-treated groups, the number of nNOS-IR cells was significantly higher than in the control groups in both areas. + means M + SIF and M + IS, # means OVX + SIF and OVX + IS, and * means OVX + E_2 + SIF and OVX + E_2 + IS difference. @ means M + IS and OVX + E_2 + IS difference. (* p in the range from 0.05 to 0.01; ** p in the range of 0.01 to 0.001; *** p <0.0001).

4. Discussion

Overall, in our experiment, the repeated administration of the IS was able to reduce the pain threshold and locomotor activity of the rats. In addition, the time spent in the light decreased in the group treated with IS, and the level of CGRP and nNOS increased in the TNC. Furthermore, estrogen treatment was able to further enhance the changes caused by IS, when compared to M + IS and OVX + IS groups.

The behavioral results showed that the infusion of IS leads to an increase in nociceptive responses. We found that the multiple administration of IS on the dura mater can cause a significant decrease in mechanical pain thresholds of both the face and hind paws in the orofacial von Frey test and the hind paw mechanical allodynia test (Figure 2B). Furthermore, we observed increased facial grooming and scratching behavior. These results may indicate pain and discomfort in the animals. During migraine attacks, many patients report cutaneous allodynia, which may be localized to the pain area of headache; however, the face and scalp may be affected as well as body and limbs [36]. In our experiment, throughout the orofacial von Frey, the pain threshold of the rats was significantly reduced (Figure 2C), which may suggest pain localized to the head area and cutaneous allodynia. The topical application of inflammatory soup to the dura mater could activate and sensitize Aδ and C fibers [5]. Multiple C fibers stimulations during repeated migraine attacks and the following activation of Aδ fibers lead to neurogenic inflammation in the trigeminovascular system [37]. As a result, hypersensitivity develops in the central trigeminal neurons, which results in an enhanced response to non-painful stimuli and an expansion of the receptive field [6]. Similar to the results obtained here, Edelmayer and colleagues described that allodynia induced by inflammatory mediators developed over several hours and was found not only on the face but also extrasegmentally on the hind paws [38]. Neuroinflammation leads to increased permeability of the blood–brain barrier, glial cell activation, and production of inflammatory mediators [39]. The activation of dorsal root ganglion neurons and microglia contributes to central sensitization [40]. The inflammatory processes and overexpression of CGRP nociceptive neurons are involved in the generation of pain hypersensitivity [41].

In addition to the decrease in the pain threshold, reduced locomotion was also observed in the open field test (Figure 2D), which might correspond to the reduced physical activity in patients with headaches because it increases the pain during migraine attacks. Worsening of migraine pain has often been perceived by patients during or after regular physical exercise [42]. In migraineurs, the throbbing pain can be aggravated by routine activities, therefore freezing and decreased locomotion might be a defense mechanism to limit the head and body movements of the animal. We hypothesized that animals experiencing a headache-like state would spend less time exploring the environment than those that are pain-free.

It should be noted that the decreased pain threshold and locomotor activity became more pronounced throughout the experiment. The behavioral changes we observed can be paralleled with human data, e.g., patients with a long history of more frequent and severe headaches may be more likely to develop sensitization and have allodynia. Bigal and colleagues described that cutaneous allodynia is more common and more severe in migraine than in other primary headaches and it is associated with the headache frequency, increased body mass index, disability, and depression [43]. Moreover, there is evidence of a direct and increasing correlation between allodynia and the duration of migraine [44]. Similar results were obtained by Louter and colleagues, namely, that there is an association between cutaneous allodynia and the number of migraine days [45]. This relationship may be explained by the repetitive activation of modulatory pain pathways. Another concept is that a noxious stimulus may lead to a sensitized state and chronification of pain. Due to the increasingly frequent attacks, the time between the attacks is decreasing, so the threshold may not be able to return to baseline. In addition, sensitization processes may further lower the threshold.

Furthermore, we found that in the IS treated group, the animals spent less time in the light part of the light–dark box (Figure 2E). This may also be related to the photophobia experienced in migraine sufferers. A study showed, that in rats the light is able to activate specifically dural-nociceptive posterior thalamic neurons, and this activation increases with increasing light intensity [46]. The processing of craniovascular nociceptive information in posterior lateral posterior and dorsal thalamic neurons relay directly to cortical areas, suggesting a role in cognitive and motor deficits during the migraine, as well as allodynia, photophobia, and phonophobia [47]. Vanagaite and colleagues found that migraineurs were more photophobic during the migraine attacks than outside the attacks, but even interictal migraine patients were more sensitive to light than controls [48]. In addition, Yalın et al. reported that a long duration of headache and a higher attack intensity correlate with more frequent incidences of nausea, vomiting, photophobia, and phonophobia [49].

Intracerebroventricular administration of CGRP causes a significant increase in light aversion, which can be prevented by the simultaneous administration of CGRP receptor antagonist, olcegepant [50].

In the trigeminal ganglia neurons, which transmit nociceptive signals from the head and face to the central nervous system, CGRP is expressed [51]. In migraine pathophysiology, CGRP is essential, especially in developing and maintaining chronic pain, and may be associated with allodynia and central sensitization [52]. An electrophysiological study described that CGRP, and its spinal receptors play a significant role in the generation and maintenance of the hyperexcitability of dorsal horn neurons caused by inflammation [53]. Greco et al. described that the level of CGRP was significantly higher in chronic migraine, or a medication-overuse headache compared to episodic migraine. Besides that, CGRP levels correlate with monthly migraine days [54]. Cernuda-Morollón and colleagues showed an increased CGRP serum level in chronic migraine compared to episodic migraine, thus CGRP may play a role in migraine chronification [55].

In our experiment, IS elevated the area covered by CGRP-IR fibers in the dorsal horn and ophthalmic nerve area (Figure 3).

Overall, these results suggest that CGRP may play a part at both the central and peripheral level in migraine mechanisms and promote the hypothesis that migraine patients have a combination of changed sensory perception of not harmful stimuli and altered brainstem and trigeminovascular activation.

In the central nervous system, CGRP and nNOS interact and may dilate meningeal vessels, presumably by the NO-inducing CGRP release of sensory fibers, resulting in vessel dilation [56]. In the central nervous system, NO plays a crucial role in central pain sensation and mediates neurotransmission and is involved in inflammatory response [57]. The activation of primary afferent neurons and CGRP release may induce nNOS by NO [58]. Berger and colleagues have shown that nNOS is present in nerve fibers of the dura mater in rats [59] and in the trigeminal nerve endings and in the TNC and the trigeminal ganglion [60]. Pradhan et al. described that chronic intermittent injection of NTG can cause an acute and chronic hypersensitivity that persists for days after the last exposure. These results are in line with clinical observations of patients with chronic migraine in whom allodynia may occur both between and during migraine attacks [61].

In our study, IS significantly increased the number of nNOS IR cells both in the whole dorsal horn and the somatotopic area of the ophthalmic nerve, responsible for the somatosensory innervation of the dura (Figure 4) [62]. This is in line with what has been described previously that nitroglycerin administration can increase the NOS-immunoreactivity in dura mater [63]. However, after three IS treatment, there was a significant difference between the two groups for the maxillary and mandibular branches as well. This can be explained by the fact, that NOS related NO diffuses freely across membranes rapidly and exert its activity in a more widespread way, not necessarily following the somatotopy, at least after three IS treatments. Thus, NO can activate signaling cascades both within the cell in which it was produced and by freely passing through membranes and activating nearby cells [30]. The increased nNOS expression in second-order trigeminal nociceptors might initiate a self-amplifying process of NO production at the basis of central sensitization [64]. Probably, the production of NO, via the increased expression of nNOS, mediates the production and release of CGRP and pituitary adenylyl-cyclase activating polypeptide as well [30]. Thus, nNOS can be considered a significant marker of the trigeminal system sensitization process in repeated episodic trigeminal activation.

In our experiment, chronic estradiol treatment significantly decreased the pain threshold, the locomotor activity and the time spent in the light (Figure 2). Since the results of male and OVX none treated animals are similar it seems valid to state that the key factor in this experimental setting is the presence or absence of estradiol. These findings are consistent with previous results, where estradiol exposure was able to increase allodynia [65,66] and the light aversion [20]. Similar results were obtained in other experimental models [67–69]. In the orofacial formalin model, after chronic estrogen treatment, the number of c-FOS IR cells in the TNC and the pain-related behavior of the animals increased, thus the high estrogen level had a pronociceptive effect in our experiment [70]. In another model, where inflammation was induced in the masseter muscle, a single treatment with estradiol-valerate increased facial allodynia [65,66]. In the model of temporomandibular joint inflammation, several days of estradiol treatment increased the inflammatory processes and reduced the appetite of the animals [71]. Others found that orofacial pain and thermal hyperalgesia induced by s.c. carrageenan injection were exacerbated by 17β-estradiol treatment [72]. Estrogen receptors are present in areas important for trigeminal nociception, including the trigeminal ganglion and TNC [73,74]. It is conceivable that estrogen may influence pain-induced neuronal processes through an increase in transient receptor potential vanilloid mRNA. 1 and anoctamine 1 in TNC. Furthermore, it cannot be ruled out that it exerts its effect by modulating the NF-κB pathway or by activating ERK in the trigeminal ganglion.

In addition to behavioral differences, we also observed that in the dorsal horn, the area covered by CGRP IR fibers, and the number of nNOS IR cells was significantly higher in chronic estrogen-treated animals compared to M + IS and OVX + IS groups (Figures 3 and 4).

All estrogen receptors are expressed in different parts of the trigeminovascular system, such as the rodent trigeminal ganglion [73,74] and dura mater [20]. Previous studies described that estrogen could positively enhance the expression of CGRP within the dorsal root ganglion [75–78], rat anterior pituitary [79], and medial preoptic nucleus [80]. Estrogen pretreatment increased dural mast cell density, suggesting that gonadal steroids can modify CGRP function [81].

García-Durán and colleagues reported that during ovulation the expression of nNOS protein in neutrophils was higher than in the follicular phase, suggesting that there may exist an association between the level of estrogen and nNOS expression in neutrophils [82]. Furthermore, Ceccatelli and colleagues described that in ovariectomized rats, the estradiol treatment increased the nNOS mRNA in the ventrolateral subdivision of the ventromedial nucleus in female rats [83].

Unfortunately, our experiment has some limitations. On one hand, our model can only mimic partial aspects of the migraine attacks, in this case, the neurogenic inflammation. On the other hand, we used animals with stable gonadal hormone levels to test the effect of estradiol, whereas normally, the female gonadal hormone levels are changing. Further experiments with cycling female animals are needed to better understand the gender difference.

5. Conclusions

Overall, in our experiment, multiple administrations of IS was able to activate and sensitize the trigeminal system and develop nociceptive behavior changes. Decreases in pain threshold and locomotor activity and the development of photophobia occurred in our experiment. Moreover, CGRP and nNOS levels increased significantly in the TNC due to the IS treatments. We found a difference between male and female animals, which reinforces the role of estrogen in migraine attacks. Based on these findings, our method may be suitable for modeling repeated episodic migraine.

Author Contributions: E.S., A.F.-S. and Z.B. carried out the experiments and E.S. analyzed the data. E.S. wrote the manuscript with support from Z.B., A.F.-S. and Á.P. Á.P. supervised the project. M.S. helped to select and perform statistical analysis. L.V. participated in the conception and design of the experiments and writing. All authors provided critical feedback and helped shape the research and manuscript. All authors have read and agreed to the published version of the manuscript.

Funding: This study was supported by GINOP (2.3.2-15-2016-00034), and the Ministry of Human Capacities, NKFIH-1279-2/2020 TKP 2020 programs.

Institutional Review Board Statement: The procedures used in our study were approved by the Committee of the Animal Research of University of Szeged (I-74-49/2017) and the Scientific Ethics Committee for Animal Research of the Protection of Animals Advisory Board (XI./1955/2020) and followed the guidelines the Use of Animals in Research of the International Association for the Study of Pain and the directive of the European Parliament (2010/63/EU).

Informed Consent Statement: No applicable.

Data Availability Statement: The data presented in this study are available on request from the corresponding author.

Acknowledgments: We thank Erzsébet Lukács for technical assistance. The graphical abstract and Figure 1 was created with BioRender.com.

Conflicts of Interest: The authors have no other relevant affiliations or financial involvement with any organization or entity with a financial interest in or financial conflict with the subject matter or materials discussed in the manuscript apart from those disclosed.

Abbreviations

CGRP	calcitonin gene-related peptide
E2	17β-estradiol
HPMA	hind paw mechanical allodynia test
IR	immunoreactive
IS	inflammatory soup
LDB	light-dark box test
NO	nitric oxide
NOS	nitric oxide synthase
NTG	nitroglycerin
OF	open field test
OVX	ovariectomized
PBS	phosphate-buffered saline
PBS-T	PBS containing 1% Triton-X-100
PFA	paraformaldehyde
SIF	synthetic interstitial fluid
TNC	transient receptor potential ankyrin 1
vF	von Frey test

References

1. Headache Classification Committee of the International Headache Society (IHS). The International Classification of Headache Disorders, 3rd edition (beta version). *Cephalalgia* **2013**, *33*, 629–808. [CrossRef] [PubMed]
2. Broner, S.W.; Bobker, S.; Klebanoff, L. Migraine in Women. *Semin Neurol.* **2017**, *37*, 601–610. [CrossRef] [PubMed]
3. Bigal, M.E.; Lipton, R.B. Migraine chronification. *Curr. Neurol. Neurosci. Rep.* **2011**, *11*, 139–148. [CrossRef] [PubMed]
4. Steen, K.H.; Steen, A.E.; Reeh, P.W. A dominant role of acid pH in inflammatory excitation and sensitization of nociceptors in rat skin, in vitro. *J. Neurosci.* **1995**, *15 (Pt 2)*, 3982–3989. [CrossRef]
5. Strassman, A.M.; Raymond, S.A.; Burstein, R. Sensitization of meningeal sensory neurons and the origin of headaches. *Nature* **1996**, *384*, 560–564. [CrossRef]
6. Burstein, R.; Yamamura, H.; Malick, A.; Strassman, A.M. Chemical stimulation of the intracranial dura induces enhanced responses to facial stimulation in brain stem trigeminal neurons. *J. Neurophysiol.* **1998**, *79*, 964–982. [CrossRef]
7. Oshinsky, M.L.; Gomonchareonsiri, S. Episodic dural stimulation in awake rats: A model for recurrent headache. *Headache* **2007**, *47*, 1026–1036. [CrossRef]

8. Jia, Z.; Tang, W.; Zhao, D.; Hu, G.; Li, R.; Yu, S. Volumetric abnormalities of the brain in a rat model of recurrent headache. *Mol. Pain* **2018**, *14*, 1744806918756466. [CrossRef]
9. Becerra, L.; Bishop, J.; Barmettler, G.; Kainz, V.; Burstein, R.; Borsook, D. Brain network alterations in the inflammatory soup animal model of migraine. *Brain Res.* **2017**, *1660*, 36–46. [CrossRef]
10. Spekker, E.; Laborc, K.F.; Bohár, Z.; Nagy-Grócz, G.; Fejes-Szabó, A.; Szűcs, M.; Vécsei, L.; Párdutz, Á. Effect of dural inflammatory soup application on activation and sensitization markers in the caudal trigeminal nucleus of the rat and the modulatory effects of sumatriptan and kynurenic acid. *J. Headache Pain* **2021**, *22*, 17. [CrossRef]
11. Wieseler, J.; Ellis, A.; Sprunger, D.; Brown, K.; McFadden, A.; Mahoney, J.; Rezvani, N.; Maier, S.F.; Watkins, L.R. A novel method for modeling facial allodynia associated with migraine in awake and freely moving rats. *J. Neurosci. Methods* **2010**, *185*, 236–245. [CrossRef]
12. Bishop, J.; Becerra, L.; Barmettler, G.; Chang, P.C.; Kainz, V.; Burstein, R.; Borsook, D. Modulation of brain networks by sumatriptan-naproxen in the inflammatory soup migraine model. *Pain* **2019**, *160*, 2161–2171. [CrossRef] [PubMed]
13. Lundblad, C.; Haanes, K.A.; Grände, G.; Edvinsson, L. Experimental inflammation following dural application of complete Freund's adjuvant or inflammatory soup does not alter brain and trigeminal microvascular passage. *J. Headache Pain* **2015**, *16*, 91. [CrossRef] [PubMed]
14. Han, X.; Ran, Y.; Su, M.; Liu, Y.; Tang, W.; Dong, Z.; Yu, S. Chronic changes in pituitary adenylate cyclase-activating polypeptide and related receptors in response to repeated chemical dural stimulation in rats. *Mol. Pain* **2017**, *13*, 1744806917720361. [CrossRef] [PubMed]
15. Zhang, M.; Liu, Y.; Zhao, M.; Tang, W.; Wang, X.; Dong, Z.; Yu, S. Depression and anxiety behaviour in a rat model of chronic migraine. *J. Headache Pain* **2017**, *18*, 27. [CrossRef] [PubMed]
16. Amin, F.M.; Aristeidou, S.; Baraldi, C.; Czapinska-Ciepiela, E.K.; Ariadni, D.D.; Di Lenola, D.; Fenech, C.; Kampouris, K.; Karagiorgis, G.; Braschinsky, M.; et al. European Headache Federation School of Advanced Studies (EHF-SAS). The association between migraine and physical exercise. *J. Headache Pain* **2018**, *19*, 83. [CrossRef] [PubMed]
17. Stucky, N.L.; Gregory, E.; Winter, M.K.; He, Y.Y.; Hamilton, E.S.; McCarson, K.E.; Berman, N.E. Sex differences in behavior and expression of CGRP-related genes in a rodent model of chronic migraine. *Headache* **2011**, *51*, 674–692. [CrossRef]
18. Yan, J.; Melemedjian, O.K.; Price, T.J.; Dussor, G. Sensitization of dural afferents underlies migraine-related behavior following meningeal application of interleukin-6 (IL-6). *Mol. Pain* **2012**, *8*, 6. [CrossRef]
19. Melo-Carrillo, A.; Lopez-Avila, A. A chronic animal model of migraine, induced by repeated meningeal nociception, characterized by a behavioral and pharmacological approach. *Cephalalgia* **2013**, *33*, 1096–1105. [CrossRef]
20. Vermeer, L.M.; Gregory, E.; Winter, M.K.; McCarson, K.E.; Berman, N.E. Behavioral effects and mechanisms of migraine pathogenesis following estradiol exposure in a multibehavioral model of migraine in rat. *Exp. Neurol.* **2015**, *263*, 8–16. [CrossRef]
21. Farajdokht, F.; Babri, S.; Karimi, P.; Alipour, M.R.; Bughchechi, R.; Mohaddes, G. Chronic ghrelin treatment reduced photophobia and anxiety-like behaviors in nitroglycerin- induced migraine: Role of pituitary adenylate cyclase-activating polypeptide. *Eur. J. Neurosci.* **2017**, *45*, 763–772. [CrossRef] [PubMed]
22. van Rossum, D.; Hanisch, U.K.; Quirion, R. Neuroanatomical localization, pharmacological characterization and functions of CGRP, related peptides and their receptors. *Neurosci. Biobehav. Rev.* **1997**, *21*, 649–678. [CrossRef] [PubMed]
23. Körtési, T.; Tuka, B.; Nyári, A.; Vécsei, L.; Tajti, J. The effect of orofacial complete Freund's adjuvant treatment on the expression of migraine-related molecules. *J. Headache Pain* **2019**, *20*, 43. [CrossRef]
24. Brain, S.D. Sensory neuropeptides: Their role in inflammation and wound healing. *Immunopharmacology* **1997**, *37*, 133–152. [CrossRef] [PubMed]
25. Sun, R.Q.; Lawand, N.B.; Willis, W.D. The role of calcitonin gene-related peptide (CGRP) in the generation and maintenance of mechanical allodynia and hyperalgesia in rats after intradermal injection of capsaicin. *Pain* **2003**, *104*, 201–208. [CrossRef]
26. Noseda, R.; Burstein, R. Advances in understanding the mechanisms of migraine-type photophobia. *Curr. Opin. Neurol.* **2011**, *24*, 197–202. [CrossRef]
27. Guzik, T.J.; Korbut, R.; Adamek-Guzik, T. Nitric oxide and superoxide in inflammation and immune regulation. *J. Physiol. Pharmacol.* **2003**, *54*, 469–487.
28. Laroux, F.S.; Lefer, D.J.; Kawachi, S.; Scalia, R.; Cockrell, A.S.; Gray, L.; Van der Heyde, H.; Hoffman, J.M.; Grisham, M.B. Role of nitric oxide in the regulation of acute and chronic inflammation. *Antioxid. Redox Signal.* **2000**, *2*, 391–396. [CrossRef]
29. Célérier, E.; González, J.R.; Maldonado, R.; Cabañero, D.; Puig, M.M. Opioid-induced hyperalgesia in a murine model of postoperative pain: Role of nitric oxide generated from the inducible nitric oxide synthase. *Anesthesiology* **2006**, *104*, 546–555. [CrossRef]
30. Pradhan, A.A.; Bertels, Z.; Akerman, S. Targeted Nitric Oxide Synthase Inhibitors for Migraine. *Neurotherapeutics* **2018**, *15*, 391–401. [CrossRef]
31. Osborne, M.G.; Coderre, T.J. Effects of intrathecal administration of nitric oxide synthase inhibitors on carrageenan-induced thermal hyperalgesia. *Br. J. Pharmacol.* **1999**, *126*, 1840–1846. [CrossRef]
32. De Alba, J.; Clayton, N.M.; Collins, S.D.; Colthup, P.; Chessell, I.; Knowles, R.G. GW274150, a novel and highly selective inhibitor of the inducible isoform of nitric oxide synthase (iNOS), shows analgesic effects in rat models of inflammatory and neuropathic pain. *Pain* **2006**, *120*, 170–181. [CrossRef] [PubMed]

33. Handy, R.L.; Moore, P.K. Effects of selective inhibitors of neuronal nitric oxide synthase on carrageenan-induced mechanical and thermal hyperalgesia. *Neuropharmacology* **1998**, *37*, 37–43. [CrossRef] [PubMed]
34. Martin, V.T. New theories in the pathogenesis of menstrual migraine. *Curr. Pain Headache Rep.* **2008**, *12*, 453–462. [CrossRef] [PubMed]
35. Kokare, D.M.; Shelkar, G.P.; Borkar, C.D.; Nakhate, K.T.; Subhedar, N.K. A simple and inexpensive method to fabricate a cannula system for intracranial injections in rats and mice. *J. Pharmacol. Toxicol. Methods* **2011**, *64*, 246–250. [CrossRef]
36. Filiz, A.; Tepe, N.; Eftekhari, S.; Boran, H.E.; Dilekoz, E.; Edvinsson, L.; Bolay, H. CGRP receptor antagonist MK-8825 attenuates cortical spreading depression induced pain behavior. *Cephalalgia* **2019**, *39*, 354–365. [CrossRef]
37. Ulrich-Lai, Y.M.; Flores, C.M.; Harding-Rose, C.A.; Goodis, H.E.; Hargreaves, K.M. Capsaicin-evoked release of immunoreactive calcitonin gene-related peptide from rat trigeminal ganglion: Evidence for intraganglionic neurotransmission. *Pain* **2001**, *91*, 219–226. [CrossRef]
38. Edelmayer, R.M.; Vanderah, T.W.; Majuta, L.; Zhang, E.-T.; Bs, B.F.; De Felice, M.; Chichorro, J.; Ossipov, M.H.; King, T.; Lai, J.; et al. Medullary pain facilitating neurons mediate allodynia in headache-related pain. *Ann. Neurol.* **2009**, *65*, 184–193. [CrossRef]
39. Ji, R.R.; Xu, Z.Z.; Gao, Y.J. Emerging targets in neuroinflammation-driven chronic pain. *Nat. Rev. Drug Discov.* **2014**, *13*, 533–548. [CrossRef]
40. Kobayashi, K.; Yamanaka, H.; Fukuoka, T.; Dai, Y.; Obata, K.; Noguchi, K. P2Y12 receptor upregulation in activated microglia is a gateway of p38 signaling and neuropathic pain. *J. Neurosci.* **2008**, *28*, 2892–2902. [CrossRef]
41. Kristiansen, K.A.; Edvinsson, L. Neurogenic inflammation: A study of rat trigeminal ganglion. *J. Headache Pain* **2010**, *11*, 485–495. [CrossRef] [PubMed]
42. Farris, S.G.; Thomas, J.G.; Abrantes, A.M.; Lipton, R.B.; Pavlovic, J.; Smitherman, T.A.; Irby, M.B.; Penzien, D.B.; Roth, J.; O'Leary, K.C.; et al. Pain worsening with physical activity during migraine attacks in women with overweight/obesity: A prospective evaluation of frequency, consistency, and correlates. *Cephalalgia* **2018**, *38*, 1707–1715. [CrossRef] [PubMed]
43. Bigal, M.E.; Ashina, S.; Burstein, R.; Reed, M.L.; Buse, D.; Serrano, D.; Lipton, R.B.; AMPP Group. Prevalence and characteristics of allodynia in headache sufferers: A population study. *Neurology* **2008**, *70*, 1525–1533. [CrossRef] [PubMed]
44. Lipton, R.B.; Bigal, M.E.; Ashina, S.; Burstein, R.; Silberstein, S.; Reed, M.L.; Serrano, D.; Stewart, W.F.; American Migraine Prevalence Prevention Advisory Group. Cutaneous allodynia in the migraine population. *Ann. Neurol.* **2008**, *63*, 148–158. [CrossRef] [PubMed]
45. Louter, M.A.; Bosker, J.E.; van Oosterhout, W.P.; van Zwet, E.W.; Zitman, F.G.; Ferrari, M.D.; Terwindt, G.M. Cutaneous allodynia as a predictor of migraine chronification. *Brain* **2013**, *136 Pt 11*, 3489–3496. [CrossRef]
46. Scher, A.I.; Stewart, W.F.; Ricci, J.A.; Lipton, R.B. Factors associated with the onset and remission of chronic daily headache in a population-based study. *Pain* **2003**, *106*, 81–89. [CrossRef]
47. Burstein, R.; Jakubowski, M.; Garcia-Nicas, E.; Kainz, V.; Bajwa, Z.; Hargreaves, R.; Becerra, L.; Borsook, D. Thalamic sensitization transforms localized pain into widespread allodynia. *Ann. Neurol.* **2010**, *68*, 81–91. [CrossRef]
48. Vanagaite, J.; Pareja, J.A.; Støren, O.; White, L.R.; Sand, T.; Stovner, L.J. Light-induced discomfort and pain in migraine. *Cephalalgia* **1997**, *17*, 733–741. [CrossRef]
49. Yalın, O.Ö.; Uluduz, D.; Özge, A.; Sungur, M.A.; Selekler, M.; Siva, A. Phenotypic features of chronic migraine. *J. Headache Pain* **2016**, *17*, 26. [CrossRef]
50. Russo, A.F.; Kuburas, A.; Kaiser, E.A.; Raddant, A.C.; Recober, A. A Potential Preclinical Migraine Model: CGRP-Sensitized Mice. *Mol. Cell. Pharmacol.* **2009**, *1*, 264–270.
51. Seybold, V.S. The role of peptides in central sensitization. *Handb. Exp. Pharmacol.* **2009**, *194*, 451–491. [CrossRef]
52. Boyer, N.; Dallel, R.; Artola, A.; Monconduit, L. General trigeminospinal central sensitization and impaired descending pain inhibitory controls contribute to migraine progression. *Pain* **2014**, *155*, 1196–1205. [CrossRef] [PubMed]
53. Neugebauer, V.; Rümenapp, P.; Schaible, H.G. Calcitonin gene-related peptide is involved in the spinal processing of mechanosensory input from the rat's knee joint and in the generation and maintenance of hyperexcitability of dorsal horn-neurons during development of acute inflammation. *Neuroscience* **1996**, *71*, 1095–1109. [CrossRef] [PubMed]
54. Greco, R.; De Icco, R.; Demartini, C.; Zanaboni, A.M.; Tumelero, E.; Sances, G.; Allena, M.; Tassorelli, C. Plasma levels of CGRP and expression of specific microRNAs in blood cells of episodic and chronic migraine subjects: Towards the identification of a panel of peripheral biomarkers of migraine? *J. Headache Pain* **2020**, *21*, 122. [CrossRef] [PubMed]
55. Cernuda-Morollón, E.; Larrosa, D.; Ramón, C.; Vega, J.; Martínez-Camblor, P.; Pascual, J. Interictal increase of CGRP levels in peripheral blood as a biomarker for chronic migraine. *Neurology* **2013**, *81*, 1191–1196. [CrossRef]
56. Iyengar, S.; Ossipov, M.H.; Johnson, K.W. The role of calcitonin gene-related peptide in peripheral and central pain mechanisms including migraine. *Pain* **2017**, *158*, 543–559. [CrossRef]
57. Neeb, L.; Reuter, U. Nitric oxide in migraine. *CNS Neurol. Disord. Drug Targets* **2007**, *6*, 258–264. [CrossRef]
58. Capuano, A.; De Corato, A.; Lisi, L.; Tringali, G.; Navarra, P.; Dello Russo, C. Proinflammatory-activated trigeminal satellite cells promote neuronal sensitization: Relevance for migraine pathology. *Mol. Pain* **2009**, *5*, 43. [CrossRef]
59. Berger, R.J.; Zuccarello, M.; Keller, J.T. Nitric oxide synthase immunoreactivity in the rat dura mater. *Neuroreport* **1994**, *5*, 519–521. [CrossRef]
60. Ramachandran, R.; Ploug, K.B.; Hay-Schmidt, A.; Olesen, J.; Jansen-Olesen, I.; Gupta, S. Nitric oxide synthase (NOS) in the trigeminal vascular system and other brain structures related to pain in rats. *Neurosci. Lett.* **2010**, *484*, 192–196. [CrossRef]

61. Pradhan, A.A.; Smith, M.L.; McGuire, B.; Tarash, I.; Evans, C.J.; Charles, A. Characterization of a novel model of chronic migraine. *Pain* 2014, *155*, 269–274. [CrossRef] [PubMed]
62. Penfield, W.; McNaughton, F.L. Dural headache and innervation of the dura mater. *Arch. Neurol. Psychiatry* 1940, *44*, 43–75. [CrossRef]
63. Knyihár-Csillik, E.; Vécsei, L. Effect of a nitric oxide donor on nitroxergic nerve fibers in the rat dura mater. *Neurosci. Lett.* 1999, *260*, 97–100. [CrossRef] [PubMed]
64. Pardutz, A.; Krizbai, I.; Multon, S.; Vecsei, L.; Schoenen, J. Systemic nitroglycerin increases nNOS levels in rat trigeminal nucleus caudalis. *Neuroreport* 2000, *11*, 3071–3075. [CrossRef]
65. Liverman, C.S.; Brown, J.W.; Sandhir, R.; Klein, R.M.; McCarson, K.; Berman, N.E. Oestrogen increases nociception through ERK activation in the trigeminal ganglion: Evidence for a peripheral mechanism of allodynia. *Cephalalgia* 2009, *29*, 520–531. [CrossRef] [PubMed]
66. Liverman, C.S.; Brown, J.W.; Sandhir, R.; McCarson, K.E.; Berman, N.E. Role of the oestrogen receptors GPR30 and ERalpha in peripheral sensitization: Relevance to trigeminal pain disorders in women. *Cephalalgia* 2009, *29*, 729–741. [CrossRef] [PubMed]
67. Bereiter, D.A. Sex differences in brainstem neural activation after injury to the TMJ region. *Cells Tissues Organs* 2001, *169*, 226–237. [CrossRef]
68. Bereiter, D.A.; Cioffi, J.L.; Bereiter, D.F. Oestrogen receptor-immunoreactive neurons in the trigeminal sensory system of male and cycling female rats. *Arch. Oral Biol.* 2005, *50*, 971–979. [CrossRef]
69. Allen, A.L.; McCarson, K.E. Estrogen increases nociception-evoked brain-derived neurotrophic factor gene expression in the female rat. *Neuroendocrinology* 2005, *81*, 193–199. [CrossRef] [PubMed]
70. Fejes-Szabó, A.; Spekker, E.; Tar, L.; Nagy-Grócz, G.; Bohár, Z.; Laborc, K.F.; Vécsei, L.; Párdutz, Á. Chronic 17β-estradiol pretreatment has pronociceptive effect on behavioral and morphological changes induced by orofacial formalin in ovariectomized rats. *J. Pain Res.* 2018, *11*, 2011–2021. [CrossRef]
71. Kou, X.X.; Wu, Y.W.; Ding, Y.; Hao, T.; Bi, R.Y.; Gan, Y.H.; Ma, X. 17β-estradiol aggravates temporomandibular joint inflammation through the NF-κB pathway in ovariectomized rats. *Arthritis Rheum.* 2011, *63*, 1888–1897. [CrossRef] [PubMed]
72. Nag, S.; Mokha, S.S. Activation of the trigeminal α2-adrenoceptor produces sex-specific, estrogen dependent thermal antinociception and antihyperalgesia using an operant pain assay in the rat. *Behav. Brain Res.* 2016, *314*, 152–158. [CrossRef]
73. Puri, V.; Cui, L.; Liverman, C.S.; Roby, K.F.; Klein, R.M.; Welch, K.M.A.; Berman, N.E. Ovarian steroids regulate neuropeptides in the trigeminal ganglion. *Neuropeptides* 2005, *39*, 409–417. [CrossRef] [PubMed]
74. Aggarwal, M.; Puri, V.; Puri, S. Effects of estrogen on the serotonergic system and calcitonin gene-related peptide in trigeminal ganglia of rats. *Ann. Neurosci.* 2012, *19*, 151–157. [CrossRef] [PubMed]
75. Vermeer, L.M.; Gregory, E.; Winter, M.K.; McCarson, K.E.; Berman, N.E. Exposure to bisphenol A exacerbates migraine-like behaviors in a multibehavior model of rat migraine. *Toxicol. Sci.* 2014, *137*, 416–427. [CrossRef]
76. Gangula, P.R.; Lanlua, P.; Wimalawansa, S.; Supowit, S.; DiPette, D.; Yallampalli, C. Regulation of calcitonin gene-related peptide expression in dorsal root ganglia of rats by female sex steroid hormones. *Biol. Reprod.* 2000, *62*, 1033–1039. [CrossRef]
77. Mowa, C.N.; Usip, S.; Collins, J.; Storey-Workley, M.; Hargreaves, K.M.; Papka, R.E. The effects of pregnancy and estrogen on the expression of calcitonin gene-related peptide (CGRP) in the uterine cervix, dorsal root ganglia and spinal cord. *Peptides* 2003, *24*, 1163–1174. [CrossRef]
78. Sarajari, S.; Oblinger, M.M. Estrogen effects on pain sensitivity and neuropeptide expression in rat sensory neurons. *Exp. Neurol.* 2010, *224*, 163–169. [CrossRef]
79. Gon, G.; Giaid, A.; Steel, J.H.; O'Halloran, D.J.; Van Noorden, S.; Ghatei, M.A.; Jones, P.M.; Amara, S.G.; Ishikawa, H.; Bloom, S.R. Localization of immunoreactivity for calcitonin gene-related peptide in the rat anterior pituitary during ontogeny and gonadal steroid manipulations and detection of its messenger ribonucleic acid. *Endocrinology* 1990, *127*, 2618–2629. [CrossRef]
80. Yuri, K.; Kawata, M. Estrogen affects calcitonin gene-related peptide- and methionine-enkephalin-immunoreactive neuron in the female rat preoptic area. *Neurosci. Lett.* 1994, *169*, 5–8. [CrossRef]
81. Labastida-Ramírez, A.; Rubio-Beltrán, E.; Villalón, C.M.; MaassenVanDenBrink, A. Gender aspects of CGRP in migraine. *Cephalalgia* 2019, *39*, 435–444. [CrossRef] [PubMed]
82. García-Durán, M.; de Frutos, T.; Díaz-Recasens, J.; García-Gálvez, G.; Jiménez, A.; Montón, M.; Farré, J.; Sánchez de Miguel, L.; González-Fernández, F.; Arriero, M.D.; et al. Estrogen stimulates neuronal nitric oxide synthase protein expression in human neutrophils. *Circ. Res.* 1999, *85*, 1020–1026. [CrossRef] [PubMed]
83. Ceccatelli, S.; Grandison, L.; Scott, R.E.; Pfaff, D.W.; Kow, L.M. Estradiol regulation of nitric oxide synthase mRNAs in rat hypothalamus. *Neuroendocrinology* 1996, *64*, 357–363. [CrossRef] [PubMed]

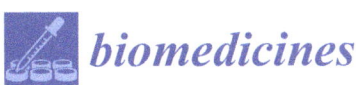

Article

A Biosafety Study of Human Umbilical Cord Blood Mononuclear Cells Transduced with Adenoviral Vector Carrying Human Vascular Endothelial Growth Factor cDNA In Vitro

Ilnur I. Salafutdinov [1,2,*], Dilara Z. Gatina [2], Maria I. Markelova [2], Ekaterina E. Garanina [2], Sergey Yu. Malanin [2], Ilnaz M. Gazizov [1], Andrei A. Izmailov [1], Albert A. Rizvanov [2], Rustem R. Islamov [1], András Palotás [2,3,4] and Zufar Z. Safiullov [1]

1. Department of Histology, Cytology and Embryology, Kazan State Medical University, Kazan 420012, Russia; ilnazaziz@mail.ru (I.M.G.); gostev.andrei@gmail.com (A.A.I.); rustem.islamov@gmail.com (R.R.I.); redblackwhite@mail.ru (Z.Z.S.)
2. Institute of Fundamental Medicine and Biology, Kazan Federal University, Kazan 420008, Russia; ekaterinaakagaranina@gmail.com (E.E.G.); sergen83@mail.ru (S.Y.M.); rizvanov@gmail.com (A.A.R.); palotas@asklepios-med.eu (A.P.)
3. Asklepios-Med (Private Medical Practice and Research Center), H-6722 Szeged, Hungary
4. Tokaj-Hegyalja University, H-3910 Tokaj, Hungary
* Correspondence: sal.ilnur@gmail.com

Abstract: The biosafety of gene therapy remains a crucial issue for both the direct and cell-mediated delivery of recombinant cDNA encoding biologically active molecules for the pathogenetic correction of congenital or acquired disorders. The diversity of vector systems and cell carriers for the delivery of therapeutic genes revealed the difficulty of developing and implementing a safe and effective drug containing artificial genetic material for the treatment of human diseases in practical medicine. Therefore, in this study we assessed changes in the transcriptome and secretome of umbilical cord blood mononuclear cells (UCB-MCs) genetically modified using adenoviral vector (Ad5) carrying cDNA encoding human vascular endothelial growth factor (VEGF165) or reporter green fluorescent protein (GFP). A preliminary analysis of UCB-MCs transduced with Ad5-VEGF165 and Ad5-GFP with MOI of 10 showed efficient transgene expression in gene-modified UCB-MCs at mRNA and protein levels. The whole transcriptome sequencing of native UCB-MCs, UCB-MC+Ad5-VEGF165, and UCB-MC+Ad5-GFP demonstrated individual sample variability rather than the effect of Ad5 or the expression of recombinant *vegf165* on UCB-MC transcriptomes. A multiplex secretome analysis indicated that neither the transduction of UCB-MCs with Ad5-GFP nor with Ad5-VEGF165 affects the secretion of the studied cytokines, chemokines, and growth factors by gene-modified cells. Here, we show that UCB-MCs transduced with Ad5 carrying cDNA encoding human VEGF165 efficiently express transgenes and preserve transcriptome and secretome patterns. This data demonstrates the biosafety of using UCB-MCs as cell carriers of therapeutic genes.

Keywords: cord blood stem cell transplantation; genetic vectors; vascular endothelial growth factor A; transcriptome; secretome; biosafety; genetic therapy

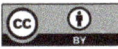

1. Introduction

Gene therapy is an actively developing area in practical medicine not only for the correction of inherited diseases [1,2], but also in regenerative medicine to activate endogenous tissue potential [3]. In vivo or direct gene therapy is based on the delivery of therapeutic genes with plasmid or viral vectors, which is predominantly systemic in nature and involves the transduction of different cells in a variety of body organs [2]. Ex vivo or cell-mediated gene therapy for the delivery of transgenes employs stem or mature cells of autogenous or allogenic origin [4]. Ex vivo gene therapy excludes the direct effect of vector antigens with a host immune system and provides temporary or permanent expression of transgenes by genetically modified cells. The rationale for the use of a particular gene therapy depends on the pathogenetic aspects of the disease [5]. However, the biosafety of direct and cell-mediated gene delivery strategies remains a critical issue in translating gene therapy potentiality from preclinical studies to clinical trials. The side effects of vector systems on the recipient organism mainly pertain to immunogenicity and mutagenicity [6], whereas little is known about the effects of transgene expression on transduced cells.

Advances in gene therapy are opening up new perspectives in the treatment of central nervous system (CNS) diseases. The natural limits of CNS regeneration pose major problems for the treatment of neurological disorders of various aetiologies [7]. The delivery of therapeutic genes encoding neurotrophic factors to the brain and spinal cord of patients with neurodegenerative diseases, traumatic injuries, or ischaemic stroke is a prospective approach to increase neuronal survival in the acute phase, as well as to stimulate directed axonal growth, remyelination, and the recovery of lost interneuronal connections in the rehabilitation period [8]. However, in clinical practice worldwide, there are no effective neuroregenerative therapies available for these patients, and symptomatic treatment has no effect on quality of life or life expectancy [9,10].

Cell-mediated gene therapy is effectively used to treat hereditary diseases. Severe combined immunodeficiency was the first hereditary disease for which the use of recombinant cDNA encoding a protein capable of restoring lost lymphocyte function was proposed for treatment. This treatment was proposed in 1990 [11]. To deliver the therapeutic gene to mature lymphocytes, hematopoietic stem cells (HSCs) are isolated from the patient's bone marrow, transduced ex vivo using a gamma retroviral vector carrying cDNA of the enzyme adenosine deaminase, and returned to the patient's blood. As a result, all HSC progeny, including lymphocytes, carry transgenes encoding the normal enzyme. A similar method has been proposed for the treatment of X-linked adrenoleukodystrophy caused by an *ABCD1* gene mutation (adenosine-triphosphate-binding cassette transporter). After the transplantation of autologous HSCs, where the mutant gene has been corrected using a lentiviral vector, the patient regained phagocyte function, including the restoration of microglia cell function, which enables normal fatty acid metabolism in the CNS [12].

In practical medicine, allogeneic HSC transplantation is the most widely used approach for the treatment of malignant and benign diseases of the hematopoietic system in clinical care [13,14]. For cell therapy, HSCs are derived from umbilical cord blood, peripheral blood, and bone marrow [15]. Umbilical cord blood mononuclear fraction contains HSCs, progenitor endothelial cells [16], multipotent mesenchymal stromal cells [17], and other even less differentiated stem cells with pluripotent properties [18–20], which gives reason to consider them as a potential source for cell therapy (in autografting and allografting) for ischemic, traumatic, and degenerative diseases [21–23]. In addition, UCB-MCs produce antioxidant, angiogenic, and neurotrophic factors, which can also have a stimulating effect on the regeneration of the target organ [24–27].

Currently, umbilical cord blood mononuclear cells (UCB-MCs) are being actively tested in the treatment of CNS disorders. It is important to note that UCB-MCs may be used for transplantation without HLA matching and immunosuppression therapy. The UCB-MC population mostly consists of immature T-cells with a higher CD4+/CD8+ T-cell ratio [28]. The biosafety of the allogenic transplantation of UCB-MCs was demonstrated in the treatment of patients with non-hematopoietic degenerative conditions [21]. The beneficial effects of UCB-MCs were shown in the aged brain [29] and in the treatment of Parkinson's disease [30], amyotrophic lateral sclerosis (ALS) [31–33], ischemic stroke [34,35], and neurotrauma [36,37]. The limited number of available cells from a single donor remains a serious problem when using UCB-MCs in clinical practice. Hence, genetic modification of UCB-MCs can increase their therapeutic potential, enabling their use in targeted pathogenetic therapy. Genetically engineered UCB-MCs can migrate to the site of degeneration and enable the local and temporary production of recombinant therapeutic molecules. In earlier studies, we demonstrated the positive effect of gene-modified UCB-MCs producing recombinant vascular endothelial growth factor (VEGF) on the symptomatic outcome and life-span of transgenic ALS mice [38].

The link between ALS and VEGF, which is involved in the survival of motor neurons, has been shown in in vitro and in vivo experiments [39]. The important role of VEGF in embryogenesis as an angiogenic and neurogenic factor suggests the potential use of recombinant VEGF to modulate neuroplasticity in various CNS diseases [40]. The VEGF family includes VEGF-A (previously simply known as VEGF), VEGF-B, VEGF-C, VEGF-D, VEGF-E, and placental growth factor (PlGF) [41]. As a result of alternative splicing of the gene encoding VEGF-A, molecules consisting of 121, 145, 165, 189, or 206 amino acids are synthesized. Mostly soluble VEGF121 (diffusing over long distances) and VEGF165 (reaching distant and nearby targets) are the focus of current intensive research [42]. Preclinical studies have demonstrated the beneficial effects of VEGF in the treatment of neurological disorders [40]. The neuroprotective effect of VEGF on the brain was shown in ischemic stroke [43,44], traumatic brain injuries [45–47], spinal cord injuries [48,49], and neurodegenerative diseases [42,50,51].

Thus, ex vivo gene modification of UCB-MCs allows us to enhance their native neuroprotective properties. In addition, this approach can be useful to obtain UCB-MCs with the therapeutic effects required for the treatment of human diseases based on the temporal synthesis and secretion of specific bioactive therapeutic molecules responsible for the correction of a particular pathological disorder. We have recently demonstrated the positive effect of UCB-MCs transduced with Ad5-LTF carrying the human lactoferrin gene on the recovery of maxillofacial phlegmon in rats [52] and the induction of angiogenesis by UCB-MCs transduced with Ad5-VEGF165 applied in an in vivo Matrigel plug assay [53]. However, the biosafety of UCB-MC transduction using an adenoviral vector and transgene overexpression on the native functional characteristics of UCB-MCs remains unclear. Therefore, in this study we assessed the transcriptome landscape and cytokine profiling of genetically modified human UCB-MCs transduced with an adenoviral vector (Ad5) carrying a cDNA encoding human VEGF165.

2. Materials and Methods

2.1. Study Design

In continuing research to develop an effective gene therapy approach to stimulate regeneration in the CNS, we have demonstrated the positive effect of genetically modified UCB-MCs in transgenic ALS mice [38] and in rats with spinal cord injuries [54] and stroke [55]. Following these reports, we expanded this study to estimate the biosafety of UCB-MCs transduced with Ad5-VEGF165 in vitro. In a preliminary independent experiment using cord blood samples ($n = 3$) we assessed the efficacy of UCB-MC transduction with Ad5-VEGF165 and Ad5-GFP at MOI = 10. The synthesis of mRNA transgenes and recombinant proteins (VEGF and GFP) was confirmed by RT-PCR, Western blot, ELISA, flow cytometry, and fluorescence microscopy. The main goal of this study was to assess the impact of an adenoviral vector (Ad5) and a transgene (*vegf165*) on the transcription and secretion patterns of genetically modified UCB-MCs derived from six cord blood samples using RNA-seq and a multiplex assay, respectively.

2.2. Preparation of Umbilical Cord Blood Mononuclear Cells

Umbilical cord blood was collected after informed consent had been obtained from the pregnant women, and prenatal testing to determine their eligibility for blood donation was carried out. The cord blood was collected in containers with citrate, phosphate, dextrose, and adenine (CDFA-1) (Baxter International Inc., Deerfield, IL, USA) in accordance with the protocol that adheres to the legitimate and ethical standards generally accepted in the stem cell bank of Kazan State Medical University and approved by the Kazan State Medical University Animal Care and Use Committee (approval No. 5 dated 26 May 2020). Over the next 12 h, umbilical cord blood mononuclear cells (UCB-MCs) were isolated by standard density barrier sedimentation using Ficoll (1.077 g/mL), as described previously [38].

2.3. Adenoviral Transduction of UCB-MCs

Recombinant serotype 5 (Ad5) adenoviral vectors carrying cDNA of the human VEGF gene and a reporter gene encoding green fluorescent protein (GFP) were generated using Gateway cloning technology according to manufacturer's instructions (Invitrogen, Carlsbad, CA, USA), as described previously [38]. The titres of Ad5-VEGF165 (2.6×10^9 PFU/mL) and Ad5-GFP (1.2×10^{10} PFU/mL) were determined by plaque formation assay in HEK-293 cells (ATCC, 293T/17 [HEK 293T/17] CRL-11268TM) [56]. Genetic modification of UCB-MCs with Ad5-VEGF165 or Ad5-GFP was performed with a multiplicity of infection (MOI) equal to 10 (MOI = 10) according to the UCB-MC count and Ad5 titre. The samples of gene-modified and native UCB-MCs and conditioned culture medium were analysed 72 h after incubation in an RPMI-1640 medium (PanEco, Moscow, Russia) supplemented with 10% FBS and a mixture of antibiotic penicillin and streptomycin (100 U/mL and 100 µg/mL, respectively) at 37 °C under 5% CO_2. All the work with cell cultures was performed under aseptic conditions in a Herasafe biological safety cabinet (Germany) with respect to the generally accepted rules of work with eukaryotic cells.

2.4. Flow Cytometry and Fluorescence Microscopy

The efficiency of UCB-MC transduction with Ad5 carrying a reporter gene encoding green fluorescent protein (Ad5-GFP) was analysed 72 h after cell transduction. The synthesis of GFP in gene-modified cells was examined using an Axio Observer Z1 inverted fluorescence microscope (Carl Zeiss, Oberkochen, Germany). The number of GFP-positive UCB-MC+Ad5-GFP was estimated using a BD FACSAria III flow cytomgraphy fluorimeter (BD Bioscience, New York, NY, USA) and BD FACS Diva7 software (BD Bioscience, New York, NY, USA) [57].

2.5. Quantitative Reverse Transcription PCR

The mRNA level of VEGF165 and GFP in UCB-MC+Ad5-VEGF and UCB-MC+Ad5-GFP was revealed using qRT-PCR. The total RNA was isolated from gene-modified UCB-MCs 72 h after transduction using the TRIzol reagent (Thermo Fisher Scientific, Waltham, MA, USA) and cDNA synthesis was performed. qRT-PCR was conducted on the Real-Time CFX96 Touch instrument (BioRad Laboratories, Hercules, CA, USA). The primer and probe sequences used in qRT-PCR are listed in Table 1. Triplicate reactions were performed for each sample, and the ∆∆Ct (Livak) method was used to calculate the average relative target gene expression normalized by β-actin rRNA [58]. Standard curves were generated using serial dilutions of plasmid DNA containing the respective inserts (VEGF and GFP). The target gene mRNA levels in native UCB-MCs were taken as 100%.

Table 1. Primer sequences used for real-time quantitative reverse transcriptase polymerase chain reaction (qRT-PCR).

Name	Nucleotide Sequence
β-actin-TM-Forward (human)	GCGAGAAGATGACCCAGGATC
β-actin-TM-Reverse (human)	CCAGTGGTACGGCCAGAGG
β-actin-TM-Probe (human)	[FAM]CCAGCCATGTACGTTGCTATCCAGGC[BH1]
hVEGF-TM49-Forward (human)	TACCTCCACCATGCCAAGTG
hVEGF-TM110-Reverse (human)	TGATTCTGCCCTCCTCCTTCT
hVEGF-TM-Probe (human)	[FAM]TCCCAGGCTGCACCCATGG[BH1]
GFP-TM-Forward	AGCAAAGACCCCAACGAGAA
GFP-TM-Reverse	GGCGGCGGTCACGAA
GFP-TM-Probe	[FAM]CGCGATCACATGGTCCTGCTGG[BH1]

2.6. Western Blotting

The ability of UCB-MC+Ad5-VEGF to synthetize recombinant VEGF was studied 72 h after the transduction of UCB-MCs with Ad5-VEGF165 using Western blot. The protein extracts obtained from native and genetically modified UCB-MCs were separated by electrophoresis in a 15% polyacrylamide gel in the presence of sodium dodecyl sulphate (SDS-PAGE) and were transferred onto PVDF (Polyvinylidene difluoride) membranes. The non-specific binding of primary antibodies (Abs) was blocked using 5% non-fat milk diluted in Twin-PBS (pH 7.4) at 21 °C for 4 h.

Afterwards, the PVDF membranes were incubated with Abs against VEGF (Sigma, Saint Louis, MO, USA, V6627, 1:1000) and β-actin (Genscript, Piscataway, NJ, USA, A00730-40, 1:3000) overnight at 4 °C. Horseradish peroxidase conjugated Abs were used to visualize the target proteins [59]. The data obtained on UCB-MC+Ad5-GFP and native UCB-MCs were used for comparative analysis. Two independent experiments were performed in order to obtain the results.

2.7. Enzyme-Linked Immunosorbent Assay

The potential of UCB-MC+Ad5-VEGF165 to secrete recombinant VEGF was investigated in supernatants collected 72 h after the incubation of gene-modified and native UCB-MCs, using an enzyme-linked immunosorbent assay (ELISA) [60] and ELISA kit for human VEGF (DuoSet, DY293B). The levels of soluble VEGF, according to the optical density, was measured using a BioRad xMark multifunctional microplate spectrophotometer (BioRad, Hercules, CA, USA) at a wavelength of 450 nm. The standard curves plotted using serial dilutions of the recombinant protein provided in the kit were used for quantification. The results were obtained from two technical repetitions.

2.8. Multiplex Secretome Profiling

Supernatants obtained 72 h after the incubation of native and gene-modified UCB-MCs (UCB-MC+Ad5-VEGF165 and UCB-MC+Ad5-GFP) that were prepared from six individual donors were used for cytokine, chemokine, and growth factor analysis with commercially available fluorophore-conjugated microspheres (fluorophore-conjugated beads), employing xMap technology (Luminex, Austin, TX, USA) [61]. Bio-Plex Pro™ Human Cytokine Screening 48-Plex was used in this study. Each sample was studied in triplicate. Standard curves for each cytokine were generated using standards provided by the manufacturer. The data collected was analysed using MasterPlex CT control software v.3 and MasterPlex QT analysis software v.3 (MiraiBio, San Bruno, CA, USA).

2.9. Transcriptome Sequencing and Bioinformatics Analysis

Whole Transcriptome Sequencing "WTS" of native UCB-MCs and gene-modified UCB-MCs (UCB-MC+Ad5-VEGF165 and UCB-MC+Ad5-GFP) obtained from six individual donors was performed using the Illumina platform [62]. Total RNA was extracted 72 h after the incubation of UCB-MCs using TRIzol (Thermo Fisher Scientific) treated with DNase I and purified using the QIAGEN RNeasy Mini Kit. The Agilent Bioanalyzer 2100 and Qubit (Thermo Fisher Scientific) were used to assess the quality and concentration of the isolated RNA samples. All the RNA samples had RNA integrity numbers of more than 8.10. The target mRNA samples were enriched from previously isolated and characterized total RNA using the NEBNext Poly(A) mRNA Magnetic Isolation Module (NEB, #E7490 S) kit (New England Biolabs, Ipswich, MA, USA). cDNA libraries from all the mRNA samples were prepared using the NEBNext Ultra II Directional RNA library prep kit and sample purification beads (NEB, #E7765 S) (New England Biolabs). The DNA sequence of each cluster in flow cells was determined in 150 cycles according to Sequencing By Synthesis (SBS) technology, employing the NextSeq 500/550 High Output v2.5 Kit (150 cycles) and the NextSeq500 Sequencing System (Illumina, San Diego, CA, USA) using the 2×75 bp mode. After evaluating the quality of the sequencing, the obtained reads were aligned with the human reference transcriptome assembly GRCh38 (hg38) from

Genome Reference Consortium (GCA_000001405.15 GCF_000001405.26) using a Kallisto pseudoaligner [63]. Differentially expressed transcripts and genes were annotated using the R "sleuth" package (www.r-project.org, www.rdocumentation.org/packages/sleuth) (accessed date on 17 November 2022). A functional enrichment analysis of the genes with >10 TPM (transcripts per million) was performed using WebGestalt (WEB-based Gene Set Analysis Toolkit) [64].

2.10. Statistics

The statistical analysis was performed using GraphPad Prism® 7 software (GraphPad, Inc., La Jolla, CA, USA). The data are presented as the mean ± standard error (SE). Statistically significant differences were assessed using a one-way analysis of variance (ANOVA) followed by Tukey's test. Statistical significance is denoted by $p < 0.05$.

3. Results

3.1. Transduction Efficacy and Expression of Transgenes in UCB-MCs

This part of the study was conducted as a preliminary task using distinct cord blood samples (n = 3). Using fluorescence microscopy in UCB-MCs transduced with Ad5-GFP, a specific green glow was detected in the cytoplasm of the gene-modified cells (Figure 1A). The flow cytometry study revealed 28.0 ± 2.3% of the GFP-positive cells (Figure 1B). The qRT-PCR analysis demonstrated an increase in GFP mRNA by 100-fold in UCB-MC+Ad5-GFP when compared with non-transduced UCB-MCs (Figure 1C). The analysis of recombinant *vegf165* expression in the UCB-MC+Ad5-VEGF165 also revealed a 100-fold elevated level of mRNA (Figure 1D). The synthesis of VEGF165 in gene-modified UCB-MCs was confirmed by Western blot analysis and showed bands corresponding to a positive reaction with Abs against VEGF (Figure 1E). Secretion of the recombinant protein was documented using ELISA, which detected 2623.0 ± 45.5 pg/mL of VEGF in the conditioned culture medium after UCB-MC+Ad5-VEGF165 incubation, compared with native UCB-MCs (22.1 ± 2.1 pg/mL) (Figure 1F).

3.2. Transcriptome Analysis of the Genetically Modified UCB-MCs

A comparative analysis of the mRNA transcription profiles in native UCB-MCs and gene-modified UCB-MCs (UCB-MC+Ad5-GFP and UCB-MC+Ad5-VEGF165) obtained from six individual samples of cord blood (donors) was performed based on 18 cDNA libraries. A bioinformatics analysis of the RNA-seq data revealed 2.4–2.8 × 10^7 paired reads per samples and transcripts of 10164 genes. The principal component analysis (PCA) of the RNA-seq data showed that samples representing the three comparison groups did not cluster together. However, the samples were grouped according to the cord blood source (donor). The results obtained from the principal component analysis are visualized on a biplot (Figure 2). Among a wide range of genes with an expression of at least 100 transcripts per million, there were no differences in the transcriptome profiles of the native and gene-modified UCB-MCs (Figure 3). At the same time, the recombinant genes *gfp* (log2(Fold change) = 7.15, q value < 0.05) and *vegf165* (log2(Fold change) = 4.41, q value < 0.05) showed increased expression in UCB-MC+Ad5-GFP and UCB-MC+Ad5-VEGF165, respectively, compared to the non-transduced UCB-MCs, as expected. Functional profiling of the detected genes was performed using a GO-based enrichment analysis, where genes whose representation was above 10 TPM in at least one of the samples studied were included. Interpretation using WebGestalt software (http://www.webgestalt.org) allowed the formation of a functional profile of native and gene-modified UCB-MCs, including three groups of annotations (biological processes, molecular functions, and cellular components) presented in the highest category of the Gene Ontology hierarchy. The findings showed that the majority of the genes associated with biological processes were related to metabolism. In the category of cellular components, the majority of the genes detected were related to the cell membrane and cell nucleus, and in the category of molecular functions, they were related to protein binding (Figure 4).

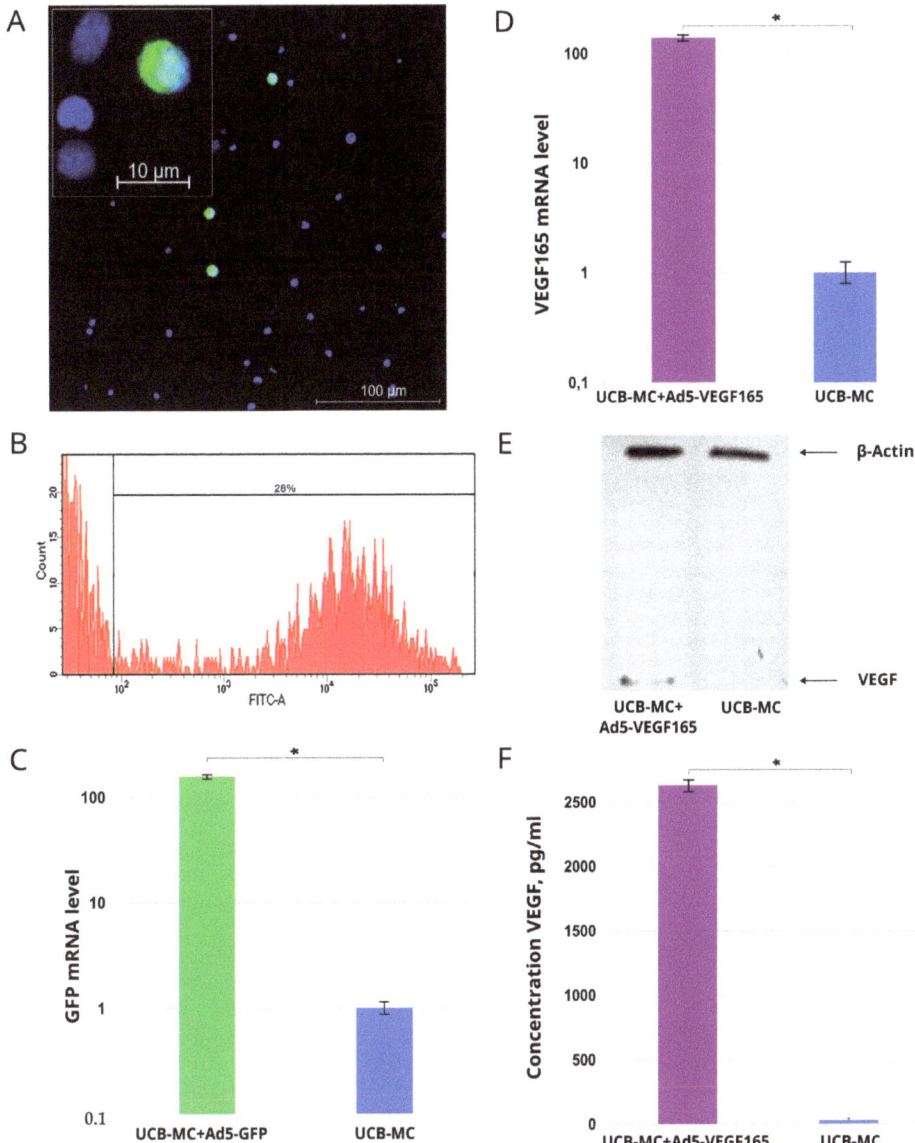

Figure 1. Expression of reporter green fluorescent protein (GFP) gene and recombinant gene encoding vascular endothelial growth factor (*vegf165*) by genetically modified human umbilical cord blood mononuclear cells (UCB-MCs) 72 h after transduction with Ad5-GFP and with Ad5-VEGF165, respectively. (**A**) Fluorescence microscopy demonstrates GFP-positive UCB-MC+Ad5-GFP (green glow). Nuclei were stained with Hoechst 33342 (blue glow). (**B**) Flow cytometry revealed 28% of UCB-MCs synthetizing GFP. (**C**) Quantitative analysis of GFP mRNA levels in UCB-MC+Ad5-GFP by qRT-PCR. (**D**) Quantitative analysis of VEGF165 mRNA levels in UCB-MC+Ad5-VEGF165 using qRT-PCR. (**E**) Western blotting analysis of recombinant VEGF165 in UCB-MC+Ad5-VEGF165. (**F**) Content of the recombinant VEGF165 in the conditioned culture medium after the incubation of UCB-MC+Ad5-VEGF165 using ELISA. *—$p < 0.05$.

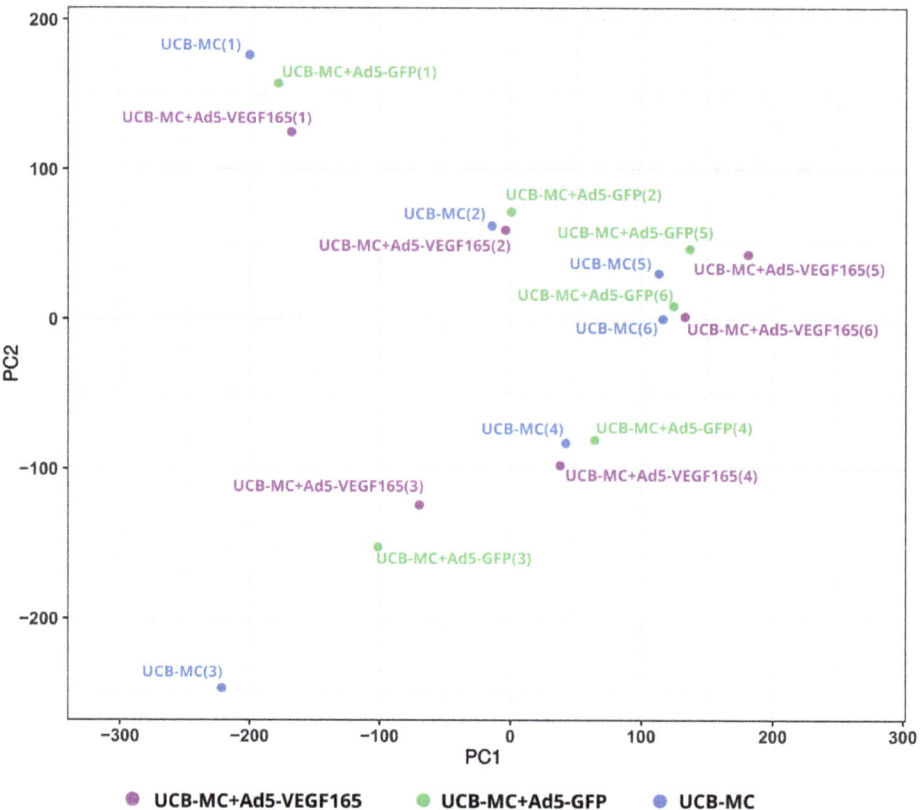

Figure 2. Principal component analysis (PCA) of gene expression data in gene-modified UCB-MCs (UCB-MC+Ad5-VEGF165 and UCB-MC+Ad5-GFP) and native UCB-MCs 72 h after incubation. The samples obtained from six individual donors are presented as numbers in parentheses (1–6).

3.3. Secretome Profiling of the Genetically Modified UCB-MCs

The multiplex secretome analysis of cytokines, chemokines, and growth factors, including 48 analytes in supernatants obtained 72 h after the incubation of native and gene-modified UCB-MCs (UCB-MC+Ad5-VEGF165 and UCB-MC+Ad5-GFP) prepared from six cord blood samples, did not reveal any differences between the groups studied. However, in UCB-MC+Ad5-VEGF165, an increase in VEGF content was observed when compared with native UCB-MCs and UCB-MC+Ad5-GFP (Figure 5).

The cluster analysis of the obtained secretomes also confirmed that the genetic modification of UCB-MCs does not affect their secretion of cytokines, chemokines, and growth factors (Figure 6). At the same time, the samples of UCB-MCs obtained from individual donors had different secretion profiles of the analytes studied, and the grouping of gene-modified cells was consistent with the UCB-MC source.

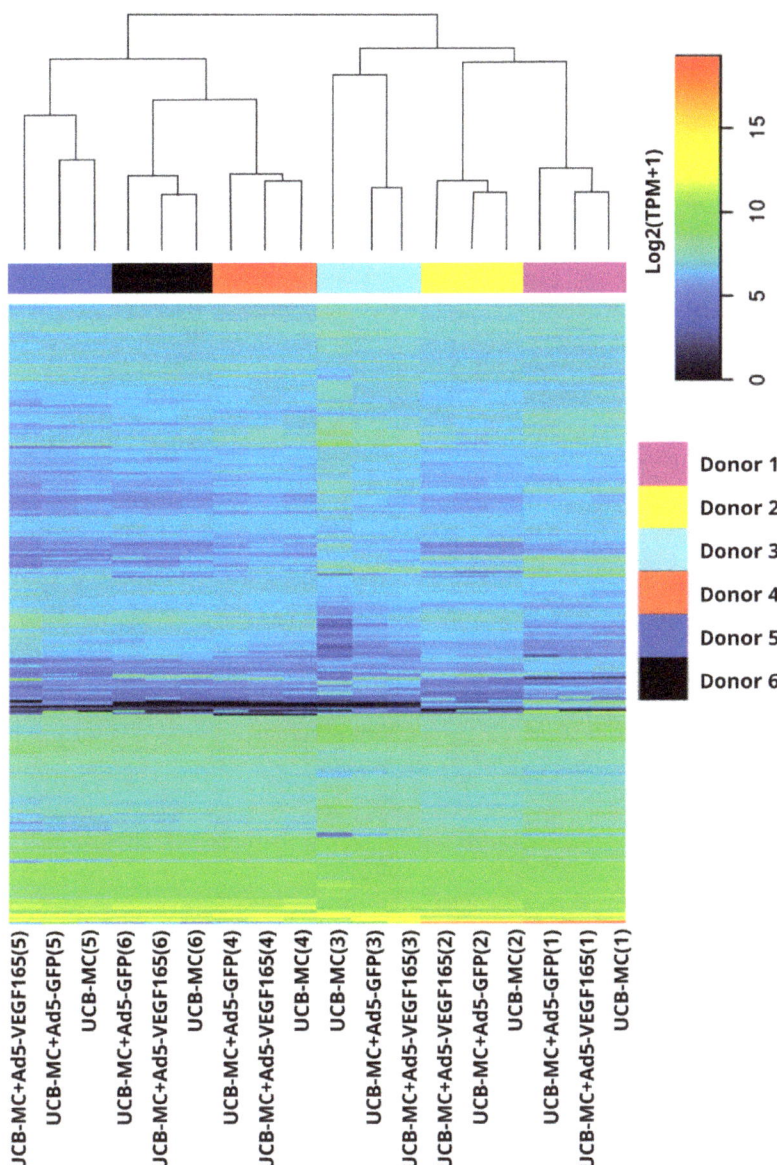

Figure 3. Heatmap representing log2 transcripts per million (TPM) in gene-modified UCB-MCs (UCB-MC+Ad5-VEGF165 and UCB-MC+Ad5-GFP) and native UCB-MCs 72 h after incubation. Data is presented for the first 1760 genes whose expression was at least 100 transcripts per million. The samples obtained from six individual donors are presented as numbers in parentheses (1–6).

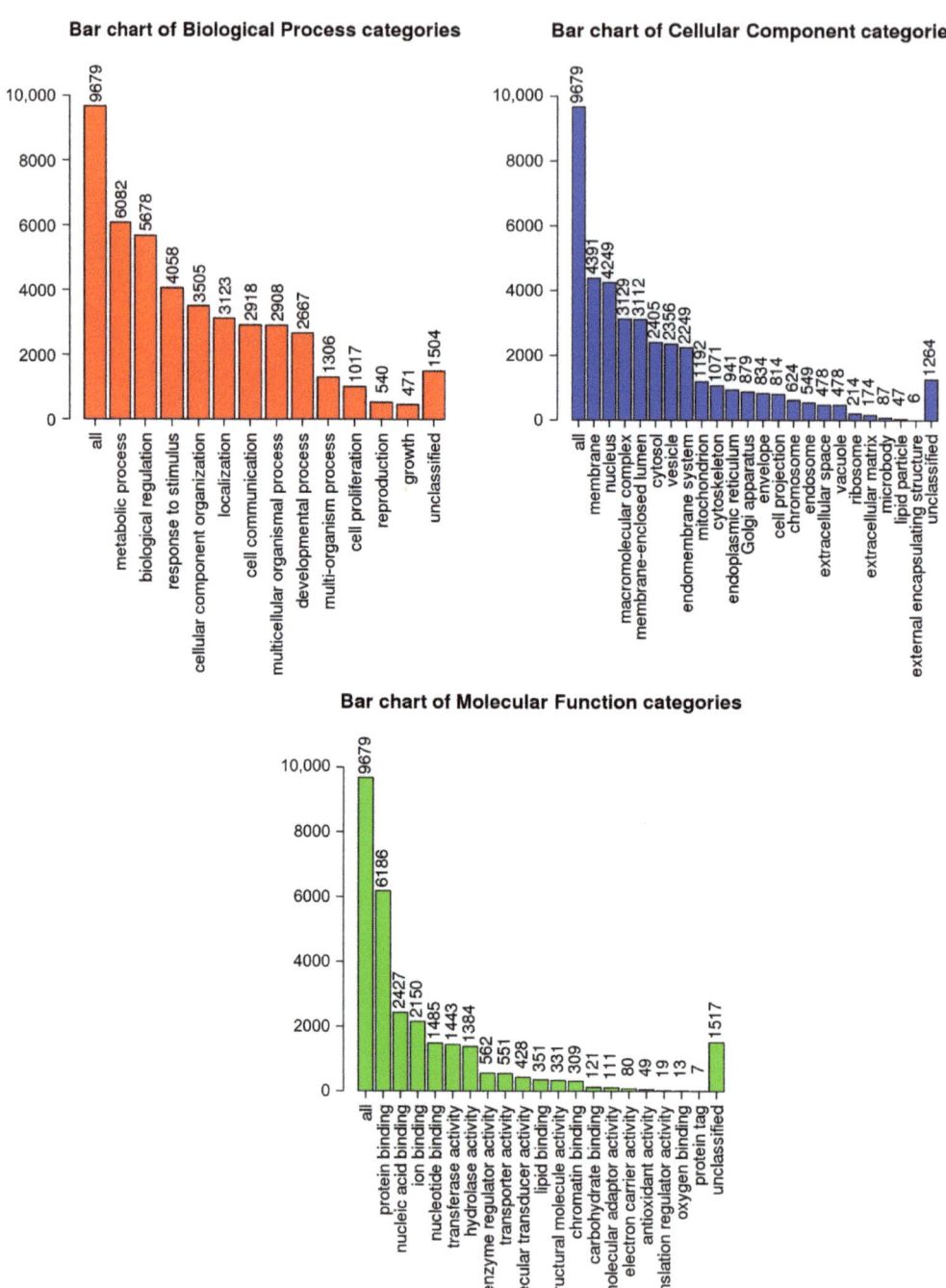

Figure 4. Gene Ontology (GO)-based enrichment analysis of native UCB-MC transcriptomes. GO terms are presented for the categories of biological processes, cellular components, and molecular functions.

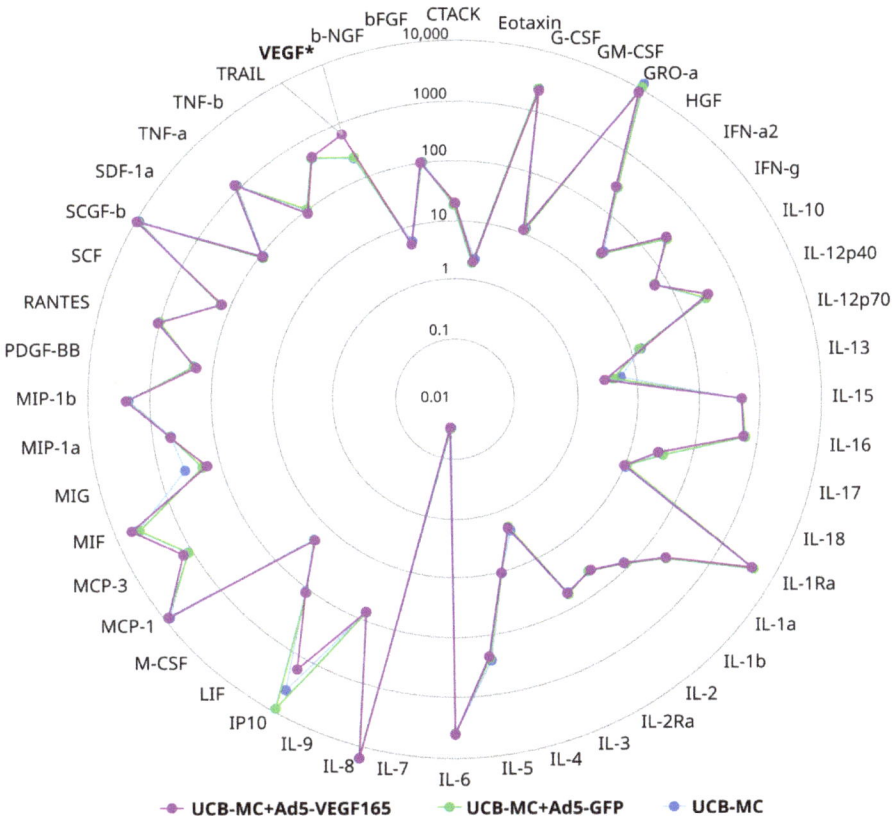

Figure 5. Radial comparative diagram of cytokine, chemokine, and growth factor representation in supernatant obtained 72 h after the incubation of gene-modified UCB-MCs (UCB-MC+Ad5-VEGF165 and UCB-MC+Ad5-GFP) and native UCB-MCs. The concentration of the analytes studied is presented in pg/mL. *—$p < 0.05$.

Thus, UCB-MC transduction with Ad5-VEGF165 and Ad5-GFP at MOI = 10 revealed effective expression of the transgenes at mRNA and protein levels. The bioinformatics analysis of the RNA-seq data obtained from the native UCB-MCs and gene-modified UCB-MCs (UCB-MC+Ad5-VEGF165 and UCB-MC+Ad5-GFP) revealed that the adenoviral construct (Ad5) or transgene (*vegf165*) had no effect on 10164 gene transcripts. The multiplex secretome analysis of 48 cytokines, chemokines, and growth factors also showed no differences in the secretion patterns of the native and genetically modified UCB-MCs and was in line with the results obtained from the bioinformatics analysis of the UCB-MC transcriptomes.

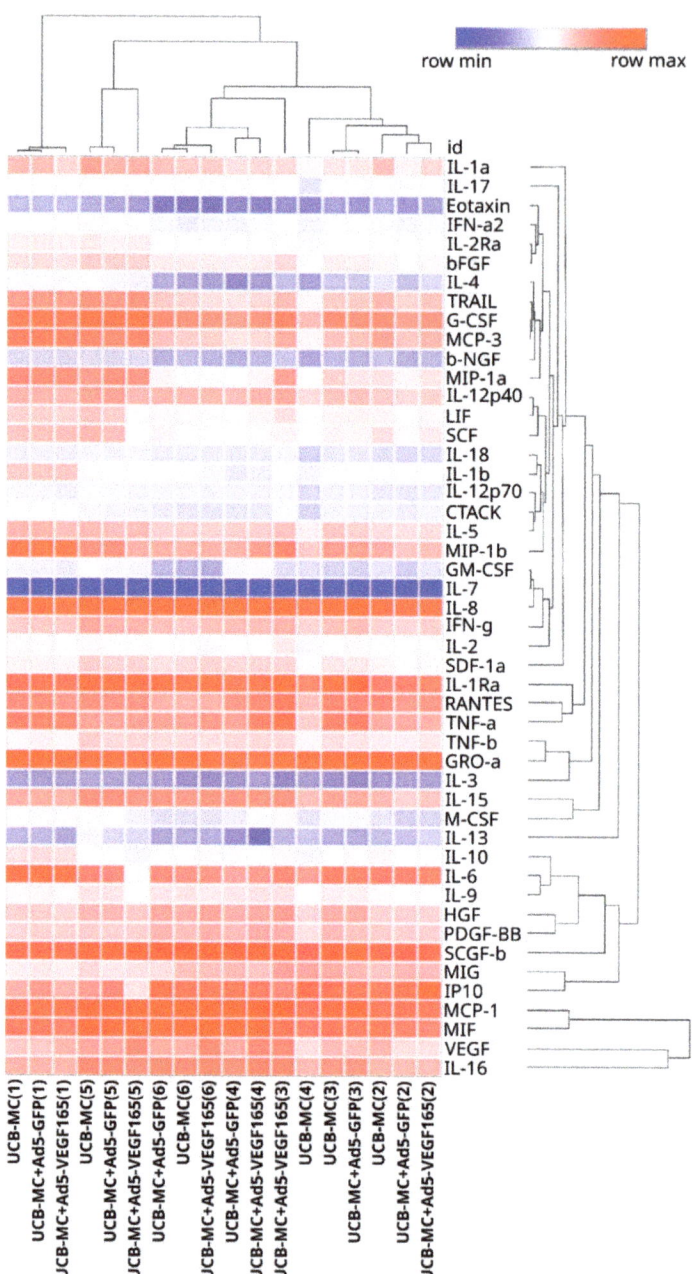

Figure 6. Heatmap of cytokine, chemokine, and growth factor representation in supernatant obtained 72 h after the incubation of gene-modified UCB-MCs (UCB-MC+Ad5-VEGF165 and UCB-MC+Ad5-GFP) and native UCB-MCs. The samples obtained from six individual donors are presented as numbers in parentheses (1–6).

4. Discussion

In recent years, the steady growth of gene therapy research has demonstrated its significant impact on regenerative therapies. Gene therapy is considered a powerful tool not only for correcting the function of a mutated gene, but also for targeting changes in cell function [65]. Despite the great promise of gene therapy for the treatment of human diseases, the risk of side effects is one of the main reasons for the slow introduction of a drug containing recombinant cDNA as a pharmaceutical product. Therefore, biosafety aspects play a crucial role in the translation of a gene therapy drug from biomedical research into clinical care [66].

Gene therapy implies the delivery of therapeutic genes into the recipient's body using non-viral or viral vectors (direct gene therapy) or on cell carriers (cell-mediated gene therapy). The advantages and disadvantages of each method of transgene delivery have been discussed in many research publications concerning gene therapy [3,67]. The choice of the vector or cell delivery system for the therapeutic gene may depend on the nature of the disease (inherited or acquired), the duration of the planned treatment (lifetime or in the acute or chronic phase of the disease), the assumed effect (local or systemic), and the intended effect (etiotropic, pathogenetic, or symptomatic).

An important focus of gene therapy is to increase the level of expression of genes encoding trophic factors and growth factors that stimulate the regenerative potential of organs associated with the disease. The method of delivery of therapeutic genes encoding biologically active molecules using ex vivo gene-modified cells, which serve as producers of these molecules, serves as an alternative to the intravenous administration of recombinant proteins. A significant disadvantage of using recombinant proteins for replacement therapy is their short half-life and the need for the repeated use of expensive drugs during the course of disease treatment. Transplantation of the genetically modified cells expressing transgenes is reasonable, not only through the production of therapeutic molecules, but also through the effect of transgene carrier cells (stem cells, progenitor cells, or mature cells) on the regenerative capacity of the damaged tissue.

In this regard, an attractive opportunity in regenerative medicine is the use of UCB-MCs to deliver recombinant genes encoding growth and trophic factors. Numerous studies have demonstrated the feasibility of using UCB-MCs, not only to correct haematological disorders, but also to stimulate the regeneration of various tissues and organs in ischemic and degenerative diseases [21]. Cord blood cells are readily available and have the lowest immunogenicity compared to other allogeneic cells [28,68]. Also of interest is the legal and ethical opportunity to apply UCB-MCs in clinical practice.

In the therapy of ischemic diseases, genetically modified UCB-MCs are used to stimulate angiogenesis. A positive therapeutic effect was achieved in an animal model of chronic hind limb skeletal muscle ischemia after the transplantation of UCB-MCs overexpressing human VEGF [69]. In a rat model of myocardial infarction, UCB isolated HSCs overexpressing VEGF and PDGF (platelet-derived growth factor gene) [70], or VEGF and angiopoietin-1 (Ang1) genes [71] inhibited the development of cardiac muscle necrosis and increased capillary density in the myocardium. In our studies, in order to stimulate regeneration in the CNS, we developed UCB-MCs simultaneously overexpressing three recombinant neuroprotective factors (VEGF, GDNF [glial-cell-line-derived neurotrophic factor], and NCAM [neural cell adhesion molecule]) [55,72,73].

The successful translation of a gene-cell pharmaceutical product into clinical practice requires the establishment of its efficacy and the conduct of preclinical studies to ensure its biosafety. The genetic modification of cells using a plasmid or viral vector, through the influence of the vector itself or its expressed products, can change the genotype and/or phenotype of genetically modified cells. In the present study, we studied the transcriptome and secretome patterns of UCB-MCs transduced with Ad5 carrying cDNA of human *vegf165* and compared them with UCB-MCs transduced with Ad5-GFP and native UCB-MCs. Preliminary molecular and cellular analyses confirmed the efficacy of UCB-MC transduction with a human adenovirus serotype 5 (Ad5) vector. At an MOI of 10, the number of UCB-MC+Ad5-GFP was 28% and the recombinant *vegf165* mRNA level in UCB-MC+Ad5-VEGF165 was 100-fold higher than in native UCB-MCs. The synthesis and secretion of recombinant VEGF in UCB-MC+Ad5-VEGF165 were also established by Western blot and ELISA, respectively.

The bioinformatics analysis of the native and genetically modified UCB-MC RNA-seq data revealed that the variability observed in the transcriptome is primarily attributed to individual donor variability rather than the genetic modification of UCB-MC transcriptomes. The three annotation groups (biological processes, molecular functions, and cellular components) presented in the highest category of the Gene Ontology hierarchy showed similar GO-based enrichment patterns in modified and native cells, which was consistent with the absence of differences in the transcriptomes. The secretome profiling (the secretion of studied cytokines, chemokines, and growth factors) of UCB-MCs did not reveal differences between native and gene-modified UCB-MCs (UCB-MC+Ad5-VEGF165 and UCB-MC+Ad5-GFP). Consequently, we found no negative effects of the adenoviral vector (the study of UCB-MC+Ad5-GFP) or transgene (*vegf165*) expression (the study of UCB-MC+Ad5-VEGF165) on the transcription activity and functional status of gene-modified UCB-MCs. The increased *vegf165* expression in UCB-MC+Ad5-VEGF165, demonstrated by transcriptome and secretome analyses, aligns with the results obtained by qRT-PCR, Western blot, and ELISA in the preliminary study. At the same time, it is important to note that transcriptomes and secretomes differed between the UCB-MC samples obtained from individual donors.

Thus, UCB-MC+Ad5-VEGF165 retain their native properties and actively secrete recombinant VEGF. These data support the rationality of using genetically modified UCB-MCs for the temporary synthesis and secretion of recombinant therapeutic molecules in the treatment of neurological diseases. Before translating gene therapy with UCB-MCs into clinical trials, more research is needed to develop a GMP protocol for the preparation of genetically engineered UCB-MCs and to study the biosafety, dosage, transplantation methods, targeting, and pharmacokinetics of recombinant molecules in large animals with morphological, functional, and biochemical characteristics similar to humans.

We believe that the results of this work provide a solid fundamental platform for biosafety research into genetically modified UCB-MCs and will enable the translation of cell-mediated gene therapies into clinical care.

5. Conclusions

The safety of pharmaceutical products containing artificial genetic material is one of the important issues when implementing gene therapy in practical medicine. Two modes of introducing transgenes into the patient, including virus-mediated and cell-mediated delivery, are currently being actively investigated. These approaches have advantages and disadvantages in terms of transgene expression efficiency and biosafety. The aim of this research was to investigate the biosafety of genetically modified UCB-MCs transduced with a human adenovirus serotype 5 (Ad5) vector carrying cDNA encoding human VEGF. The efficacy of *vegf165* expression has been proven at the level of mRNA transcription, recombinant protein synthesis, and secretion. It is worth noting that the efficient production of recombinant VEGF165 does not negatively affect the transcriptome profile and secretion of the studied cytokines, chemokines, and growth factors by genetically modified UCB-MCs. At the same time, the UCB-MC samples obtained from six donors had different transcriptome and secretion patterns, indicating individual variability. Thus, we propose that the data on effective transgene expression and preservation of the native properties of genetically modified UCB-MCs brings us closer to the possibility of using UCB-MCs as cell carriers of artificial genetic materials and as producers of recombinant therapeutic molecules in ex vivo gene therapy.

Author Contributions: Conceptualization, I.I.S., A.A.R. and Z.Z.S.; formal analysis, I.I.S., M.I.M. and A.A.I.; funding acquisition, I.I.S. and Z.Z.S.; investigation, D.Z.G., M.I.M., E.E.G. and S.Y.M.; methodology, I.I.S., S.Y.M., I.M.G. and Z.Z.S.; supervision, I.I.S., R.R.I. and A.P.; visualization, A.A.I.; writing—review and editing, I.I.S. and Z.Z.S. All authors have read and agreed to the published version of the manuscript.

Funding: This research was funded by a grant from the Russian Science Foundation, No. 19-75-10030 (Z.Z.S.).

Institutional Review Board Statement: The study was conducted according to the guidelines of the Declaration of Helsinki. Umbilical cord blood was collected from healthy women in labour at 39–40 weeks of pregnancy, after obtaining informed consent for pregnant and prenatal screening for contraindications to blood donation in maternity hospitals in Kazan in accordance with protocol that adheres to the legitimate and ethical standards generally accepted in the stem cell bank of Kazan State Medical University and approved by the Kazan State Medical University Animal Care and Use Committee (approval No. 5 dated 26 May 2020).

Informed Consent Statement: Informed consent was obtained from each study subject according to the guidelines approved under this protocol (article 20, Federal Law "Protection of Health Rights of Citizens of Russian Federation" N323-FZ, 21 November 2011).

Data Availability Statement: The data presented in this study is available on request from the corresponding author.

Acknowledgments: This paper has been supported by the Kazan Federal University Strategic Academic Leadership Programme (PRIORITY-2030).

Conflicts of Interest: The authors declare no conflict of interest.

References

1. Aiuti, A.; Roncarolo, M.G.; Naldini, L. Gene Therapy for ADA-SCID, the First Marketing Approval of an Ex Vivo Gene Therapy in Europe: Paving the Road for the next Generation of Advanced Therapy Medicinal Products. *EMBO Mol. Med.* **2017**, *9*, 737–740. [CrossRef] [PubMed]
2. Mendell, J.R.; Al-Zaidy, S.A.; Rodino-Klapac, L.R.; Goodspeed, K.; Gray, S.J.; Kay, C.N.; Boye, S.L.; Boye, S.E.; George, L.A.; Salabarria, S.; et al. Current Clinical Applications of In Vivo Gene Therapy with AAVs. *Mol. Ther.* **2021**, *29*, 464–488. [CrossRef] [PubMed]
3. Sudhakar, V.; Sudhakar, R.M. Gene Therapy for Neurodegenerative Diseases. *Neurotherapeutics* **2019**, *16*, 166–175. [CrossRef] [PubMed]
4. Naldini, L. Ex Vivo Gene Transfer and Correction for Cell-Based Therapies. *Nat. Rev. Genet.* **2011**, *12*, 301–315. [CrossRef]
5. Arjmand, B.; Larijani, B.; Sheikh Hosseini, M.; Payab, M.; Gilany, K.; Goodarzi, P.; Parhizkar Roudsari, P.; Amanollahi Baharvand, M.; Hoseini Mohammadi, N.S. The Horizon of Gene Therapy in Modern Medicine: Advances and Challenges. *Adv. Exp. Med. Biol.* **2020**, *1247*, 33–64. [CrossRef]
6. Gonin, P.; Buchholz, C.J.; Pallardy, M.; Mezzina, M. Gene Therapy Bio-Safety: Scientific and Regulatory Issues. *Gene Ther.* **2005**, *12* (Suppl. S1), S146–S152. [CrossRef]
7. Kovacs, G.G. Molecular Pathology of Neurodegenerative Diseases: Principles and Practice. *J. Clin. Pathol.* **2019**, *72*, 725–735. [CrossRef]
8. Ahuja, C.S.; Nori, S.; Tetreault, L.; Wilson, J.; Kwon, B.; Harrop, J.; Choi, D.; Fehlings, M.G. Traumatic Spinal Cord Injury—Repair and Regeneration. *Neurosurgery* **2017**, *80*, S9–S22. [CrossRef]
9. Feske, S.K. Ischemic Stroke. *Am. J. Med.* **2021**, *134*, 1457–1464. [CrossRef]
10. Niziolek, G.; Sandsmark, D.K.; Pascual, J.L. Neurotrauma. *Curr. Opin. Crit. Care* **2022**, *28*, 715–724. [CrossRef]
11. Blaese, R.M.; Culver, K.W.; Miller, A.D.; Carter, C.S.; Fleisher, T.; Clerici, M.; Shearer, G.; Chang, L.; Chiang, Y.; Tolstoshev, P.; et al. T Lymphocyte-Directed Gene Therapy for ADA-SCID: Initial Trial Results after 4 Years. *Science* **1995**, *270*, 475–480. [CrossRef] [PubMed]
12. Cartier, N.; Hacein-Bey-Abina, S.; Bartholomae, C.C.; Veres, G.; Schmidt, M.; Kutschera, I.; Vidaud, M.; Abel, U.; Dal-Cortivo, L.; Caccavelli, L.; et al. Hematopoietic Stem Cell Gene Therapy with a Lentiviral Vector in X-Linked Adrenoleukodystrophy. *Science* **2009**, *326*, 818–823. [CrossRef]
13. Morgan, R.A.; Gray, D.; Lomova, A.; Kohn, D.B. Hematopoietic Stem Cell Gene Therapy: Progress and Lessons Learned. *Cell Stem Cell* **2017**, *21*, 574–590. [CrossRef] [PubMed]
14. Bujko, K.; Kucia, M.; Ratajczak, J.; Ratajczak, M.Z. Hematopoietic Stem and Progenitor Cells (HSPCs). *Adv. Exp. Med. Biol.* **2019**, *1201*, 49–77. [CrossRef] [PubMed]
15. Yu, V.W.C.; Scadden, D.T. Hematopoietic Stem Cell and Its Bone Marrow Niche. *Curr. Top. Dev. Biol.* **2016**, *118*, 21–44. [CrossRef] [PubMed]

16. Orlando, N.; Pellegrino, C.; Valentini, C.G.; Bianchi, M.; Barbagallo, O.; Sparnacci, S.; Forni, F.; Fontana, T.M.; Teofili, L. Umbilical Cord Blood: Current Uses for Transfusion and Regenerative Medicine. *Transfus. Apher. Sci.* **2020**, *59*, 102952. [CrossRef] [PubMed]
17. Shi, P.A.; Luchsinger, L.L.; Greally, J.M.; Delaney, C.S. Umbilical Cord Blood: An Undervalued and Underutilized Resource in Allogeneic Hematopoietic Stem Cell Transplant and Novel Cell Therapy Applications. *Curr. Opin. Hematol.* **2022**, *29*, 317–326. [CrossRef]
18. Verina, T.; Fatemi, A.; Johnston, M.V.; Comi, A.M. Pluripotent Possibilities: Human Umbilical Cord Blood Cell Treatment after Neonatal Brain Injury. *Pediatr. Neurol.* **2013**, *48*, 346–354. [CrossRef]
19. Erices, A.; Conget, P.; Minguell, J.J. Mesenchymal Progenitor Cells in Human Umbilical Cord Blood. *Br. J. Haematol.* **2000**, *109*, 235–242. [CrossRef]
20. Ding, D.-C.; Shyu, W.-C.; Lin, S.-Z. Mesenchymal Stem Cells. *Cell Transplant.* **2011**, *20*, 5–14. [CrossRef]
21. Yang, W.Z.; Zhang, Y.; Wu, F.; Min, W.P.; Minev, B.; Zhang, M.; Luo, X.L.; Ramos, F.; Ichim, T.E.; Riordan, N.H.; et al. Safety Evaluation of Allogeneic Umbilical Cord Blood Mononuclear Cell Therapy for Degenerative Conditions. *J. Transl. Med.* **2010**, *8*, 75. [CrossRef]
22. Dasari, V.R.; Spomar, D.G.; Li, L.; Gujrati, M.; Rao, J.S.; Dinh, D.H. Umbilical Cord Blood Stem Cell Mediated Downregulation of Fas Improves Functional Recovery of Rats after Spinal Cord Injury. *Neurochem. Res.* **2008**, *33*, 134–149. [CrossRef] [PubMed]
23. Sun, J.M.; Kurtzberg, J. Cord Blood for Brain Injury. *Cytotherapy* **2015**, *17*, 775–785. [CrossRef] [PubMed]
24. Newman, M.B.; Davis, C.D.; Kuzmin-Nichols, N.; Sanberg, P.R. Human Umbilical Cord Blood (HUCB) Cells for Central Nervous System Repair. *Neurotox. Res.* **2003**, *5*, 355–368. [CrossRef] [PubMed]
25. Allan, D.S. Using Umbilical Cord Blood for Regenerative Therapy: Proof or Promise? *Stem Cells* **2020**, *38*, 590–595. [CrossRef] [PubMed]
26. Newman, M.B.; Emerich, D.F.; Borlongan, C.V.; Sanberg, C.D.; Sanberg, P.R. Use of Human Umbilical Cord Blood (HUCB) Cells to Repair the Damaged Brain. *Curr. Neurovasc. Res.* **2004**, *1*, 269–281. [CrossRef]
27. Fan, C.-G.; Zhang, Q.-J.; Tang, F.-W.; Han, Z.-B.; Wang, G.-S.; Han, Z.-C. Human Umbilical Cord Blood Cells Express Neurotrophic Factors. *Neurosci. Lett.* **2005**, *380*, 322–325. [CrossRef]
28. Pranke, P.; Failace, R.R.; Allebrandt, W.F.; Steibel, G.; Schmidt, F.; Nardi, N.B. Hematologic and Immunophenotypic Characterization of Human Umbilical Cord Blood. *Acta Haematol.* **2001**, *105*, 71–76. [CrossRef]
29. Bachstetter, A.D.; Pabon, M.M.; Cole, M.J.; Hudson, C.E.; Sanberg, P.R.; Willing, A.E.; Bickford, P.C.; Gemma, C. Peripheral Injection of Human Umbilical Cord Blood Stimulates Neurogenesis in the Aged Rat Brain. *BMC Neurosci.* **2008**, *9*, 22. [CrossRef]
30. Ende, N.; Chen, R. Parkinson's Disease Mice and Human Umbilical Cord Blood. *J. Med.* **2002**, *33*, 173–180.
31. Garbuzova-Davis, S.; Sanberg, C.D.; Kuzmin-Nichols, N.; Willing, A.E.; Gemma, C.; Bickford, P.C.; Miller, C.; Rossi, R.; Sanberg, P.R. Human Umbilical Cord Blood Treatment in a Mouse Model of ALS: Optimization of Cell Dose. *PLoS ONE* **2008**, *3*, e2494. [CrossRef] [PubMed]
32. Ende, N.; Weinstein, F.; Chen, R.; Ende, M. Human Umbilical Cord Blood Effect on Sod Mice (Amyotrophic Lateral Sclerosis). *Life Sci.* **2000**, *67*, 53–59. [CrossRef] [PubMed]
33. Knippenberg, S.; Thau, N.; Schwabe, K.; Dengler, R.; Schambach, A.; Hass, R.; Petri, S. Intraspinal Injection of Human Umbilical Cord Blood-Derived Cells Is Neuroprotective in a Transgenic Mouse Model of Amyotrophic Lateral Sclerosis. *Neurodegener. Dis.* **2012**, *9*, 107–120. [CrossRef] [PubMed]
34. Ramli, Y.; Alwahdy, A.S.; Kurniawan, M.; Juliandi, B.; Wuyung, P.E. Intra-Arterial Transplantation of Human Umbilical Cord Blood Mononuclear Cells in Sub-Acute Ischemic Stroke Increases VEGF Expression in Rats. *J. Stem Cells Regen. Med.* **2018**, *14*, 69–79. [CrossRef] [PubMed]
35. Chen, J.; Sanberg, P.R.; Li, Y.; Wang, L.; Lu, M.; Willing, A.E.; Sanchez-Ramos, J.; Chopp, M. Intravenous Administration of Human Umbilical Cord Blood Reduces Behavioral Deficits after Stroke in Rats. *Stroke* **2001**, *32*, 2682–2688. [CrossRef]
36. Xi, Y.; Yue, G.; Gao, S.; Ju, R.; Wang, Y. Human Umbilical Cord Blood Mononuclear Cells Transplantation for Perinatal Brain Injury. *Stem Cell Res. Ther.* **2022**, *13*, 458. [CrossRef]
37. Zhu, H.; Poon, W.; Liu, Y.; Leung, G.K.-K.; Wong, Y.; Feng, Y.; Ng, S.C.P.; Tsang, K.S.; Sun, D.D.T.F.; Yeung, D.K.; et al. Phase I-II Clinical Trial Assessing Safety and Efficacy of Umbilical Cord Blood Mononuclear Cell Transplant Therapy of Chronic Complete Spinal Cord Injury. *Cell Transplant.* **2016**, *25*, 1925–1943. [CrossRef]
38. Islamov, R.R.; Rizvanov, A.A.; Mukhamedyarov, M.A.; Salafutdinov, I.I.; Garanina, E.E.; Fedotova, V.Y.; Solovyeva, V.V.; Mukhamedshina, Y.O.; Safiullov, Z.Z.; Izmailov, A.A.; et al. Symptomatic Improvement, Increased Life-Span and Sustained Cell Homing in Amyotrophic Lateral Sclerosis after Transplantation of Human Umbilical Cord Blood Cells Genetically Modified with Adeno-Viral Vectors Expressing a Neuro-Protective Factor and a Neur. *Curr. Gene Ther.* **2015**, *15*, 266–276. [CrossRef]
39. Sathasivam, S. VEGF and ALS. *Neurosci. Res.* **2008**, *62*, 71–77. [CrossRef]
40. Lange, C.; Storkebaum, E.; De Almodóvar, C.R.; Dewerchin, M.; Carmeliet, P. Vascular Endothelial Growth Factor: A Neurovascular Target in Neurological Diseases. *Nat. Rev. Neurol.* **2016**, *12*, 439–454. [CrossRef]
41. Ferrara, N.; Gerber, H.-P.; LeCouter, J. The Biology of VEGF and Its Receptors. *Nat. Med.* **2003**, *9*, 669–676. [CrossRef] [PubMed]
42. De Almodovar, C.R.; Lambrechts, D.; Mazzone, M.; Carmeliet, P.; Ruiz de Almodovar, C.; Lambrechts, D.; Mazzone, M.; Carmeliet, P. Role and Therapeutic Potential of VEGF in the Nervous System. *Physiol. Rev.* **2009**, *89*, 607–648. [CrossRef] [PubMed]
43. Ma, Y.; Zechariah, A.; Qu, Y.; Hermann, D.M. Effects of Vascular Endothelial Growth Factor in Ischemic Stroke. *J. Neurosci. Res.* **2012**, *90*, 1873–1882. [CrossRef]

44. Chen, B.; Zhang, Y.; Chen, S.; Xuran, L.; Dong, J.; Chen, W.; Tao, S.; Yang, W.; Zhang, Y. The Role of Vascular Endothelial Growth Factor in Ischemic Stroke. *Pharmazie* **2021**, *76*, 127–131. [CrossRef] [PubMed]
45. Zhou, Z.; Gao, S.; Li, Y.; Peng, R.; Zheng, Z.; Wei, W.; Zhao, Z.; Liu, X.; Li, L.; Zhang, J. VEGI Improves Outcomes in the Early Phase of Experimental Traumatic Brain Injury. *Neuroscience* **2020**, *438*, 60–69. [CrossRef]
46. Thau-Zuchman, O.; Shohami, E.; Alexandrovich, A.G.; Leker, R.R. Vascular Endothelial Growth Factor Increases Neurogenesis after Traumatic Brain Injury. *J. Cereb. Blood Flow Metab.* **2010**, *30*, 1008–1016. [CrossRef]
47. Siddiq, I.; Park, E.; Liu, E.; Spratt, S.K.; Surosky, R.; Lee, G.; Ando, D.; Giedlin, M.; Hare, G.M.T.; Fehlings, M.G.; et al. Treatment of Traumatic Brain Injury Using Zinc-Finger Protein Gene Therapy Targeting VEGF-A. *J. Neurotrauma* **2012**, *29*, 2647–2659. [CrossRef]
48. Li, J.; Chen, S.; Zhao, Z.; Luo, Y.; Hou, Y.; Li, H.; He, L.; Zhou, L.; Wu, W. Effect of VEGF on Inflammatory Regulation, Neural Survival, and Functional Improvement in Rats Following a Complete Spinal Cord Transection. *Front. Cell. Neurosci.* **2017**, *11*, 381. [CrossRef]
49. Liu, X.; Xu, W.; Zhang, Z.; Liu, H.; Lv, L.; Han, D.; Liu, L.; Yao, A.; Xu, T. Vascular Endothelial Growth Factor-Transfected Bone Marrow Mesenchymal Stem Cells Improve the Recovery of Motor and Sensory Functions of Rats With Spinal Cord Injury. *Spine* **2020**, *45*, E364–E372. [CrossRef]
50. Pronto-Laborinho, A.C.; Pinto, S.; de Carvalho, M. Roles of Vascular Endothelial Growth Factor in Amyotrophic Lateral Sclerosis. *Biomed. Res. Int.* **2014**, *2014*, 947513. [CrossRef]
51. Lambrechts, D.; Storkebaum, E.; Morimoto, M.; Del-Favero, J.; Desmet, F.; Marklund, S.L.; Wyns, S.; Thijs, V.; Andersson, J.; van Marion, I.; et al. VEGF Is a Modifier of Amyotrophic Lateral Sclerosis in Mice and Humans and Protects Motoneurons against Ischemic Death. *Nat. Genet.* **2003**, *34*, 383–394. [CrossRef] [PubMed]
52. Agatieva, E.; Ksembaev, S.; Sokolov, M.; Markosyan, V.; Gazizov, I.; Tsyplakov, D.; Shmarov, M.; Tutykhina, I.; Naroditsky, B.; Logunov, D.; et al. Evaluation of Direct and Cell-Mediated Lactoferrin Gene Therapy for the Maxillofacial Area Abscesses in Rats. *Pharmaceutics* **2021**, *13*, 58. [CrossRef] [PubMed]
53. Gatina, D.Z.; Gazizov, I.M.; Zhuravleva, M.N.; Arkhipova, S.S.; Golubenko, M.A.; Gomzikova, M.O.; Garanina, E.E.; Islamov, R.R.; Rizvanov, A.A.; Salafutdinov, I.I. Induction of Angiogenesis by Genetically Modified Human Umbilical Cord Blood Mononuclear Cells. *Int. J. Mol. Sci.* **2023**, *24*, 4396. [CrossRef] [PubMed]
54. Islamov, R.R.; Izmailov, A.A.; Sokolov, M.E.; Fadeev, F.O.; Bashirov, F.V.; Eremeev, A.A.; Shmarov, M.M.; Naroditskiy, B.S.; Chelyshev, Y.A.A.; Lavrov, I.A.; et al. Evaluation of Direct and Cell-Mediated Triple-Gene Therapy in Spinal Cord Injury in Rats. *Brain Res. Bull.* **2017**, *132*, 44–52. [CrossRef]
55. Markosyan, V.; Safiullov, Z.; Izmailov, A.; Fadeev, F.; Sokolov, M.; Kuznetsov, M.; Trofimov, D.; Kim, E.; Kundakchyan, G.; Gibadullin, A.; et al. Preventive Triple Gene Therapy Reduces the Negative Consequences of Ischemia-Induced Brain Injury after Modelling Stroke in a Rat. *Int. J. Mol. Sci.* **2020**, *21*, 6858. [CrossRef]
56. Baer, A.; Kehn-Hall, K. Viral Concentration Determination through Plaque Assays: Using Traditional and Novel Overlay Systems. *J. Vis. Exp.* **2014**, *4*, e52065. [CrossRef]
57. Chu, Y.W.; Wang, R.; Schmid, I.; Sakamoto, K.M. Analysis with Flow Cytometry of Green Fluorescent Protein Expression in Leukemic Cells. *Cytometry* **1999**, *36*, 333–339. [CrossRef]
58. Livak, K.J.; Schmittgen, T.D. Analysis of Relative Gene Expression Data Using Real-Time Quantitative PCR and the 2(-Delta Delta C(T)) Method. *Methods* **2001**, *25*, 402–408. [CrossRef]
59. Garanina, E.E.; Mukhamedshina, Y.O.; Salafutdinov, I.I.; Kiyasov, A.P.; Lima, L.M.; Reis, H.J.; Palotás, A.; Islamov, R.R.; Rizvanov, A.A. Construction of Recombinant Adenovirus Containing Picorna-Viral 2A-Peptide Sequence for the Co-Expression of Neuro-Protective Growth Factors in Human Umbilical Cord Blood Cells. *Spinal Cord* **2016**, *54*, 423–430. [CrossRef]
60. Clark, M.F.; Lister, R.M.; Bar-Joseph, M. ELISA Techniques. In *Plant Molecular Biology*; Methods in Enzymology; Academic Press: Cambridge, MA, USA, 1986; Volume 118, pp. 742–766.
61. Valekova, I.; Skalnikova, H.K.; Jarkovska, K.; Motlik, J.; Kovarova, H. Multiplex Immunoassays for Quantification of Cytokines, Growth Factors, and Other Proteins in Stem Cell Communication. *Methods Mol. Biol.* **2015**, *1212*, 39–63. [CrossRef]
62. Kukurba, K.R.; Montgomery, S.B. RNA Sequencing and Analysis. *Cold Spring Harb. Protoc.* **2015**, *2015*, 951–969. [CrossRef] [PubMed]
63. Bray, N.L.; Pimentel, H.; Melsted, P.; Pachter, L. Near-Optimal Probabilistic RNA-Seq Quantification. *Nat. Biotechnol.* **2016**, *34*, 525–527. [CrossRef] [PubMed]
64. Liao, Y.; Wang, J.; Jaehnig, E.J.; Shi, Z.; Zhang, B. WebGestalt 2019: Gene Set Analysis Toolkit with Revamped UIs and APIs. *Nucleic Acids Res.* **2019**, *47*, W199–W205. [CrossRef] [PubMed]
65. Steffin, D.H.M.; Hsieh, E.M.; Rouce, R.H. Gene Therapy: Current Applications and Future Possibilities. *Adv. Pediatr.* **2019**, *66*, 37–54. [CrossRef]
66. Blind, J.E.; McLeod, E.N.; Brown, A.; Patel, H.; Ghosh, S. Biosafety Practices for In Vivo Viral-Mediated Gene Therapy in the Health Care Setting. *Appl. Biosaf.* **2020**, *25*, 194–200. [CrossRef]
67. High, K.A.; Roncarolo, M.G. Gene Therapy. *N. Engl. J. Med.* **2019**, *381*, 455–464. [CrossRef]
68. Berglund, S.; Magalhaes, I.; Gaballa, A.; Vanherberghen, B.; Uhlin, M. Advances in Umbilical Cord Blood Cell Therapy: The Present and the Future. *Expert Opin. Biol. Ther.* **2017**, *17*, 691–699. [CrossRef]

69. Ikeda, Y.; Fukuda, N.; Wada, M.; Matsumoto, T.; Satomi, A.; Yokoyama, S.-I.; Saito, S.; Matsumoto, K.; Kanmatsuse, K.; Mugishima, H. Development of Angiogenic Cell and Gene Therapy by Transplantation of Umbilical Cord Blood with Vascular Endothelial Growth Factor Gene. *Hypertens. Res.* **2004**, *27*, 119–128. [CrossRef]
70. Das, H.; George, J.C.; Joseph, M.; Das, M.; Abdulhameed, N.; Blitz, A.; Khan, M.; Sakthivel, R.; Mao, H.-Q.; Hoit, B.D.; et al. Stem Cell Therapy with Overexpressed VEGF and PDGF Genes Improves Cardiac Function in a Rat Infarct Model. *PLoS ONE* **2009**, *4*, e7325. [CrossRef]
71. Chen, H.K.; Hung, H.F.; Shyu, K.G.; Wang, B.W.; Sheu, J.R.; Liang, Y.J.; Chang, C.C.; Kuan, P. Combined Cord Blood Stem Cells and Gene Therapy Enhances Angiogenesis and Improves Cardiac Performance in Mouse after Acute Myocardial Infarction. *Eur. J. Clin. Investig.* **2005**, *35*, 677–686. [CrossRef]
72. Islamov, R.R.; Rizvanov, A.A.; Fedotova, V.Y.; Izmailov, A.A.; Safiullov, Z.Z.; Garanina, E.E.; Salafutdinov, I.I.; Sokolov, M.E.; Mukhamedyarov, M.A.; Palotás, A. Tandem Delivery of Multiple Therapeutic Genes Using Umbilical Cord Blood Cells Improves Symptomatic Outcomes in ALS. *Mol. Neurobiol.* **2017**, *54*, 4756–4763. [CrossRef] [PubMed]
73. Islamov, R.; Bashirov, F.; Fadeev, F.; Shevchenko, R.; Izmailov, A.; Markosyan, V.; Sokolov, M.; Kuznetsov, M.; Davleeva, M.; Garifulin, R.; et al. Epidural Stimulation Combined with Triple Gene Therapy for Spinal Cord Injury Treatment. *Int. J. Mol. Sci.* **2020**, *21*, 8896. [CrossRef] [PubMed]

Disclaimer/Publisher's Note: The statements, opinions and data contained in all publications are solely those of the individual author(s) and contributor(s) and not of MDPI and/or the editor(s). MDPI and/or the editor(s) disclaim responsibility for any injury to people or property resulting from any ideas, methods, instructions or products referred to in the content.

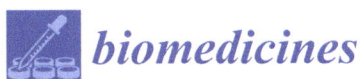

Article

Genetic Association Study and Machine Learning to Investigate Differences in Platelet Reactivity in Patients with Acute Ischemic Stroke Treated with Aspirin

Anna Ikonnikova [1,*], Anastasia Anisimova [2], Sergey Galkin [2], Anastasia Gunchenko [2], Zhabikai Abdukhalikova [2], Marina Filippova [1], Sergey Surzhikov [1], Lidia Selyaeva [1], Valery Shershov [1], Alexander Zasedatelev [1], Maria Avdonina [1] and Tatiana Nasedkina [1]

1. Engelhardt Institute of Molecular Biology, Russian Academy of Sciences, 119991 Moscow, Russia
2. Department of Neurology, Neurosurgery and Medical Genetics, Faculty of Medicine, Pirogov Russian National Research Medical University, Ministry of Health of the Russian Federation, 117997 Moscow, Russia
* Correspondence: anyuik@gmail.com

Abstract: Aspirin resistance (AR) is a pressing problem in current ischemic stroke care. Although the role of genetic variations is widely considered, the data still remain controversial. Our aim was to investigate the contribution of genetic features to laboratory AR measured through platelet aggregation with arachidonic acid (AA) and adenosine diphosphate (ADP) in ischemic stroke patients. A total of 461 patients were enrolled. Platelet aggregation was measured via light transmission aggregometry. Eighteen single-nucleotide polymorphisms (SNPs) in *ITGB3*, *GPIBA*, *TBXA2R*, *ITGA2*, *PLA2G7*, *HMOX1*, *PTGS1*, *PTGS2*, *ADRA2A*, *ABCB1* and *PEAR1* genes and the intergenic *9p21.3* region were determined using low-density biochips. We found an association of rs1330344 in the *PTGS1* gene with AR and AA-induced platelet aggregation. Rs4311994 in *ADRA2A* gene also affected AA-induced aggregation, and rs4523 in the *TBXA2R* gene and rs12041331 in the *PEAR1* gene influenced ADP-induced aggregation. Furthermore, the effect of rs1062535 in the *ITGA2* gene on NIHSS dynamics during 10 days of treatment was found. The best machine learning (ML) model for AR based on clinical and genetic factors was characterized by AUC = 0.665 and F1-score = 0.628. In conclusion, the association study showed that *PTGS1*, *ADRA2A*, *TBXA2R* and *PEAR1* polymorphisms may affect laboratory AR. However, the ML model demonstrated the predominant influence of clinical features.

Keywords: aspirin resistance; genetic markers; genetics; machine learning; CatBoost; ischemic stroke; SNP; pharmacogenetics; platelet aggregation; biochip

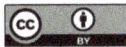

1. Introduction

Aspirin is a key drug widely used for ischemic stroke patients as antiplatelet therapy to prevent recurrent ischemic events [1]. This drug acts by irreversibly blocking the activity of the cyclooxygenases (COX)-1 and -2 also known as prostaglandin G/H synthases 1 and 2 (PTGS1 and PTGS2), respectively [2]. While the COX-1 enzyme is produced constitutively, the COX-2 form is highly inducible, mainly by inflammation. The COX-1 enzyme is expressed in mature platelets and catalyzes the conversion of arachidonic acid (AA) to prostaglandins G2 and H2, with a subsequent production of thromboxane A2 (TXA2) [3,4]. Thromboxane A2 is released into the bloodstream and binds to TXA2 receptors on the surface of neighboring platelets, causing their activation. Additionally, TXA2 acts synergistically with other substances released by activated platelets (adenosine diphosphate (ADP), fibrinogen, factor V) to increase the process. The main antithrombotic effect of low-dose (75–125 mg) aspirin is mediated by selective inhibition of COX-1 [5]. As a result of aspirin action, the production of TXA2, which is the main compound in platelet activation and aggregation, is suppressed for the lifetime of the platelet (7–10 days) [2]. The pathway of TXA2 production and the antiplatelet effect of aspirin are shown in Figure S1.

The response to aspirin varies between individuals, and up to 57% of patients show the so-called aspirin resistance (AR) [6]. AR is classified into clinical and laboratory resistance. Clinical AR is established by the inability of aspirin to prevent the subsequent acute vascular events [7]. Laboratory AR can be defined as ex vivo high on-treatment platelet reactivity (HTPR) such as the insufficient antiplatelet effect of aspirin measured by different laboratory tests [7,8]. Tests measure inactive metabolites of TXA2 in serum or urine [9,10] or analyze platelet aggregation and adhesion. Among the assays that determine platelet function, light transmission aggregometry (LTA) is considered as the gold standard in platelet function testing [11]. Automated (point-of-care) assays such as VerifyNow®, PFA-100®, Multiplate®, Plateletworks® and others are widely used for monitoring platelet response to antiplatelet agents including aspirin [6,12,13]. HTPR was shown to increase the risk of recurrent vascular events and long-term clinical outcomes for patients with cerebrovascular pathology [14–17]. Nevertheless, platelet function tests differ in their ability to predict the risk of cardiovascular outcomes [12].

AR seems to be a complex phenomenon with a number of factors potentially contributing to it, but its causes and mechanisms are still unclear [18]. One of these factors that might underlie AR is heredity, having a profound impact on the variability in residual platelet function during aspirin therapy [19]. Genes encoding key platelet aggregation proteins are under the most intense scrutiny.

A number of genetic markers have already been studied to assess their possible contribution to AR [6,20]. First, single-nucleotide polymorphisms (SNPs) in the genes encoding COX enzymes (*PTGS1* and *PTGS2*) were found to influence AR [21–28]. Polymorphisms in the *TBXA2R* gene, encoding the specific TXA2 receptor, were associated with the effect of aspirin in a number of studies [29–31]. The genes involved in the COX-independent platelet activation pathways as well as platelet glycoprotein genes might also be involved in AR. The effect of polymorphisms in the genes *HMOX1* [24], *PLA2G7* [30], *ADRA2A* [30], *ITGB3* [22,32], *GPIBA* [33], *ITGA2* [34] and *PEAR1* [35–37] on inter-individual variations in the aspirin response has been discussed. A locus on chromosome *9p21.3*, associated with CVD and ischemic stroke, was also connected with AR [30,38]. P-glycoprotein (also known as MDR1) plays a crucial role in the intestinal epithelial cell permeability to aspirin [39] and might be involved in aspirin absorption. The TT rs1045642 genotype in the gene *ABCB1* encoding P-glycoprotein was shown to protect against AR [29]. Therefore, the molecular changes in the pathways involving various genes appear to influence the AR development. However, the impact of genetic markers on the risk for an individual patient is poorly understood. Implementing the identified genetic risk factors to predict aspirin failure in clinical practice still remains challenging.

One problem lies in the inconsistency of the results from genetic studies. This may be explained by the differences in the diagnoses (ischemic stroke, cardiovascular disease, diabetes mellitus), ethnic groups, platelet function tests, sample sizes, etc. [6]. There is a noticeable lack of replication studies analyzing AR genetic background in patients with ischemic stroke from the Eastern European populations.

Another problem is the multiplicity of influencing factors that determine the ultimate success or failure of aspirin therapy. The clinical features of the disease, comorbidities, co-medications and non-modifiable risk factors such as age should be taken into account [6]. Moreover, the interaction of genetic polymorphisms as well as clinical factors may influence sensitivity to aspirin [40]. Over the past several years, machine learning (ML) models have been proven to be able to solve various problems in the medical and biological fields, including pharmacogenetics [41,42]. One of the key advantages of the ML approaches lies in their ability to find unobvious relationships and make inferences from the complex data.

The purpose of this study was to investigate genetic features associated with laboratory AR in a cohort of patients with ischemic stroke taking aspirin as antiplatelet therapy to be used in pharmacogenetic testing. We have developed a biochip assay to identify 18 SNPs previously described as markers affecting AR. To establish the connection between the patients' clinical data, genotype and laboratory response to aspirin treatment, we applied the multiple ML approaches.

2. Materials and Methods

2.1. Patients

The study included 461 Caucasian patients with primary ischemic stroke treated in the Stroke Center of City Clinical Hospital No.1 named N.I. Pirogov. The inclusion criterion was a verified ischemic stroke. Exclusion criteria comprised hemorrhagic transformation, cancer and severe liver disease, as well as other diseases and conditions affecting the parameters of platelet hemostasis. The pathogenetic variant of stroke was established according to the TOAST criteria [43] based on the clinical data, computed tomography and magnetic resonance imaging of the brain, Doppler ultrasound of the cerebral arteries and electrocardiography. The study population included 109 patients with cardioembolism, 98 patients with large artery atherosclerosis (LAA, $\geq$50% stenosis) and 250 patients with undetermined etiology (of which 53 had both LAA and cardioembolism, 197 had neither LAA nor cardioembolism). All patients received the antiplatelet, lipid-lowering, antihypertensive or anticoagulant therapy according to the clinical guidelines. For early prevention of recurrent stroke, all patients took aspirin at a dose of 125 mg daily, starting within 24 h of the stroke onset. Patients with cardioembolic stroke received the anticoagulant treatment starting on day 3, 6 or 12 depending on the stroke severity [44]. Dynamics of the NIHSS score estimated at admission and after 10 days of aspirin therapy was considered as the short-term clinical outcome.

The study was approved by the local ethics committee of the Pirogov Russian National Research Medical University (protocol no. 181 dated 28 January 2019). All participants provided a written informed consent. The study adhered to the World Medical Association Declaration of Helsinki. With a 95% confidence level, a standard deviation of 0.5 and a confidence interval (margin of error) of $\pm$5%, the sample size was estimated to be 391 patients.

2.2. Platelet Aggregation

Blood samples from the vein of the non-paretic limb were collected in the morning of the third day of aspirin intake. The region of the cubital fossa was usually selected as the venipuncture area. A tourniquet was applied to the middle third of the shoulder, while the pulse was taken on the nearest radial artery. After that, the patient clenched the hand into a fist and unclenched it several times. The skin in the venipuncture area was stretched, fixing the vein. Next, the skin was pierced next to the vein; the needle was moved 1.5 cm deep into the subcutaneous fat, and the vein was punctured. A total of 9 mL of blood was collected in the 14 mL plastic test tubes "Greiner" with 1 mL of 3.8% trisubstituted sodium citrate using 21 G $\times$ 1 1/2"/0.8 $\times$ 40 mm needles. The blood in the tube was mixed immediately. Stabilized blood was stored at room temperature for no more than 30 min prior to centrifugation. The samples were centrifuged at 200$\times$ g for 7 min. Then, 2.5 mL of the supernatant containing platelet-rich plasma was carefully taken for analysis in the aggregometer. Platelet aggregation was measured by LTA using the laser analyzer of platelet aggregation ALAT-2 (Biola Scientific, Moscow, Russia) based on the method of Born and O'Brien.

To identify a group of patients with AR, we relied on the criteria proposed by Gum et al. [45]. AR was defined as aggregation of $\geq$70% with 10 μm ADP and aggregation of $\geq$20% with 0.5 mM AA. Aspirin semi-resistance (ASR) was defined as aggregation of $\geq$70% with 10 μM ADP or aggregation of $\geq$20% with 0.5 mM AA [45]. The patients with AR and ASR were pooled into the AR group. Patients with ADP-induced aggregation <70% and AA-induced aggregation <20% were considered aspirin-sensitive (AS) and were assigned to the AS group [22].

2.3. DNA Extraction

Genomic DNA was extracted from the blood collected into the EDTA-containing tubes using the QIamp DNA Mini kit (Qiagen, Hilden, Germany) according to the manufacturer's instructions. DNA was isolated from 200 µL of the whole blood. The procedure included cell lysis, sorption on the silica gel membrane of the column, washing and elution (in 100 µL of elution buffer). The DNA concentration was measured using the NanoDrop 1000 spectrophotometer (Thermo Fisher Scientific, Waltham, MA, USA). DNA samples were subjected to further analysis if DNA concentration was at least 10 ng/µL and its 260/280 ratio was in the range of 1.75 to 1.95.

2.4. Selection of SNPs and Genotyping

Genetic markers in ten genes (*ITGB3*, *GPIBA*, *TBXA2R*, *ITGA2*, *PLA2G7*, *HMOX1*, *PTGS1*, *PTGS2*, *ADRA2A*, *ABCB1*, *PEAR1*) and one intergenic region (*9p21.3*) were selected (Table 1).

Table 1. A list of studied genetic markers.

Gene	rs ID	Wild-Type Allele	Minor Allele	Protein
ITGB3	rs5918	T	C	Platelet glycoprotein IIIa/Integrin subunit-Beta3
GPIBA	rs2243093	T	C	Glycoprotein Ib platelet subunit alpha
	rs6065	C	T	
TBXA2R	rs1131882	C	T	Thromboxane A2 receptor
	rs4523	C	T	
ITGA2	rs1126643	C	T	GPIa/IIa- Integrin alpha 2
	rs1062535	G	A	
PLA2G7	rs1051931	C	T	Lipoprotein-associated phospholipase A2/ Plasma platelet-activating factor acetylhydrolase
	rs7756935	A	C	
HMOX1	rs2071746	A	T	Heme oxygenase 1
PTGS1	rs10306114	A	G	Prostaglandin G/H synthase 1 (cyclooxygenase-1)
	rs1330344	T	C	
PTGS2	rs20417	G	C	Prostaglandin G/H synthase 2 (cyclooxygenase-2)
	rs689466	T	C	
ADRA2A	rs4311994	C	T	Alpha-2A-adrenergic receptor
9p21.3	rs10120688	G	A	Intergenic
ABCB1	rs1045642	T	C	MDR1, ATP-binding cassette subfamily B member 1
PEAR1	rs12041331	G	A	Platelet endothelial aggregation receptor-1

Genotyping involved the multiplex one-step PCR followed by allele-specific hybridization on a biochip as described before [46]. 2′-deoxyuridine 5′-triphosphate (dUTP) derivatives containing the Cy7 cyanine dye were used as fluorophores [47]. The sequences of primers and allele-specific oligonucleotide probes are listed in the Supplementary Tables S1 and S2. The biochip scheme and an example of the hybridization picture are shown in Figure S2. Genotyping results were verified by direct sequencing and high-resolution melting analysis.

2.5. Statistical Analysis

The online service SNPStats (https://www.snpstats.net/ (accessed on 26 April 2022)) [48] was used to evaluate the association of genotypes with aspirin resistance and aggregation with AA and ADP as well as the NIHSS score dynamics (adjusted by clinical variables). We used individual SNPs' data for co-dominant, dominant, recessive and log-additive models. Comparison of baseline characteristics in groups with different genotypes was performed using the Kruskal–Wallis test and the chi-square test. Allele frequencies between AS and AR groups were compared using the two-sided Fisher exact test. Statistical analysis was performed in R (version 4.1.1; R Foundation for Statistical Computing, Vienna, Austria). The differences were considered statistically significant if the p-value was below 0.05. The boxplots display the median, two hinges which correspond to the first and third quartiles and two whiskers. The upper and lower whiskers extend from the hinges to the largest value no further than 1.5×IQR from the corresponding hinge (where IQR is the inter-quartile range). Points beyond the whiskers indicate the outliers.

2.6. Machine Learning

To build a predictive machine learning model, several approaches have been tested using the following Python 3.8 libraries: sklearn.linear_model.LogisticRegression, sklearn.svm.SVC, sklearn.ensemble.RandomForestClassifier [49], XGBoost [50] and CatBoost [51]. All models were trained in a five-fold cross validation (CV) setting with folds stratified to keep the proportion of studies similar to the whole data set. Each model parameter was optimized in order to increase the classification metrics: accuracy, AUC and F1-score, paying the most attention to the latter metric. The array of features consisted of all 16 genetic markers along with the age, gender, NHISS score at admission, body mass index (BMI), atrial fibrillation (AF), stenosis, high-density lipoproteins (HDLs), low-density lipoproteins (LDLs), cholesterol and triglycerides. Feature importance ranking was obtained using Shapley additive explanations (SHAP) values, a game theoretic approach to explain the output of any machine learning model [52]. The sequence of the ML procedure pipeline is shown in Figure 1.

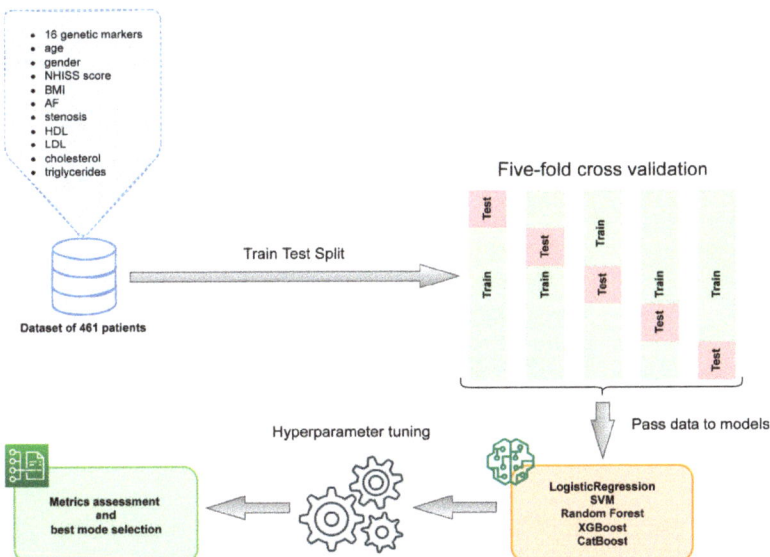

Figure 1. The machine learning pipeline.

3. Results

3.1. Baseline Characteristics of AR and AS Patients

The baseline clinical characteristics of patients are shown in Table 2. A total of 461 patients were included in the analysis. Full AR and ASR were established in 28 patients (6.1%) and 192 patients (41.6%), respectively, and these two groups were pooled into one AR group. Another 241 patients (52.3%) were AS.

Table 2. The clinical characteristics and laboratory parameters in the AS and AR groups.

Characteristics	AS Group (n = 241)	AR Group (n = 220)	p-Value
Age, (mean ± sd)	68.72 ± 14.56	73.21 ± 14.52	<0.001
Sex, n (%)			
women	117 (48.5%)	119 (54.1%)	0.235
Type of stroke according to TOAST criteria, n (%):			
LAA	55 (12.04%)	43 (9.41%)	0.0859
Cardioembolism	49 (10.72%)	60 (13.13%)	
Undetermined etiology (with LAA and Cardioembolism)	22 (4.81%)	31 (6.78%)	
Undetermined etiology (without LAA and Cardioembolism)	113 (24.73%)	84 (18.38%)	
NHISS score at admission, (mean ± sd)	10.45 ± 6.49	12.35 ± 6.67	<0.001
AF, n (%)	71 (29.58%)	91 (41.74%)	0.0088
Stenosis, % (mean ± sd)	11.53 ± 7.18	12.01 ± 7.15	0.5408
BMI, mmol/L (mean ± sd)	27.64 ± 4.83	28.17 ± 4.99	0.2219
HDL, mmol/L (mean ± sd)	1.18 ± 0.34	1.15 ± 0.35	0.3584
LDL, mmol/L (mean ± sd)	2.96 ± 0.97	2.98 ± 0.99	0.9437
Cholesterol, mmol/L (mean ± sd)	4.84 ± 1.24	4.84 ± 1.32	0.9882
Triglycerides, mmol/L (mean ± sd)	1.52 ± 1.15	1.47 ± 0.85	0.4851
Atherogenic coefficient (mean ± sd)	3.22 ± 1.1	3.37 ± 1.24	0.2309

AF—atrial fibrillation, BMI—body mass index, HDL—high-density lipoproteins, LDL—low-density lipoproteins, LAA—large artery atherosclerosis, sd—standard deviation.

The AS and AR groups differed in some clinical parameters (Table 2). AR patients were significantly older: the mean age of 73.21 years in the AR group vs. 68.72 years in the AS group ($p < 0.001$). AR patients had a more severe stroke: the mean NHISS score at admission was 12.35 and 10.45 in the AR and AS group, respectively ($p < 0.001$). Moreover, atrial fibrillation was more frequent in the AR group (41.74%) compared to the AS group (29.58%) ($p = 0.0088$).

3.2. The Association of SNPs with Aspirin Resistance in Whole Cohort of Patients

A total of 461 samples were genotyped for selected SNPs (Table 3). Genotype frequencies in the total sample, AR and AS groups conformed to the Hardy–Weinberg equilibrium (data not shown). The rs1126643 and rs1062535 markers in the *ITGA2* gene as well as rs1051931 and rs7756935 in the *PLA2G7* gene were in strong linkage disequilibrium (D' = 1.0, R2 = 1.0), and only one of them in each pair was included in the analysis.

Table 3. Genotype and allele frequencies in the AS and AR groups.

Gene	rs ID	AS Group					AR Group					p-Value *
		wt, n	het, n	mut, n	Wild-Type Allele, %	Minor Allele, %	wt, n	het, n	mut, n	Wild-Type Allele, %	Minor Allele, %	
ITGB3	rs5918	164	68	9	82	18	148	63	9	82	18	0.864
GPIba	rs2243093	167	68	6	83	17	154	61	5	84	16	0.859
GPIba	rs6065	211	29	1	94	6	182	37	1	91	9	0.173
TBXA2R	rs1131882	162	72	7	82	18	164	50	6	86	14	0.127
TBXA2R	rs4523	92	114	35	62	38	91	99	30	64	36	0.54
ITGA2	rs1062535	87	114	40	60	40	84	109	27	63	37	0.343
PLA2G7	rs1051931	159	75	6	82	18	150	64	6	83	17	0.795
HMOX1	rs2071746	74	120	47	56	44	57	115	48	52	48	0.29
PTGS1	rs10306114	213	28	0	94	6	195	24	1	94	6	1
PTGS1	rs1330344	147	85	8	79	21	119	84	17	73	27	0.044 **
PTGS2	rs20417	166	67	8	83	17	150	62	8	82	18	0.862
PTGS2	rs689466	176	58	7	85	15	163	54	3	86	14	0.638
ADRA2A	rs4311994	188	2	51	78	22	174	41	5	88	12	1
9p21.3	rs10120688	65	131	45	54	46	68	115	37	57	43	0.389
ABCB1	rs1045642	64	120	57	51	49	61	106	53	52	48	0.947
PEAR1	rs12041331	202	37	2	91	9	179	39	2	90	10	0.567

* p-value for comparison of alleles between the AS and AR groups; ** p-value < 0.05

Allele and genotype frequencies for sixteen SNPs in the AS and AR groups are listed in Table 3. The frequency of the minor allele C for rs1330344 *PTGS1* was significantly higher in the AR group than in the AS group (27% vs. 21%, $p = 0.044$).

The association of genotypes with the response to aspirin was investigated using the SNPStats online service. We included age, AF and the NHISS score at admission as covariates in the analysis, since they showed a different distribution between AR and AS groups (Table 2). The results for all studied markers are in Supplementary Table S1 (for AR and AS groups) and Supplementary Table S2 (for AA- and ADP-induced aggregation). We revealed the following associations.

The CC genotype of rs1330344 in the *PTGS1* gene was more frequent in the AR group than in the AS group (OR = 2.75, 95% CI = 1.14–6.63, p = 0.019). Data are shown in Supplementary Table S3.

We compared the association of different genotypes with AA- and ADP-induced aggregation. For *PTGS1* rs1330344, mean AA-induced aggregation was 40.5% higher in the CC genotype compared to the TT + CT genotypes (p = 0.038). For rs4311994 in the *ADRA2A* gene, mean AA-induced aggregation was 72.7% higher in patients with the TT genotype compared to the CC + CT genotypes (p = 0.043). Data are shown in Figure 2 and in Supplementary Table S4.

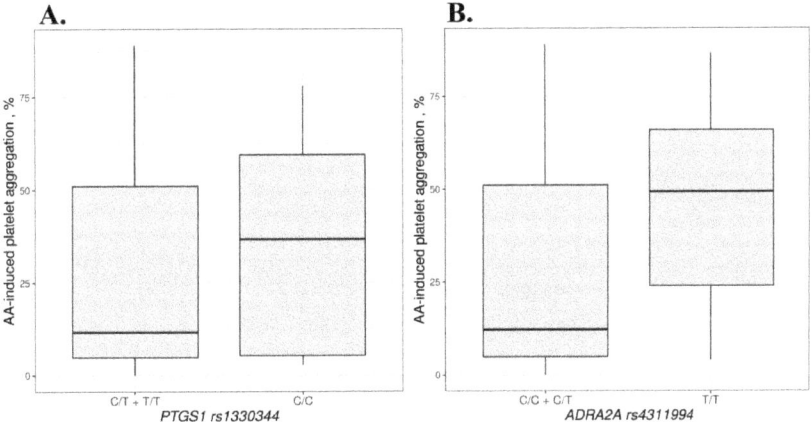

Figure 2. AA-induced aggregation based on the *PTGS1* rs1330344 (**A**) and *ADRA2A* rs4311994 (**B**) genotypes.

Mean ADP-induced aggregation was 9.2% higher in the TT + CT genotypes of *TBXA2R* rs4523 compared to the CC genotype (p = 0.043). For rs12041331 in the *PEAR1* gene, mean ADP-induced aggregation was 59.5% lower in AA homozygotes compared to the GG + GA genotypes (p = 0.017). Data are shown in Figure 3 and in Supplementary Table S2.

3.3. The Association of SNPs with AR and Platelet Reactivity in Patients with Noncardioembolic Ischemic Stroke

In total, 296 patients had noncardioembolic ischemic stroke, with 127 (43%) and 169 (57%) patients being assigned to the AR and AS groups, respectively. We analyzed the frequency of different genotypes for sixteen SNPs in the AR and AS groups. Although the CC genotype of rs1330344 in the *PTGS1* gene was more frequent in the AR group than in the AS group (OR = 2.48, 95% CI = 0.93–6.60, p = 0.062), the difference is not statistically significant.

The CC homozygotes of *PTGS1* rs1330344 had 55.4% higher mean AA-induced aggregation compared to the TT + CT genotypes (p = 0.026). Mean ADP-induced aggregation was 14.8% higher in the TT + CT genotypes of rs4523 *TBXA2R* than in the CC genotypes (p = 0.031) and 11.6% lower in the AA + GA genotypes of *ITGA2* rs1062535 comparing to GG homozygotes (p = 0.051).

Note that p-values are given before the correction for multiple comparisons; after the Bonferroni correction, all p-values were >0.05.

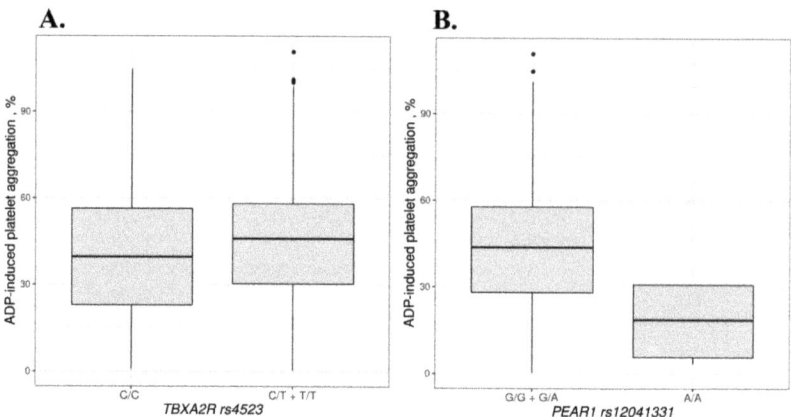

Figure 3. ADP-induced aggregation based on the *TBXA2R* rs4523 (**A**) and *PEAR1* rs12041331 (**B**) genotypes. Dots beyond the whiskers indicate the outliers.

3.4. Clinical Outcome Evaluation

We evaluated the clinical outcomes of patients with noncardioembolic ischemic stroke within the first 10 days after admission and their association with aspirin resistance. Five patients died and were excluded from the analysis. The NIHSS score on day 10 was compared with the admission NIHSS score. We found no statistically significant association of the NIHSS score dynamics analyzed with the groups of AR and AS patients.

Furthermore, the NIHSS score dynamics was evaluated in patients with different genotypes adjusted by age and the NIHSS score at admission. The AA + GA genotypes of rs1062535 in the *ITGA2* gene had worse dynamics in the NIHSS score compared to the GG genotype (5.3 vs. 6.57, $p = 0.0008$).

3.5. Machine Learning Model

To investigate the contribution of clinical and genetic features to AR, we created ML models. The overall best performance was achieved after utilizing CatBoost algorithm, high-performance open-source library for gradient boosting on decision trees. The parameters of the model that showed best performance in CV are listed in the Appendix A. For ML model generation, the total cohort of patients with ischemic stroke was included.

The ML models did not have enough predictive power if they were based only on genetic features. To overcome this limitation, we included anthropometric and clinical data in the model.

After training several models in a five-fold cross-validation setting, we compared the output metrics in order to choose the classification method with the best performance. As expected, the gradient boosting on the decision tree algorithm, CatBoost, outperformed logistic regression, the support vector machine and random forest classifiers since it was designed to leverage the information gained from categorical features. The average values of classification metrics were as follows: AUC = 0.665, F1-score = 0.628, specificity = 0.773, sensitivity = 0.60, precision = 0.63. The ML model is in the Supplementary Files (Model S1).

To assess the impact of each feature on the model performance and identify the most important factors, we conducted the Shapley additive explanations analysis (Figure 4), which allowed us to study the relationships between variables for the predicted case and their contribution to the final score. Shapley values indicate the importance of a feature by comparing model predictions with and without this feature.

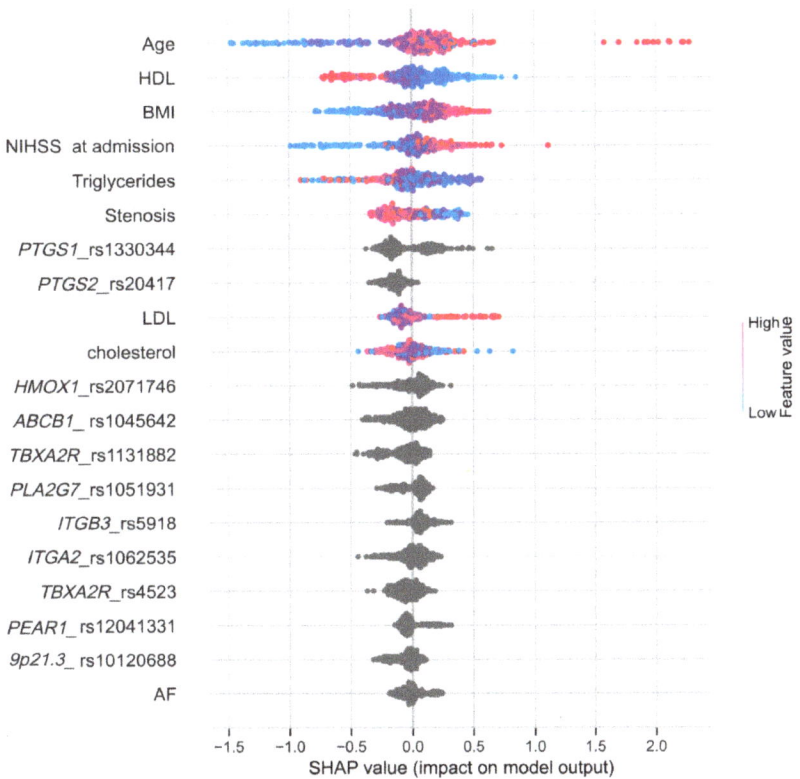

Figure 4. Feature importance ranking obtained using SHAP values. Variables are listed in order of significance from top to bottom on the *y*-axis. Each point represents a patient, and its color indicates the value of corresponding variable. The position of the points on the *x*-axis represents SHAP values, indicating the changes in log odds, and the probability of success can be extracted from this value.

4. Discussion

In the present study, we used a biochip-based assay to analyze 18 SNPs in patients with acute ischemic stroke and variable response to aspirin treatment. The SNPs were selected based on the literature data. All of them are involved in platelet activation and aggregation, and their contribution to aspirin resistance is discussed in numerous studies [6,21–37]. We evaluated the distribution of 16 genetic markers in the AS and AR groups in a cohort of 461 patients with acute ischemic stroke.

The aspirin resistance was associated with the following clinical parameters: age, the NIHSS score at admission and atrial fibrillation (Table 2). Aging is known to be associated with an elevated platelet activity [53] as well as aspirin resistance [45,54], which is consistent with our results. The initial NIHSS score was also higher in the AR patients [55]. In several studies concerning AR, ischemic stroke patients with atrial fibrillation (cardioembolism) were excluded from the analysis since they had anticoagulant therapy prescribed earlier [21,22]. In our study, all patients with all stroke variants received aspirin at least for the first 3 days, while laboratory AR was estimated during this period. This allowed us to enroll all the patients in the study, which aimed at identifying the associations between genetic markers and aspirin non-sensitivity. In addition, we performed the association studies in a cohort of non-embolic patients and evaluated clinical recovery for 10 days based on the NIHSS score dynamics. Determining the prognostic genetic markers of AR in this group can be very helpful given that the long-term aspirin treatment is recommended for these patients.

Among 16 SNPs studied, four genetic variants showed a significant association with aspirin non-sensitivity in the whole cohort: *PTGS1* (rs1330344), *ADRA2A* (rs4311994), *TBXA2R* (rs4523) and *PEAR1* (rs12041331).

The C allele and CC genotype (rs1330344) of the *PTGS1* gene encoding COX-1 were associated with AR and a higher level of AA-induced aggregation. A similar observation was made in the study by Li et.al. [23]. The CC genotype was associated with poor functional outcomes in Chinese patients with a stroke during aspirin therapy [40,56]. However, the obtained results were not always consistent [24,30,57,58]. This polymorphism is located in the regulatory region (T-1676C), and this substitution may lead to an increase in COX-1 activity and contribute to a decreased or absent response to aspirin [6]. The C allele was also found to be associated with an increased risk of ischemic stroke in the Chinese population [59]. However, in our study, rs10306114 in this gene, most frequently associated with AR [6], showed no association with AR.

Another polymorphism that demonstrated an association with AA-induced aggregation in our study, rs4311994, is also located in the regulatory region downstream (63 kb) of the 3′ end of the *ADRA2A* gene; its effect may arise from the regulation of gene expression or linkage disequilibrium with the other variants. In our study, the minor allele T of the *ADRA2A* gene (rs4311994) was associated with a higher level of AA-induced aggregation. The *ADRA2A* gene encodes the alpha-2A-adrenergic receptor involved in epinephrine-induced platelet aggregation and shear-dependent platelet function. This allele was associated with increased platelet reactivity to aspirin in the population with type 2 diabetes mellitus. [30]. However, these results were not always reproducible [60].

Notably, the alleles of the *PTGS1* and *ADRA2A* genes, associated with AR and/or high AA-induced aggregation in our study, correlated with a reduced risk of complications from the gastrointestinal tract when taking aspirin in other studies [61–63]. This may indicate a role in stimulating platelet activity in carriers of these alleles.

The *TBXA2R* rs4523 (T924C) affected ADP-induced aggregation: the aggregation was higher in the TT and CT genotypes than in the CC genotype. In other studies, the TT homozygotes also showed increased platelet reactivity [64,65]. It is a synonymous nucleotide change that can affect splicing or mRNA stabilization and translation efficiency. Otherwise, this SNP may be in linkage disequilibrium with other clinically relevant polymorphisms [64,65]. The other SNP (rs1131882) in the *TBXA2R* gene showed no association with AR in our study.

The ADP-induced aggregation was affected by intronic rs12041331 in the *PEAR1* gene being lower in the AA homozygote as compared to the GG and GA genotypes. These data are consistent with some other studies [19,37,66,67]. The *PEAR1* gene encodes the type 1 membrane protein expressed in platelets and endothelial cells. Its phosphorylation appears to promote platelet aggregation [68,69]. The rs12041331 polymorphism results in a G to A substitution in intron 1 and was previously shown to be implicated in reducing *PEAR1* expression [19]. According to Faraday et al. [19], the major G allele of rs12041331 was associated with a higher platelet aggregation both in the presence and absence of aspirin treatment. Thus, the influence of the *PEAR1* gene may not be specific to the aspirin action. The AA genotype of *PEAR1* rs12041331 was shown to be associated with an increased response to ticagrelor in healthy people [70]. However, some studies revealed no such association for this SNP [71].

In patients with noncardioembolic stroke, the polymorphism *PTGS1* rs1330344 showed a significant association with AA-induced aggregation. Thus, *PTGS1* rs1330344 might be considered as the strongest predictor of laboratory AR among the analyzed SNPs, both in the whole cohort of ischemic stroke and noncardioembolic patients. The second genetic marker associated with laboratory AR in both cohorts was rs4523 in *TBXA2R* gene. The T allele acted as a risk factor for increased ADP-induced aggregation during aspirin treatment.

An ambiguous association for *ITGA2* rs1062535 was revealed in noncardioembolic patients. The *ITGA2* gene encodes the alpha chain of the platelet collagen receptor integrin α2β1 (glycoprotein IA/IIa, GPIa/IIa), which promotes an initial interaction between platelets and collagen with further platelet activation and aggregation. The A allele of rs1062535 was suggested to stimulate the protein expression and increase affinity to collagen, which in turn facilitated platelet reactivity. The A allele of *ITGA2* rs1062535 was significantly associated with reduced post-operative bleeding after cardiac surgery [72]. In our study, on the contrary, the AA + GA genotypes correlated with lower ADP-induced aggregation. In contrast, in previously published data, the A allele was considered as a possible risk factor for thromboischaemic events [73]. This suggestion is in agreement with our findings implying a strong relationship between the A allele and negative NIHSS dynamics in noncardioembolic patients.

Thus, the role of genetic factors underlying the inter-individual differences in aspirin action is of immense interest, but further research is required to understand how genetic data can be efficiently applied to personalized therapy. Different approaches, such as general multifactor dimensionality reduction (GMDR), were employed to study the potential contribution of multiple genetic factors along with the single-locus analysis [22].

We applied the ML method to predict the risk of AR development using clinical and genetic factors. This is the first attempt to bring in the ML approach to the analysis of genetics of AR. We obtained an AUC = 0.665 for our best model (Model S1, Figure 4). On the one hand, this value seems to be modest, but on the other hand, it is in agreement with the parameters of other models based on ML for multifactorial processes. For example, similar sensitivity and specificity values were obtained for antidepressants [74,75]. However, in those studies, these parameters were obtained only from the genetic factors, whereas in our study they mainly depended on clinical factors. The developed ML model may be considered as a first approximation aimed at dealing with the problem of AR prediction. The relevance of the developed model for clinical practice is still to be confirmed. We assume that further studies involving larger and more clinically uniform cohorts of patients are required to shed light on the genetic background contributing to the resistance to aspirin treatment. Another approach relies on searching for more relevant genetic markers utilizing throughput methods of genetic analysis such as the next-generation sequencing. The assessment of polygenic risk score might prove promising as well.

As there is an alternative to aspirin for secondary stroke prevention, such as dual antiplatelet therapy or ticagrelor [76], identifying patients with a predisposition to AR can be used for personalized therapy to reduce the risk of adverse events. However, it is possible that the risk alleles for AR might also be associated with platelet aggregation when taking other antiplatelet drugs requiring special attention for such patients.

The current study has several limitations. First, when choosing genetic polymorphisms, we relied on the published studies focusing on certain candidate genetic markers. Searching for more relevant genetic markers using such high-throughput methods of genetic analysis as next-generation sequencing may prove promising. Moreover, given the complex nature of aspirin resistance, the polygenic risk score may be introduced for identifying patients with a high risk of aspirin treatment failure. The second limitation is related to the size of the studied population. It seems to be large enough compared with other studies in the field [21,24–34]. However, clarifying the genetic background of aspirin treatment failure, which is affected by numerous clinical parameters and studied SNPs, requires further studies including larger and more clinically uniform cohorts of patients. The third limitation may be related to clinical outcome assessment. A number of studies confirmed an increased risk of adverse outcomes in patients with laboratory AR [14–17]. However, the underlying mechanism of a poor response to aspirin is still unclear. The ex vivo platelet reactivity tests do not always clearly correlate with the therapeutic effect of the drug [77]. Our study focused on analyzing laboratory AR, but the most important results can be obtained from the long-term follow-up of patients and assessing the influence of genetic and clinical factors and laboratory measurements of AR on clinical outcomes. Finally, in our study, we were not always able to take into account the potential impact of other drugs used by our patients, such as anticoagulants or statins, which are usually prescribed for the secondary prevention of a stroke. The drug–drug interactions as well as malabsorption or renal dysfunction could also affect aspirin pharmacokinetics or pharmacodynamics and thus lead to a number of subsequent pharmacological effects [78,79].

5. Conclusions

Early detection of aspirin resistance in ischemic stroke patients is important for timely prescription of other antiaggregant drugs when possible. Therefore, searching for predictive markers of aspirin treatment failure is of great importance. In our study, we revealed the association between clinical parameters (age, NIHSS score, atrial fibrillation), as well as SNPs in the *PTGS1*, *ADRA2A*, *TBXA2R* and *PEAR1* genes, and laboratory indicators of platelet activity in ischemic stroke patients taking aspirin for secondary stroke prevention. The ML model of AR in the studied cohort of patients showed the prevailing contribution of clinical parameters. However, we assume that the genetic factors are a promising predictor of aspirin resistance. The ML approach revealed the prospective future directions of predicting the risk of AR development. Further replication studies including more homogeneous groups of patients, the implementation of high-throughput genotyping technologies and development of risk-predictive models based both on clinical and genetic features may be considered as key steps towards better understanding aspirin resistance in patients with an ischemic stroke.

Supplementary Materials: The following supporting information can be downloaded at: https://www.mdpi.com/article/10.3390/biomedicines10102564/s1. Figure S1: The pathway of TXA2 production and the antiplatelet effect of aspirin.; Figure S2: The biochip scheme and an example of analysis.; Table S1: Primer sequences.; Table S2: Allele-specific oligonucleotide probe sequences.; Table S3: Distribution of genetic markers in AS- and AR-groups.; Table S4: AA- and ADP-induced aggregation based on genotypes.; Model S1: ML model for aspirin resistance.

Author Contributions: Conceptualization, A.A. and T.N.; methodology, A.I., S.G., A.G., Z.A., M.F., S.S., V.S. and L.S.; validation, A.I., L.S., V.S. and Z.A.; formal analysis, A.I., S.G., Z.A. and A.G.; investigation, A.I., S.G., A.A. and T.N; resources, A.A. and S.G.; writing—original draft preparation, A.I., M.A. and S.G.; writing—review and editing, A.A., T.N. and A.Z.; visualization, A.I.; supervision, A.Z.; project administration, A.A., T.N. and A.Z.; funding acquisition, T.N. and A.Z. All authors have read and agreed to the published version of the manuscript.

Funding: The work was carried out with the support of the state program 0103-2018-0003.

Institutional Review Board Statement: The study was approved by the local ethics committee of the Pirogov Russian National Research Medical University (protocol number 181 dated 28 January 2019).

Informed Consent Statement: Informed consent was obtained from all subjects involved in the study.

Data Availability Statement: The data presented in this study are available on request from the corresponding author.

Conflicts of Interest: The authors declare no conflict of interest.

Appendix A Parameters of the Best-Performing Model

```
loss_function = 'Logloss'
learning_rate = 0.01
Iterations = 500
depth = 10
grow_policy = 'Lossguide'
max_leaves = 30
od_type = 'IncToDec'
od_pval = 0.05
od_wait = 10
```

References

1. Rothwell, P.M.; Algra, A.; Chen, Z.; Diener, H.-C.; Norrving, B.; Mehta, Z. Effects of aspirin on risk and severity of early recurrent stroke after transient ischaemic attack and ischaemic stroke: Time-course analysis of randomised trials. *Lancet* **2016**, *388*, 365–375. [CrossRef] [PubMed]
2. Capodanno, D.; Angiolillo, D.J. Aspirin for Primary Cardiovascular Risk Prevention and Beyond in Diabetes Mellitus. *Circulation* **2016**, *134*, 1579–1594. [CrossRef] [PubMed]
3. Zhao, J.; Zheng, L.; Fei, Q.; Fu, Y.; Weng, Y.; Wu, H.; Li, H.; Jun, Q.; Shao, J.; Xu, Y. Association of thromboxane A2 receptor gene polymorphisms with cerebral infarction in a Chinese population. *Neurol. Sci.* **2013**, *34*, 1791–1796. [CrossRef] [PubMed]
4. Goodman, T.; Ferro, A.; Sharma, P. Pharmacogenetics of aspirin resistance: A comprehensive systematic review. *Br. J. Clin. Pharmacol.* **2008**, *66*, 222–232. [CrossRef] [PubMed]
5. SSantos-Gallego, C.G.; Badimon, J. Overview of Aspirin and Platelet Biology. *Am. J. Cardiol.* **2021**, *144*, S2–S9. [CrossRef]
6. Ferreira, M.; Freitas-Silva, M.; Assis, J.; Pinto, R.; Nunes, J.P.; Medeiros, R. The emergent phenomenon of aspirin resistance: Insights from genetic association studies. *Pharmacogenomics* **2020**, *21*, 125–140. [CrossRef]
7. Kuliczkowski, W.; Witkowski, A.; Polonski, L.; Watala, C.; Filipiak, K.; Budaj, A.; Golanski, J.; Sitkiewicz, D.; Pregowski, J.; Gorski, J.; et al. Interindividual variability in the response to oral antiplatelet drugs: A position paper of the Working Group on antiplatelet drugs resistance appointed by the Section of Cardiovascular Interventions of the Polish Cardiac Society, endorsed by the Working Group on Thrombosis of the European Society of Cardiology. *Eur. Heart J.* **2008**, *30*, 426–435. [CrossRef]
8. Grinstein, J.; Cannon, C.P. Aspirin resistance: Current status and role of tailored therapy. *Clin. Cardiol.* **2012**, *35*, 673–680. [CrossRef]
9. Lordkipanidzé, M.; Pharand, C.; Schampaert, E.; Turgeon, J.; Palisaitis, D.A.; Diodati, J.G. A comparison of six major platelet function tests to determine the prevalence of aspirin resistance in patients with stable coronary artery disease. *Eur. Heart J.* **2007**, *28*, 1702–1708. [CrossRef]
10. Van Oosterom, N.; Barras, M.; Cottrell, N.; Bird, R. Platelet Function Assays for the Diagnosis of Aspirin Resistance. *Platelets* **2021**, *33*, 329–338. [CrossRef]
11. Le Blanc, J.; Mullier, F.; Vayne, C.; Lordkipanidzé, M. Advances in Platelet Function Testing—Light Transmission Aggregometry and Beyond. *J. Clin. Med.* **2020**, *9*, 2636. [CrossRef]
12. Venketasubramanian, N.; Agustin, S.J.; Padilla, J.L.; Yumul, M.P.; Sum, C.; Lee, S.H.; Ponnudurai, K.; Gan, R.N. Comparison of Different Laboratory Tests to Identify "Aspirin Resistance" and Risk of Vascular Events among Ischaemic Stroke Patients: A Double-Blind Study. *J. Cardiovasc. Dev. Dis.* **2022**, *9*, 156. [CrossRef] [PubMed]
13. Khan, H.; Jain, S.; Gallant, R.C.; Syed, M.H.; Zamzam, A.; Al-Omran, M.; Rand, M.L.; Ni, H.; Abdin, R.; Qadura, M. Plateletworks® as a Point-of-Care Test for ASA Non-Sensitivity. *J. Pers. Med.* **2021**, *11*, 813. [CrossRef] [PubMed]
14. Fiolaki, A.; Katsanos, A.H.; Kyritsis, A.P.; Papadani, S.; Kosmidou, M.; Moschonas, I.C.; Tselepis, A.D.; Giannopoulos, S. High on treatment platelet reactivity to aspirin and clopidogrel in ischemic stroke: A systematic review and meta-analysis. *J. Neurol. Sci.* **2017**, *376*, 112–116. [CrossRef]
15. Lv, H.; Yang, Z.; Wu, H.; Liu, M.; Mao, X.; Liu, X.; Ding, H.; Shi, Z.; Zhou, Y.; Liu, Q.; et al. High On-Treatment Platelet Reactivity as Predictor of Long-term Clinical Outcomes in Stroke Patients with Antiplatelet Agents. *Transl. Stroke Res.* **2021**, *13*, 391–398. [CrossRef]
16. Sikora, J.; Karczmarska-Wódzka, A.; Bugieda, J.; Sobczak, P. The Importance of Platelets Response during Antiplatelet Treatment after Ischemic Stroke—Between Benefit and Risk: A Systematic Review. *Int. J. Mol. Sci.* **2022**, *23*, 1043. [CrossRef]
17. Wiśniewski, A.; Filipska, K.; Sikora, J.; Kozera, G. Aspirin Resistance Affects Medium-Term Recurrent Vascular Events after Cerebrovascular Incidents: A Three-Year Follow-up Study. *Brain Sci.* **2020**, *10*, 179. [CrossRef]
18. Wiśniewski, A. Multifactorial Background for a Low Biological Response to Antiplatelet Agents Used in Stroke Prevention. *Medicina* **2021**, *57*, 59. [CrossRef]
19. Faraday, N.; Yanek, L.R.; Mathias, R.; Herrera-Galeano, J.E.; Vaidya, D.; Moy, T.F.; Fallin, M.D.; Wilson, A.F.; Bray, P.F.; Becker, L.C.; et al. Heritability of platelet responsiveness to aspirin in activation pathways directly and indirectly related to cyclooxygenase-1. *Circulation* **2007**, *115*, 2490–2496. [CrossRef]
20. Strisciuglio, T.; Franco, D.; Di Gioia, G.; De Biase, C.; Morisco, C.; Trimarco, B.; Barbato, E. Impact of genetic polymorphisms on platelet function and response to anti platelet drugs. *Cardiovasc. Diagn. Ther.* **2018**, *8*, 610–620. [CrossRef]
21. Yi, X.; Cheng, W.; Lin, J.; Zhou, Q.; Wang, C. Interaction between COX-1 and COX-2 Variants Associated with Aspirin Resistance in Chinese Stroke Patients. *J. Stroke Cerebrovasc. Dis.* **2016**, *25*, 2136–2144. [CrossRef] [PubMed]
22. Yi, X.; Wang, C.; Zhou, Q.; Lin, J. Interaction among COX-2, P2Y1 and GPIIIa gene variants is associated with aspirin resistance and early neurological deterioration in Chinese stroke patients. *BMC Neurol.* **2017**, *17*, 4. [CrossRef] [PubMed]
23. Li, X.-L.; Cao, J.; Fan, L.; Wang, Q.; Ye, L.; Cui, C.-P.; Wang, Y.-Z.; Liu, L.; Li, B.; Wu, R.-J.; et al. Genetic polymorphisms of *ho-1* and *cox-1* are associated with aspirin resistance defined by light transmittance aggregation in chinese han patients. *Clin. Appl. Thromb.* **2012**, *19*, 513–521. [CrossRef] [PubMed]
24. Xu, Z.-H.; Jiao, J.-R.; Yang, R.; Luo, B.-Y.; Wang, X.-F.; Wu, F. Aspirin resistance: Clinical significance and genetic polymorphism. *J. Int. Med. Res.* **2012**, *40*, 282–292. [CrossRef]
25. Halushka, M.; Walker, L.P. Genetic variation in cyclooxygenase 1: Effects on response to aspirin. *Clin. Pharmacol. Ther.* **2003**, *73*, 122–130. [CrossRef]

26. Kunicki, T.J.; Williams, S.A.; Nugent, D.J.; Harrison, P.; Segal, H.C.; Syed, A.; Rothwell, P.M. Lack of association between aspirin responsiveness and seven candidate gene haplotypes in patients with symptomatic vascular disease. *Thromb. Haemost.* **2009**, *101*, 123–133.
27. Ulehlova, J.; Slavik, L.; Kucerova, J.; Krcova, V.; Vaclavik, J.; Indrak, K. Genetic polymorphisms of platelet receptors in patients with acute myocardial infarction and resistance to antiplatelet therapy. *Genet. Test. Mol. Biomark.* **2014**, *18*, 599–604. [CrossRef]
28. Maree, A.O.; Curtin, R.J.; Chubb, A.; Dolan, C.; Cox, D.; O'Brien, J.; Crean, P.; Shields, D.C.; Fitzgerald, D.J. Cyclooxygenase-1 haplotype modulates platelet response to aspirin. *J. Thromb. Haemost.* **2005**, *3*, 2340–2345. [CrossRef]
29. Peng, L.-L.; Zhao, Y.-Q.; Zhou, Z.-Y.; Jin, J.; Zhao, M.; Chen, X.-M.; Chen, L.; Cai, Y.-F.; Li, J.-L.; Huang, M. Associations of MDR1, TBXA2R, PLA2G7, and PEAR1 genetic polymorphisms with the platelet activity in Chinese ischemic stroke patients receiving aspirin therapy. *Acta Pharmacol. Sin.* **2016**, *37*, 1442–1448. [CrossRef]
30. Postula, M.; Kaplon-Cieslicka, A.; Rosiak, M.; Kondracka, A.; Serafin, A.; Filipiak, K.J.; Członkowski, A.; Opolski, G.; Janicki, P.K. Genetic determinants of platelet reactivity during acetylsalicylic acid therapy in diabetic patients: Evaluation of 27 polymorphisms within candidate genes. *J. Thromb. Haemost.* **2011**, *9*, 2291–2301. [CrossRef]
31. Milanowski, L.; Pordzik, J.; Janicki, P.K.; Kaplon-Cieslicka, A.; Rosiak, M.; Peller, M.; Tyminska, A.; Ozieranski, K.; Filipiak, K.J.; Opolski, G.; et al. New single-nucleotide polymorphisms associated with differences in platelet reactivity and their influence on survival in patients with type 2 diabetes treated with acetylsalicylic acid: An observational study. *Geol. Rundsch.* **2016**, *54*, 343–351. [CrossRef]
32. Szczeklik, A.; Undas, A.; Sanak, M.; Frołow, M.; Węgrzyn, W. Relationship between bleeding time, aspirin and the PlA1/A2 polymorphism of platelet glycoprotein IIIa. *Br. J. Haematol.* **2000**, *110*, 965–967. [CrossRef]
33. Al-Azzam, S.I.; Alzoubi, K.H.; Khabour, O.F.; Tawalbeh, D.; Al-Azzeh, O. The contribution of platelet glycoproteins (GPIa C807T and GPIba C-5T) and cyclooxygenase 2 (COX-2G-765C) polymorphisms to platelet response in patients treated with aspirin. *Gene* **2013**, *526*, 118–121. [CrossRef]
34. Wang, H.; Sun, X.; Dong, W.; Cai, X.; Zhou, Y.; Zhang, Y.; Jiang, W.; Fang, Q. Association of GPIa and COX-2 gene polymorphism with aspirin resistance. *J. Clin. Lab. Anal.* **2017**, *32*, e22331. [CrossRef]
35. Xiang, Q.; Zhou, S.; Lewis, J.P.; Shuldiner, A.R.; Ren, G.; Cui, Y. Genetic Variants of PEAR1 are Associated with Platelet Function and Antiplatelet Drug Efficacy: A Systematic Review and Meta-Analysis. *Curr. Pharm. Des.* **2018**, *23*, 6815–6827. [CrossRef] [PubMed]
36. Li, Z.; Jiang, H.; Ding, Y.; Zhang, D.; Zhang, X.; Xue, J.; Ma, R.; Hu, L.; Yue, Y. Platelet Endothelial Aggregation Receptor 1 Polymorphism Is Associated With Functional Outcome in Small-Artery Occlusion Stroke Patients Treated With Aspirin. *Front. Cardiovasc. Med.* **2021**, *8*, 664012. [CrossRef] [PubMed]
37. Lewis, J.P.; Ryan, K.; O'Connell, J.R.; Horenstein, R.B.; Damcott, C.M.; Gibson, Q.; Pollin, T.I.; Mitchell, B.D.; Beitelshees, A.L.; Pakzy, R.; et al. Genetic variation in PEAR1 is associated with platelet aggregation and cardiovascular outcomes. *Circ. Cardiovasc. Genet.* **2013**, *6*, 184–192. [CrossRef]
38. Musunuru, K.; Post, W.S.; Herzog, W.; Shen, H.; O'Connell, J.R.; McArdle, P.F.; Ryan, K.A.; Gibson, Q.; Cheng, Y.-C.; Clearfield, E.; et al. Association of single nucleotide polymorphisms on chromosome 9p21.3 with platelet reactivity: A potential mechanism for increased vascular disease. Circ Cardiovasc Genet. *Circ. Cardiovasc. Genet.* **2010**, *3*, 445–453. [CrossRef]
39. Kugai, M.; Uchiyama, K.; Tsuji, T.; Yoriki, H.; Fukui, A.; Qin, Y.; Higashimura, Y.; Mizushima, K.; Yoshida, N.; Katada, K.; et al. MDR1 is Related to intestinal epithelial injury induced by acetylsalicylic acid. *Cell. Physiol. Biochem.* **2013**, *32*, 942–950. [CrossRef] [PubMed]
40. Cai, H.; Cai, B.; Sun, L.; Zhang, H.; Zhou, S.; Cao, L.; Guo, H.; Sun, W.; Yan, B.; Davis, S.M.; et al. Association between PTGS1 polymorphisms and functional outcomes in Chinese patients with stroke during aspirin therapy: Interaction with smoking. *J. Neurol. Sci.* **2017**, *376*, 211–215. [CrossRef] [PubMed]
41. Cilluffo, G.; Fasola, S.; Ferrante, G.; Malizia, V.; Montalbano, L.; La Grutta, S. Machine Learning: An Overview and Applications in Pharmacogenetics. *Genes* **2021**, *12*, 1511. [CrossRef] [PubMed]
42. Wei, W.; Zhao, J.; Roden, D.M.; Peterson, J.F. Machine Learning Challenges in Pharmacogenomic Research. *Clin. Pharmacol. Ther.* **2021**, *110*, 552–554. [CrossRef]
43. Madden, K.P.; Karanjia, P.N.; Adams, H.P.; Clarke, W.R. Accuracy of initial stroke subtype diagnosis in the TOAST study. Trial of ORG 10172 in Acute Stroke Treatment. *Neurology* **1995**, *45*, 1975–1979. [CrossRef]
44. Kirchhof, P.; Benussi, S.; Kotecha, D.; Ahlsson, A.; Atar, D.; Casadei, B.; Castella, M.; Diener, H.-C.; Heidbuchel, H.; Hendriks, J.; et al. 2016 ESC Guidelines for the management of atrial fibrillation developed in collaboration with EACTS. *Eur. Heart J.* **2016**, *37*, 2893–2962. [CrossRef]
45. Gum, P.A.; Kottke-Marchant, K.; Welsh, P.A.; White, J.; Topol, E.J. A prospective, blinded determination of the natural history of aspirin resistance among stable patients with cardiovascular disease. *J. Am. Coll. Cardiol.* **2003**, *41*, 961–965. [CrossRef]
46. Ikonnikova, A.Y.; Filippova, M.A.; Surzhikov, S.A.; Pozhitnova, V.O.; Kazakov, R.E.; Lisitsa, T.S.; Belkov, S.A.; Nasedkina, T.V. Biochip-based approach for comprehensive pharmacogenetic testing. *Drug Metab. Drug Interact.* **2020**, *36*, 33–40. [CrossRef]
47. Shershov, V.E.; Ikonnikova, A.Y.; Vasiliskov, V.A.; Lapa, S.A.; Miftakhov, R.A.; Kuznetsova, V.E.; Chudinov, A.V.; Nasedkina, T.V. The Efficiency of DNA Labeling with Near-Infrared Fluorescent Dyes. *Biophysics* **2020**, *65*, 736–741. [CrossRef]
48. Solé, X.; Guinó, E.; Valls, J.; Iniesta, R.; Moreno, V. SNPStats: A web tool for the analysis of association studies. *Bioinformatics* **2006**, *22*, 1928–1929. [CrossRef] [PubMed]

49. Pedregosa, F.; Varoquaux, G.; Gramfort, A.; Michel, V.; Thirion, B.; Grisel, O.; Duchesnay, E. Scikit-learn: Machine learning in Python. *J. Mach. Learn. Res.* **2011**, *12*, 2825–2830.
50. Chen, T.; Guestrin, C. Xgboost: A scalable tree boosting system. In Proceedings of the 22nd Acm Sigkdd International Conference on Knowledge Discovery and Data Mining, San Francisco, CA, USA, 13–17 August 2016.
51. Dorogush; Veronika, A.; Ershov, V.; Gulin, A. CatBoost: Gradient boosting with categorical features support. *arXiv* **2018**, arXiv:1810.11363.
52. Lundberg; Scott, M.; Lee, S. A unified approach to interpreting model predictions. *Adv. Neural Inf. Process. Syst.* **2017**, *30*, 4768–4777.
53. Le Blanc, J.; Lordkipanidzé, M. Platelet Function in Aging. *Front. Cardiovasc. Med.* **2019**, *6*, 109. [CrossRef]
54. Oh, M.S.; Yu, K.-H.; Lee, J.-H.; Jung, S.; Kim, C.; Jang, M.U.; Lee, J.; Lee, B.C. Aspirin resistance is associated with increased stroke severity and infarct volume. *Neurology* **2016**, *86*, 1808–1817. [CrossRef]
55. Ghorbani-Shirkouhi, S.; Ashouri, F.; Neshin, S.A.S.; Saberi, A.; Hasanzadeh, B.; Shahshahani, P. The prevalence and associated factors of aspirin resistance among prophylactic aspirin users. *Rom. J. Neurol.* **2021**, *20*, 50–56. [CrossRef]
56. Cao, L.; Zhang, Z.; Sun, W.; Bai, W.; Sun, W.; Zhang, Y.; Wang, X.; Cai, B.; Xie, X.; Duan, Z.; et al. Impacts of COX-1 gene polymorphisms on vascular outcomes in patients with ischemic stroke and treated with aspirin. *Gene* **2014**, *546*, 172–176. [CrossRef]
57. Pettinella, C.; Romano, M.; Stuppia, L.; Santilli, F.; Liani, R.; Davì, G. Cyclooxygenase-1 haplotype C50T/A-842G does not affect platelet response to aspirin. *Thromb. Haemost.* **2009**, *101*, 687–690. [CrossRef] [PubMed]
58. Li, Q.; Chen, B.-L.; Ozdemir, V.; Ji, W.; Mao, Y.-M.; Wang, L.-C.; Lei, H.-P.; Fan, L.; Zhang, W.; Liu, J.; et al. Frequency of genetic polymorphisms of COX1, GPIIIa and P2Y1 in a Chinese population and association with attenuated response to aspirin. *Pharmacogenomics* **2007**, *8*, 577–586. [CrossRef] [PubMed]
59. Zhao, L.; Fang, J.; Zhou, M.; Zhou, J.; Yu, L.; Chen, N.; He, L. Interaction between COX-1 and COX-2 increases susceptibility to ischemic stroke in a Chinese population. *BMC Neurol.* **2019**, *19*, 291. [CrossRef]
60. Johnson, A.D.; Yanek, L.R.; Chen, M.-H.; Faraday, N.; Larson, M.; Tofler, G.; Lin, S.J.; Kraja, A.T.; Province, M.A.; Yang, Q.; et al. Genome-wide meta-analyses identifies seven loci associated with platelet aggregation in response to agonists. *Nat. Genet.* **2010**, *42*, 608–613. [CrossRef] [PubMed]
61. Forgerini, M.; Urbano, G.; de Nadai, T.R.; Batah, S.S.; Fabro, A.T.; Mastroianni, P.D.C. Genetic Variants in PTGS1 and NOS3 Genes Increase the Risk of Upper Gastrointestinal Bleeding: A Case-Control Study. *Front. Pharmacol.* **2021**, *12*, 671835. [CrossRef] [PubMed]
62. Mallah, N.; Zapata-Cachafeiro, M.; Aguirre, C.; Ibarra-García, E.; Palacios–Zabalza, I.; Macías-García, F.; Domínguez-Muñoz, J.E.; Piñeiro-Lamas, M.; Ibáñez, L.; Vidal, X.; et al. Influence of Polymorphisms Involved in Platelet Activation and Inflammatory Response on Aspirin-Related Upper Gastrointestinal Bleeding: A Case-Control Study. *Front. Pharmacol.* **2020**, *11*, 860. [CrossRef]
63. Wu, Y.; Hu, Y.; You, P.; Chi, Y.-J.; Zhou, J.-H.; Zhang, Y.-Y.; Liu, Y.-L. Study of Clinical and Genetic Risk Factors for Aspirin-induced Gastric Mucosal Injury. *Chin. Med. J.* **2016**, *129*, 174–180. [CrossRef]
64. Fujiwara, T.; Ikeda, M.; Esumi, K.; Fujita, T.D.; Kono, M.; Tokushige, H.; Hatoyama, T.; Maeda, T.; Asai, T.; Ogawa, T.; et al. Exploratory aspirin resistance trial in healthy Japanese volunteers (J-ART) using platelet aggregation as a measure of thrombogenicity. *Pharm. J.* **2007**, *7*, 395–403. [CrossRef]
65. Wang, Z.; Gao, F.; Men, J.; Yang, J.; Modi, P.; Wei, M. Polymorphisms and high on-aspirin platelet reactivity after off-pump coronary artery bypass grafting. *Scand. Cardiovasc. J.* **2013**, *47*, 194–199. [CrossRef]
66. Würtz, M.; Nissen, P.H.; Grove, E.L.; Kristensen, S.D.; Hvas, A.-M. Genetic determinants of on-aspirin platelet reactivity: Focus on the influence of pear1. *PLoS ONE* **2014**, *9*, e111816. [CrossRef]
67. Hu, X.; Liu, C.; Zhang, M.; Zhang, W. Impact of the *PEAR 1* polymorphism on clinical outcomes in Chinese patients receiving dual antiplatelet therapy after percutaneous coronary intervention. *Pharmacogenomics* **2022**, *23*, 639–648. [CrossRef]
68. Nanda, N.; Bao, M.; Lin, H.; Clauser, K.; Komuves, L.; Quertermous, T.; Conley, P.B.; Phillips, D.R.; Hart, M.J. Platelet endothelial aggregation receptor 1 (pear1), a novel epidermal growth factor repeat-containing transmembrane receptor, participates in platelet contact-induced activation. *J. Biol. Chem.* **2005**, *280*, 24680–24689. [CrossRef]
69. Kauskot, A.; Di Michele, M.; Loyen, S.; Freson, K.; Verhamme, P.; Hoylaerts, M.F. A novel mechanism of sustained platelet αIIbβ3 activation via PEAR1. *Blood* **2012**, *119*, 4056–4065. [CrossRef]
70. Li, M.; Hu, Y.; Wen, Z.; Li, H.; Hu, X.; Zhang, Y.; Zhang, Z.; Xiao, J.; Tang, J.; Chen, X. Association of PEAR1 rs12041331 polymorphism and pharmacodynamics of ticagrelor in healthy Chinese volunteers. *Xenobiotica* **2017**, *47*, 1130–1138. [CrossRef]
71. Lewis, J.P.; Riaz, M.; Xie, S.; Polekhina, G.; Wolfe, R.; Nelson, M.; Tonkin, A.M.; Reid, C.M.; Murray, A.M.; McNeil, J.J.; et al. Genetic Variation in PEAR1, Cardiovascular Outcomes and Effects of Aspirin in a Healthy Elderly Population. *Clin. Pharmacol. Ther.* **2020**, *108*, 1289–1298. [CrossRef]
72. Greiff, G.; Pleym, H.; Stenseth, R.; Wahba, A.; Videm, V. Genetic variation influences the risk of bleeding after cardiac surgery: Novel associations and validation of previous findings. *Acta Anaesthesiol. Scand.* **2015**, *59*, 796–806. [CrossRef] [PubMed]
73. Rath, D.; Schaeffeler, E.; Winter, S.; Levertov, S.; Müller, K.; Droppa, M.; Stimpfle, F.; Langer, H.F.; Gawaz, M.; Schwab, M.; et al. GPIa Polymorphisms Are Associated with Outcomes in Patients at High Cardiovascular Risk. *Front. Cardiovasc. Med.* **2017**, *4*, 52. [CrossRef] [PubMed]

74. Maciukiewicz, M.; Marshe, V.S.; Hauschild, A.-C.; Foster, J.A.; Rotzinger, S.; Kennedy, J.L.; Kennedy, S.H.; Müller, D.J.; Geraci, J. GWAS-based machine learning approach to predict duloxetine response in major depressive disorder. *J. Psychiatr. Res.* **2018**, *99*, 62–68. [CrossRef] [PubMed]
75. Fabbri, C.; Corponi, F.; Albani, D.; Raimondi, I.; Forloni, G.; Schruers, K.; Kasper, S.; Kautzky, A.; Zohar, J.; Souery, D.; et al. Pleiotropic genes in psychiatry: Calcium channels and the stress-related FKBP5 gene in antidepressant resistance. *Prog. Neuro-Psychopharmacol. Biol. Psychiatry* **2018**, *81*, 203–210. [CrossRef]
76. Shah, J.; Liu, S.; Yu, W. Contemporary antiplatelet therapy for secondary stroke prevention: A narrative review of current literature and guidelines. *Stroke Vasc. Neurol.* **2022**; *ahead of print*. [CrossRef]
77. Agayeva, N.; Gungor, L.; Topcuoglu, M.A.; Arsava, E.M. Pathophysiologic, rather than laboratory-defined resistance drives aspirin failure in ischemic stroke. *J. Stroke Cerebrovasc. Dis.* **2015**, *24*, 745–750. [CrossRef]
78. Rocca, B.; Petrucci, G. Variability in the Responsiveness to low-dose aspirin: Pharmacological and disease-related mechanisms. *Thrombosis* **2012**, *2012*, 376721. [CrossRef]
79. Gonzalez-Conejero, R.; Rivera, J.; Corral, J.; Acuña, C.; Guerrero, J.A.; Vicente, V. Biological assessment of aspirin efficacy on healthy individuals: Heterogeneous response or aspirin failure? *Stroke* **2005**, *36*, 276–280. [CrossRef]

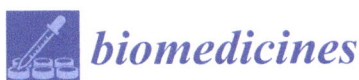

Review

Exploring the Heart–Mind Connection: Unraveling the Shared Pathways between Depression and Cardiovascular Diseases

Justyna Sobolewska-Nowak [1,*], Katarzyna Wachowska [1], Artur Nowak [2], Agata Orzechowska [1], Agata Szulc [3], Olga Płaza [3] and Piotr Gałecki [1]

1. Department of Adult Psychiatry, Medical Univeristy of Lodz, 90-419 Lodz, Poland; katarzyna.wachowska@umed.lodz.pl (K.W.); agata.orzechowska@umed.lodz.pl (A.O.); piotr.galecki@umed.lodz.pl (P.G.)
2. Department of Immunopathology, Medical Univeristy of Lodz, 90-419 Lodz, Poland; artur.nowak@stud.umed.lodz.pl
3. Psychiatric Clinic of the Faculty of Health Sciences, Medical University of Warsaw, 02-091 Warsaw, Poland; agata.szulc@wum.edu.pl (A.S.); olga.w.plaza@gmail.com (O.P.)
* Correspondence: justyna.sobolewska@stud.umed.lodz.pl

Abstract: Civilization diseases are defined as non-communicable diseases that affect a large part of the population. Examples of such diseases are depression and cardiovascular disease. Importantly, the World Health Organization warns against an increase in both of these. This narrative review aims to summarize the available information on measurable risk factors for CVD and depression based on the existing literature. The paper reviews the epidemiology and main risk factors for the coexistence of depression and cardiovascular disease. The authors emphasize that there is evidence of a link between depression and cardiovascular disease. Here, we highlight common risk factors for depression and cardiovascular disease, including obesity, diabetes, and physical inactivity, as well as the importance of the prevention and treatment of CVD in preventing depression and other mental disorders. Conversely, effective treatment of CVD can also help prevent depression and improve mental health outcomes. It seems advisable to introduce screening tests for depression in patients treated for cardiac reasons. Importantly, in patients treated for mood disorders, it is worth controlling CVD risk factors, for example, by checking blood pressure and pulse during routine visits. It is also worth paying attention to the mental condition of patients with CVD. This study underlines the importance of interdisciplinary co-operation.

Keywords: depression; cardiovascular disease; obesity; diabetes; civilization diseases; mental disorders; risk factors; inflammation; interleukins; comorbidity

1. Introduction

Depression and cardiovascular disease are both serious, growing problems in the modern world. They belong to group of diseases known as civilization diseases, meaning that they affect many people worldwide. As stated by the WHO, depression affects around 5% of adult people, an estimated 280 million people. Depression might lead to suicide and 700,000 people die by suicide every year [1]. When it comes to cardiovascular disease, it has been estimated that 17.9 million people died from CVDs in 2019, which account for 32% of all global deaths. Of these deaths, 85% were due to heart attack and stroke [2]. It is, therefore, easy to understand that both of these diseases are strongly associated with not only severe impairment in everyday functioning but also the risk of premature death. Depressive disorder has been generally associated with CVD [3] and it has been observed that depression with atypical features is linked even more strongly with cardiac risk [4]. Depression has been observed as an independent risk factor for cardiac health problems [5] as well as a consequence of CVD [6]. It was also associated with the morbidity and mortality of cardiovascular disease [7]. When gender is taken into account, it has been observed that

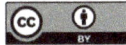

depression causes a greater increase in CVD incidence in women, and females suffering from CVD experience higher levels of depression than men [6]. Although well-observed associations between depression and CVD have been described, it has not been clearly established how these disorders interact yet. Possible risk factors combining these two very different states have been described and involve, among others, inflammation [8]. The presented article explores common risk factors between these two seemingly very different states, but starts off with basic information about the discussed disorders.

Civilization diseases are defined as non-communicable diseases that affect a large proportion of the population. They are considered to pose a serious, still-growing problem that affect people in low- and middle-income countries disproportionately strongly, where more than three quarters of global NCD deaths (31.4 million) occur. We can point out examples of conditions such as obesity, diabetes, cardiovascular disease, cancer, Alzheimer's disease, and depression [9,10].

The frequent occurrence of these diseases is characteristic of highly developed areas in terms of economy and civilization. Anti-health behaviors and other risk factors among citizens of wealthy countries are the main causes of a poor health condition [11]. It should be remembered that these diseases significantly reduce the quality of life and, in the long run, can lead to death.

Depression is a common chronic mental disorder that affects thoughts, mood and physical health [12]. To be diagnosed with a major depressive episode according to the DSM-V (Diagnostic and Statistical Manual of Mental Disorders) classification, a patient should have at least five of the symptoms presented in Table 1 that have been present over the same 2-week period and which indicate a change from previous functioning:

Table 1. Common symptoms of depression.

Depressed mood, or loss of interest or pleasure.
Depressed most of the day, almost every day, as indicated by subjective feelings (e.g., feeling sad, empty, hopeless) or observations of others (e.g., crying).
Markedly decreased interest or pleasure in all or nearly all activities most of the day, almost every day (according to subjective report or observation).
Significant weight loss when not dieting or gaining weight (e.g., change of more than 5% of body weight in a month) or a decrease or increase in appetite almost every day.
Insomnia or hypersomnia almost daily. Psychomotor agitation or retardation almost daily (observed by others, not just a subjective feeling of restlessness or slowness).
Fatigue or loss of energy almost every day.
Feelings of worthlessness or excessive or inappropriate guilt (which may be delusional) almost daily (not just remorse or guilt about illness).
Decreased ability to think or concentrate, or indecisiveness almost every day (according to subjective accounts or observed by others).
Recurrent thoughts of death (not just fear of death), recurrent suicidal thoughts without a specific plan, or suicide attempts or a specific plan to commit suicide. Symptoms cause clinically significant distress or impairment in social, occupational, or other important areas of functioning.

Please note that an episode cannot be attributed to the physiological effects of a substance or to any other medical condition. The occurrence of a major depressive episode is not better explained by the presence of schizoaffective disorder, schizophrenia, schizophrenia-like disorder, delusional disorder or other schizophrenia spectrum disorder, and other psychotic disorders. There also must be no history of a manic or hypomanic episode [13].

As we can see, the symptoms of depressive disorders vary from person to person. For many years, researchers have mainly focused on the causes of mental illness, including mood disorders. In the late 1990s, a link between a reduced brain activity and reduced cortical volume in patients suffering from bipolar and unipolar depression was discovered [14]. Later, histopathological examination of the brains of patients with mood disorders showed a lower cortical thickness and cell density in the prefrontal cortex [15]. Volumetric magnetic resonance imaging studies of patients with major depressive disorders compared to healthy controls suggested a complete reduction in brain volume, especially in the anterior cingulate and orbitofrontal cortex [16]. Additionally, of interest are the results of a meta-analysis performed by Hamilton et al. who observed significant differences in amygdala volume between treated and untreated depressed patients [17]. Ménard et al., in their paper, summarized the findings and insights for which parallel results were obtained in people with depression and models of mood disorders in rodents to investigate the potential etiology of depression. It has been discovered that several factors may be responsible for the development of depressive disorders: immunological, immune and inflammatory factors, psychological factors (e.g., stressful life events, childhood and adolescence), and neurobiological factors (participation of astrocytes in neurovascular coupling and neuronal functioning) [18].

All these discoveries can help us understand the so-called neuropathology of depressive syndrome. However, the complexity of the neurobiological processes involved in the disease make depression a conundrum of a syndrome and raise important questions regarding the importance of different brain regions (e.g., limbic structures) in the neuropathology of the disease [19]. It is a global health problem, as it is estimated that up to 5.0% of adults suffer from depression [20]. Among people suffering from depression, 40–80% of patients have suicidal thoughts, 20–60% make suicide attempts, and as many as 15% of patients successfully take their own lives. Every year, one million people worldwide die of depression, and 3800 people die from it every day [21]. According to statistics published in 2021 by the World Health Organization, more than 700,000 people die by suicide each year. This problem also affects young people; suicide is the fourth-most common cause of death at the age of 15–29 [1].

Cardiovascular disease (CVD) is the collection of diseases of the heart and circulatory system. It is a group of heterogeneous diseases sharing a common main cause of development, namely atherosclerosis. CVDs are chronic diseases that develop gradually throughout life and are asymptomatic for a long time [22]. The first group of causes includes ischemic heart disease, coronary artery disease (e.g., myocardial infarction), cerebrovascular diseases (e.g., stroke), and aortic and arterial diseases, including hypertension and peripheral vascular diseases. Other causes of CVD include congenital heart defects, rheumatic heart diseases, cardiomyopathies, and arrhythmias [23]. Cardiovascular diseases are the most common cause of death in both developed and underdeveloped countries [20]. According to statistics published in 2021 by the World Health Organization, an estimated 17.9 million people died from cardiovascular disease in 2019, accounting for 32% of all deaths worldwide. Of these deaths, 85% were due to heart attack and stroke. Of the 17 million premature deaths (under the age of 70) due to NCDs in 2019, 38% were due to CVD [7]. As risk factors, we recognize personal characteristics or a set of these, situations, conditions and potentially life events as well as diseases occurring in the patient, which have an impact on the emergence of further health problems. CVD risk factors can be divided into three large groups: biochemical, lifestyle-related, and those related to individual predispositions [2]. In the same way, factors affecting the development of depression can be classified.

Although it is well known that depression and CVD are common comorbidities, their interactions are not fully understood. Such co-morbidity brings not only increased suffering among patients but also generates high treatment costs. Understanding this relationship seems very important given the growing problem of both depression and CVD.

This review is an attempt to answer the question of whether the following guidelines can help in coping with everyday practice or whether a different approach is needed for specific patients. It also explores ways to prevent these diseases. The authors attempt to answer the questions in Table 2.

Table 2. Objectives of the review article.

The questions:
Do depression and CVD have common risk factors?
Are depression and CVD related to diabetes?
Are depression and CVD related to physical activity?
Are depression and CVD related to obesity?
Is it worth conducting CVD prophylaxis in patients with depression?
Is it worth conducting depression prevention in patients with CVD?
Is it advisable and necessary to conduct further research in this field?

2. Depression and Cardiovascular Disease

Since depression and CVD symptoms often co-occur, we conducted a literature review to determine the prevalence of both conditions and the impact of comorbidity on diagnosis, clinical outcomes, and treatment. This review aims to summarize the available information on measurable risk factors for CVD and depression based on the existing literature. The authors of this paper wish to draw clinicians' attention to the problems of patients suffering from or at risk of comorbidities. The objectives of studying the links between depression and cardiovascular disease (CVD) can be summarized as follows. Understanding the association: The first objective is to investigate and understand the relationship between depression and CVD. This involves determining the prevalence of depression among individuals with CVD and identifying potential risk factors that contribute to the development of both conditions. Additionally, it aims to explore the impact of CVD on the onset or worsening of depression.

Identifying common mechanisms: The second objective is to uncover the shared biological, physiological, and behavioral pathways that connect depression and CVD. This includes examining factors such as inflammation, oxidative stress, hormonal imbalances, and lifestyle factors such as diet, exercise, and smoking. Understanding these mechanisms can provide insights into the underlying processes and help develop targeted interventions.

Improving risk assessment and screening: The third objective aims to enhance the identification and assessment of individuals at risk for both depression and CVD. It involves developing and validating screening tools that can identify individuals who may be susceptible to developing both conditions. Incorporating depression as a risk factor for CVD seeks to improve risk-assessment models and identify subgroups that may require specific interventions.

Enhancing treatment and prevention strategies: This objective focuses on improving treatment and prevention approaches for individuals with comorbid depression and CVD. It involves evaluating the efficacy of interventions that target both conditions and developing integrated care models that address the complex interplay between mental and physical health. Furthermore, it aims to explore the impact of treating depression on CVD outcomes, and vice versa, as well as the effectiveness of lifestyle modifications and psychosocial interventions in reducing the risk and progression of both conditions.

Informing Public Health Policies and Practices: The final objective is to inform public health policies and practices regarding depression and CVD. This involves providing evidence-based recommendations for prevention and management strategies. It also seeks to influence healthcare policies to prioritize integrated care for individuals with comorbid depression and CVD, promote mental health awareness, reduce stigma, and foster collaboration between mental health and cardiovascular care providers.

By pursuing these objectives, researchers and healthcare professionals can gain a deeper understanding of the links between depression and CVD, leading to improved patient care, early intervention, and better overall health outcomes. In our review, we decided to highlight common risk factors between depression and cardiovascular disease. Particular attention was paid to obesity, diabetes, physical activity, and inflammation.

Evidence of a link between depression and cardiovascular disease is still being sought. Studies have been conducted to prove the bi-directional relationship between these diseases. A number of studies have established evidence of cardiovascular autonomic dysfunction in depressed patients. Increased mortality in heart disease, especially in specific sections of the population such as myocardial infarction patients, is also associated with multiple markers of autonomic dysregulation of the cardiovascular system. These include an increase in the resting and circadian heart rate, acceleration or deceleration of the heart rate in response to physical stressors, variability in the pace and sensitivity of baroreceptors, and high variability in ventricular repolarization [24].

In 2008, the Scientific Advisory Committee on Depression and Coronary Heart Disease of Americans, in conjunction with The Heart Association (AHA), recommended screening for depression in patients diagnosed with heart disease [25]. In March 2014, the AHA recommended elevating depression to a risk factor for adverse outcomes in patients with acute coronary syndrome [26].

Matthews et al. (2005) found in their research that there is a relationship between the severity of depressive symptoms and systemic vascular resistance (SVR). In particular, in the SVR, the effect of interaction between the severity of the depressive episode and stress was observed, and the severe course of depression was associated with a significantly higher SVR at rest [27]. Additionally, Whang et al. conducted a large prospective study on the health of nurses in the USA, the results of which showed that the symptoms of depression are associated with a higher probability of subsequent cardiovascular events, and even worse, sudden cardiac death [28]. Interestingly, depressed patients treated for a long time with selective serotonin reuptake inhibitors (SSRIs) had a lower risk of myocardial infarction than depressed patients not taking antidepressants [29].

3. Obesity

Overweight and obesity are defined as abnormal or excessive fat accumulation that presents a risk to health. A body mass index (BMI) over 25 is considered overweight, and over 30 is obese. The issue has grown to epidemic proportions, with over 4 million people dying each year as a result of being overweight or obese in 2017 according to the global burden of disease [30]. Obesity is one of the main causes of lifestyle diseases. Depression and obesity often coexist in individuals. They are common diseases with serious public health consequences. The relationship between these conditions is two-way: the presence of one increases the risk of developing the other [31]. Numerous studies have shown a strong association between obesity and the development of depressive symptoms and clinical depression. Several longitudinal studies have also shown a higher incidence of depression among individuals with obesity [32,33]. The relationship between obesity and depression is complex and multifaceted, influenced by various biological, psychological, and social factors [34]. Psychosocial factors play a role in the association between obesity and depression. Stigmatization, discrimination, and low self-esteem related to obesity can contribute to the development of depressive symptoms [35]. It is important to note that not all individuals who are obese will develop depression, and not all individuals with depression will be obese. Shared biological mechanisms may contribute to the relationship between obesity and depression. Chronic low-grade inflammation, dysregulation of the hypothalamic–pituitary–adrenal axis, and altered brain neurotransmitter systems have been implicated in both conditions [36,37]. However, the strong association between the two conditions highlights the need for comprehensive care that addresses both physical and mental well-being when managing obesity and depression. Integrated treatment approaches, including psychological support, lifestyle modifications, and appropriate medical interventions, can help improve outcomes for individuals dealing with obesity and depression. Depression has also been identified as a risk factor for the development of obesity. Depressive symptoms can lead to unhealthy behaviors, such as a sedentary lifestyle, poor dietary choices, and emotional eating, which contribute to weight gain [38]. Obesity can complicate the management of depression. Studies have shown that obesity is associated with a poorer response to antidepressant treatment and a higher risk of treatment resistance [39]. Additionally, obesity-related health problems and physical discomfort may contribute to reduced mobility and impaired self-esteem, affecting the overall well-being of individuals with depression. Depression can hinder weight-management efforts in individuals with obesity. Depressive symptoms can lead to reduced motivation, low energy levels, and decreased adherence to healthy lifestyle behaviors, such as physical activity and dietary modifications [40]. Addressing the underlying depression is essential to support successful weight management efforts.

Obesity is not only a risk factor for depression but also for cardiovascular disease (CVD). Obesity is widely recognized as a significant risk factor for cardiovascular disease (CVD). Excessive body weight, particularly when it is characterized by excess fat accumulation, places strain on the cardiovascular system and increases the likelihood of developing various cardiovascular conditions [31,41]. The relationship between obesity, depression, and cardiovascular disease is complex, with each condition influencing the development and progression of the others. Obesity significantly increases the risk of developing cardiovascular diseases. A meta-analysis performed by Whitlock et al. involving over 900,000 participants showed that obesity was associated with a higher risk of coronary heart disease, stroke, and heart failure [42]. Several other studies have consistently demonstrated the increased risk of hypertension, dyslipidemia, coronary artery disease, and other cardiovascular conditions in individuals with obesity [43,44].

Du et al. in a study showed that the prevalence of depression was 17.83% in patients with central obesity and 12.6% in non-obese patients. Thus, there is a noticeable difference in the incidence of depression between the two groups. This leads to the conclusion that the occurrence of depression is positively related to the degree of obesity [45]. Fox et al. found that depression and anxiety were associated with more severe obesity among adolescents seeking treatment [46].

Obesity contributes to cardiovascular diseases through various mechanisms. Excess adipose tissue leads to the release of pro-inflammatory cytokines and adipokines, which promote systemic inflammation and endothelial dysfunction [47]. Obesity is also associated with insulin resistance, dyslipidemia, and metabolic abnormalities, all of which contribute to the development of atherosclerosis and cardiovascular risk [48,49]. On the one hand, obesity itself contributes to this risk, and on the other hand, the risk is also affected by diseases associated with it, such as hypertension, diabetes, insulin resistance, and sleep apnea [50]. Obesity adversely affects the cardiovascular (CV) system in several ways. It may also depend on the distribution of body fat. These complex obesity issues remain the greatest challenge for clinicians dealing with multiple obesity phenotypes. Due to the prevalence of obesity, physicians and nutritionists should have the skills and tools to recognize high-risk forms of obesity. It is important to quickly identify patients with visceral obesity and patients with severe obesity. Imaging and cardiometabolic studies have clearly shown that reducing BMI lowers also the risk of CVD, at least in overweight or moderately obese patients [51]. Interestingly, a study conducted by Rogge et al. in 2013, in patients with initially asymptomatic aortic stenosis, being overweight or obese had no effect on disease progression or related cardiovascular or ischemic events, but both were associated with increased mortality [52]. In 2019, Pagidipati et al. in their work concluded that those who were overweight or obese class I had a lower cardiovascular risk than those who were underweight/normal weight. These results suggest the presence of an obesity paradox, but this paradox may reflect an epidemiological artifact rather than a true negative relationship between normal body weight and clinical outcomes [53]. Daumit et al. showed that behavioral counseling, care coordination, and care management intervention statistically significantly reduced the overall risk of cardiovascular disease in adults with major mental health conditions [54]. In a study conducted by Faulconbridge et al. the authors tested whether a combination treatment targeting obesity and depression at the same time would produce greater improvements in weight, mood, and CVD risk factors than a treatment targeting each disease individually. The results showed that behavioral weight management resulted in short-term improvements in weight, mood, and CVD risk, comparable to a combination treatment of cognitive behavioral therapy for depression [55]. Weight loss has been shown to have significant cardiovascular benefits. Studies have demonstrated that intentional weight loss through lifestyle modifications or bariatric surgery can improve multiple cardiovascular risk factors, including blood pressure, lipid profiles, and insulin sensitivity [56,57]. Weight-loss interventions have also been associated with a reduction in the incidence of cardiovascular events [58]. The increasing prevalence of obesity worldwide has significant public health implications for cardiovascular disease burden. Addressing obesity through prevention efforts, lifestyle modifications, and interventions targeting weight loss is crucial in reducing the incidence and impact of cardiovascular diseases [59].

4. Physical Activity

Physical inactivity is a known risk factor for many diseases, including cardiovascular disease. Regular physical activity is proven to help prevent and manage noncommunicable diseases (NCDs) such as heart disease, stroke, diabetes, and several cancers. It also helps prevent hypertension, maintain healthy body weight and can improve mental health, quality of life, and well-being. Physical activity refers to all movement. Popular ways to be active include walking, cycling, wheeling, sports, active recreation, and play, and can be performed at any level of skill and for enjoyment by everybody [60]. As a preventive measure, it is recommended to exercise three times a week for at least 30 min continuously with a heart rate of at least 130 beats per minute. Thanks to physical activity, it is also possible to relieve stress. Exercise is a physiological stressor that can benefit the cardiovascular system in many ways. The evidence collected so far is sufficient to consider exercise an essential tool in the prevention of cardiovascular disease, if properly prescribed and supervised [61]. Physical inactivity refers to a lack of regular physical activity or exercise. It involves a sedentary lifestyle and a minimal amount of movement or engagement in physical activities. Research has shown that physical inactivity can be considered a risk factor for depression [62]. Sedentary behavior has been associated with an increased risk of developing depression. Individuals who engage in high levels of sedentary behavior, such as excessive TV watching or computer use, have shown higher rates of depression compared to those with lower sedentary behavior levels [63]. It is important to note that while physical inactivity can be considered a risk factor for depression, it is not the sole determinant of the condition. Depression is a complex disorder influenced by a variety of genetic, environmental, and psychological factors. However, incorporating regular physical activity into one's routine can be beneficial for both physical and mental well-being, potentially reducing the risk of depression and promoting overall health. Sedentary behavior has been associated with negative effects on mental health markers, such as increased levels of stress, anxiety, and symptoms of depression. Prolonged sitting and physical inactivity can disrupt neurotransmitter regulation and impair brain functioning, leading to mood disturbances [64]. Lack of physical activity is a well-established risk factor for cardiovascular diseases (CVD). It is important to note that physical inactivity is just one of several risk factors for CVD, and its impact on cardiovascular health can be influenced by other factors such as genetics, diet, and smoking. However, adopting a physically active lifestyle can significantly reduce the risk of developing CVD and improve overall cardiovascular health [65].

Exercise is considered a non-pharmacological intervention that may delay obesity-related comorbidities, improve cardiovascular fitness, and modulate inflammation. These lead to an improvement in the immune response and the attenuation of low-grade chronic inflammation, characterized by the release of cytokines, which provides benefits at a systemic level. Many studies report that this happens by reducing visceral adipose tissue mass, with a subsequent reduction in the release of adipokines from adipose tissue (AT) and/or by inducing an anti-inflammatory environment [66]. Cattadori et al. provided a comprehensive review of the impact of physical fitness and physical activity on the risk, management and prognosis of heart failure (HF). Exercise is a basic preventive tool in patients with HF. So, exercise training is a form of therapy. Good physical condition, i.e., normal exercise capacity, is a strong prognostic parameter in patients with HF [67].

Lapmanee et al. found in rats that voluntary jogging was effective in reducing anxiety and depression-like behavior. Intense effort and forced effort did not give such a result. On the contrary—they caused stress by intensifying the symptoms of anxiety and depression [68]. Danielsson et al. in their randomized study showed that physical exercise in a physiotherapeutic setting seems to have an effect on depressive severity and performance in major depression. Their findings suggest that physical therapy may be a viable clinical strategy that inspires and guides people with major depression to exercise [69].

Schuch et al. in a meta-analysis showed a strong antidepressant effect of exercise. In studies of participants diagnosed with major depressive disorder (MDD), the positive effect of exercise was greater. This effect was more pronounced in outpatients who did not have other comorbidities and exercised under the supervision of qualified trainers [70]. Soucy et al. (2017) in their work noted that activities such as behavioral activation (BA) and physical activity (PA) can reduce the severity of depressive symptoms in adults. Improvement may persist for up to two months of follow-up. Both types of activity had a large and statistically significant effect. Physical activity was more effective in relieving symptoms. Their findings suggest that various forms of activation, whether physical or daily activity, reduce symptoms of depression [71]. Sedentary behavior has been consistently linked to an increased risk of developing CVD, including coronary heart disease, stroke, and cardiovascular mortality. Sedentary individuals have shown a higher incidence of these conditions compared to those who engage in regular physical activity [72]. Prolonged sitting and sedentary behavior have been associated with detrimental effects on cardiovascular health markers, such as increased blood pressure, unfavorable lipid profiles (elevated triglycerides and reduced high-density lipoprotein cholesterol), impaired glucose metabolism, and increased levels of inflammatory markers [73]. The work of Reed et al. found that for patients with coronary heart disease, exercise programs were well attended, safe, and beneficial in improving physical and mental health [74]. Johansson et al. in their project, they evaluated the effects of a 9-week online cognitive behavioral therapy program compared to an online discussion forum on depressive symptoms in patients with cardiovascular disease. The results showed that in the online cognitive behavioral therapy group, a significant correlation was found between changes in depressive symptoms and changes in physical activity [75]. A study conducted by Peterson et al. showed that patients with severe depressive symptoms who achieved the primary outcome of the study, which was an increase in physical activity of ≥ 336 kcal/week, had significantly lower rates of cardiovascular morbidity and mortality at 12 months [76].

5. Diabetes

Diabetes is a chronic, metabolic disease characterized by elevated levels of blood glucose (or blood sugar), which leads over time to serious damage to the heart, blood vessels, eyes, kidneys, and nerves. The most common is type 2 diabetes, usually in adults, which occurs when the body becomes resistant to insulin or does not make enough insulin. In the past three decades, the prevalence of type 2 diabetes has risen dramatically in countries of all income levels [77]. Diabetes mellitus diabetes management and self-care behaviors, leading to poorer glycemic control and an increased risk of complications. Therefore, addressing both the physical and mental health needs of individuals with diabetes is essential to promote overall well-being and improve outcomes [78]. It is well-established that diabetes is a significant risk factor for cardiovascular diseases (CVD). In fact, individuals with diabetes are at a much higher risk of developing heart disease compared to those without diabetes. Managing diabetes effectively can help reduce the risk of cardiovascular diseases. Controlling blood sugar levels through medication, adopting a healthy diet, engaging in regular physical activity, managing blood pressure and cholesterol levels, and avoiding smoking are key steps in preventing or minimizing the impact of diabetes on cardiovascular health. Regular check-ups with healthcare providers are crucial for monitoring and addressing any potential risks or complications [79]. In developed countries such as the United States (US) and the United Kingdom, many epidemiological studies have been conducted on depression and diabetes and their comorbidities. Existing reports indicate that the situation is also similar in other countries, although it is not as well documented [80]. The prevalence of depressive disorders in diabetics generally ranges from 10% to 15%. This means that there is about twice the incidence of depression in people without diabetes. The coexisting disease significantly worsens the prognosis for both diseases and increases their mortality [81]. Individuals with diabetes are at a higher risk of developing depression compared to the general population. A systematic review and meta-analysis performed by Ali et al. found that the prevalence of depression in people with diabetes was nearly double that of those without diabetes [82]. Other studies have reported similar findings, highlighting the increased vulnerability to depression among individuals with diabetes [83]. Several biological and psychosocial mechanisms contribute to the association between diabetes and depression. The chronic inflammation and oxidative stress associated with diabetes can impact brain function and increase the risk of depressive symptoms [83]. Additionally, the psychosocial stressors related to diabetes management, such as dietary restrictions, medication adherence, and fear of complications, can lead to emotional distress and depression [84]. Depression can have a detrimental effect on the management and outcomes of diabetes. A meta-analysis performed by Gonzalez et al. demonstrated that depression was associated with poorer glycemic control among individuals with diabetes [85]. Depression can hinder self-care behaviors, such as medication adherence, regular physical activity, and healthy eating, leading to suboptimal diabetes control and an increased risk of complications [86]. The presence of diabetes can also complicate the treatment of depression. People with diabetes and comorbid depression may have a poorer response to antidepressant medications compared to those without diabetes [87]. Additionally, diabetes-related symptoms, such as fatigue and decreased motivation, can overlap with depressive symptoms, making it challenging to differentiate and manage both conditions effectively [88]. Diabetes and depression share several common risk factors, including obesity, sedentary lifestyle, and genetic predisposition [89,90]. Joseph and Golden (2016) hypothesized that the dysregulation of the hypothalamic-pituitary-adrenal (HPA) axis is an important biological link between stress, depression, and diabetes. A flatter or blunted circadian cortisol curve that is relatively maintained throughout life is associated with a risk of developing depression. Suppression of the circadian cortisol curve is a specific predictor of diabetes and higher glycated hemoglobin levels in diabetic patients. This variable is an important characteristic of cardiometabolic risk. Dysregulation of the HPA axis has been found to be a critical link in the high incidence of depression and comorbid diabetes [91].

Diabetes significantly increases the risk of developing cardiovascular disease. A meta-analysis performed by Sarwar et al. involving more than 450,000 individuals demonstrated that individuals with diabetes have approximately twice the risk of developing CVD compared to those without diabetes [92]. Several other studies have confirmed this association and have shown that diabetes is an independent risk factor for the development of CVD [93]. Chronic hyperglycemia and insulin resistance, key features of diabetes, contribute to the development and progression of cardiovascular disease. Prolonged exposure to elevated blood glucose levels can damage blood vessels, leading to atherosclerosis and increased risk of coronary artery disease, myocardial infarction, and stroke [94,95]. Insulin resistance, commonly observed in type 2 diabetes, is also associated with endothelial dysfunction and impaired cardiac function [96]. Diabetes and cardiovascular disease share common risk factors, such as obesity, hypertension, dyslipidemia, and a sedentary lifestyle. These risk factors often cluster together and contribute to the development of both conditions [97]. The presence of diabetes can further amplify the impact of these risk factors, leading to a higher cardiovascular risk. Diabetes can also lead to a specific form of heart disease known as diabetic cardiomyopathy. It is characterized by structural and functional changes in the heart muscle, independent of coronary artery disease or hypertension. Diabetic cardiomyopathy is associated with impaired cardiac function, diastolic dysfunction, and an increased risk of heart failure [98]. Medications commonly used for CVD management, such as beta-blockers and thiazide diuretics, can affect glycemic control and insulin sensitivity, requiring adjustments in diabetes treatment [99]. Furthermore, the presence of CVD can complicate self-care behaviors, such as physical activity, leading to difficulties in glycemic control and diabetes management [100]. Given the strong association between diabetes and cardiovascular disease, comprehensive management strategies should address both conditions simultaneously. Lifestyle modifications, including healthy eating, regular physical activity, and weight management, are crucial for reducing cardiovascular risk in individuals with diabetes [101]. Additionally, aggressive management of cardiovascular risk factors, such as blood pressure, cholesterol, and glycemic control, is essential to prevent or delay the onset of CVD complications [102].

6. Inflammation

Inflammation is the body's natural response to protect itself from damage. It is the body's immune system response to an irritant. There are two types: acute and chronic [103]. Inflammation is a complex physiological response by the immune system to protect the body from harmful stimuli, such as pathogens, toxins, or tissue damage. While inflammation is a crucial defense mechanism, chronic or persistent inflammation can have negative effects on various aspects of health, including mental health. There is increasing evidence suggesting that inflammation may play a role in the development and progression of depression. The presence of chronic inflammation can increase the risk of developing depression, particularly in individuals who may be genetically predisposed or have other risk factors. Understanding the relationship between inflammation and depression can potentially lead to new treatment approaches targeting inflammation as a way to manage or prevent depressive symptoms [104]. Inflammation is increasingly recognized as a significant risk factor for cardiovascular disease (CVD). While inflammation is a natural response of the immune system to injury or infection, chronic inflammation can contribute to the development and progression of various cardiovascular conditions. Inflammation has also been implicated in the development and progression of other cardiovascular conditions such as peripheral artery disease (narrowing of blood vessels outside the heart), heart valve disease, and arrhythmias [105]. Managing inflammation is crucial for reducing the risk of cardiovascular disease. In some cases, anti-inflammatory medications may be prescribed by healthcare professionals to manage chronic inflammation associated with specific conditions. Early detection and intervention are essential to prevent or mitigate the inflammatory processes that contribute to cardiovascular disease. However, when inflammation becomes chronic or lasts too long, it can prove harmful and can lead to disease. The role of pro-inflammatory cytokines, chemokines, adhesion molecules, and inflammatory enzymes has been linked to chronic inflammation. Chronic inflammation has been found to mediate a wide variety of diseases, including cardiovascular disease, cancer, diabetes, arthritis, Alzheimer's disease, lung disease, and autoimmune disease [106]. Inflammation is a biological process that protects the body from threatening factors in order to maintain homeostasis. Excessive inflammation contributes to the pathophysiology of various diseases [107].

Many modern studies show that even low levels of chronic inflammation contribute to depression. From a scientific point of view, depression is increasingly often defined as a complex pathophysiological condition associated with excessive inflammation. Elevated levels of pro-inflammatory cytokines in patients have been cited as evidence. Another important aspect is the cellular response of the immune system. In the body of people with this mood disorder, mechanisms related to inflammation occur, which results in an increase in the activity of platelet activating factors, oxidative and nitrogen stress, and mitochondrial dysfunction. This information may initiate new trends in treatment [108]. The inflammatory process and the secondary activation of the immune system in depression are seen in the peripheral and central nervous systems. This explains the relationship between immune and inflammatory mood disorders [109]. Moludi et al. in studies tested the anti-inflammatory and antidepressant effect of Lactobacillus Rhamnosus G (LGG), a probiotic strain, alone or in combination with the prebiotic, inulin, in patients with ischemic heart disease. The effects of synbiotics have been shown to control both chronic inflammation and depression. These results suggest that a probiotic plus a prebiotic may exert at least some of their effect on depression through inflammatory cytokines [110]. Kiecolt-Glaser et al. decided to investigate increased intestinal permeability ("leaky gut") as one potential mechanistic pathway from marital distress and depression to increased inflammation. Two endotoxin biomarkers, LPS-binding protein (LBP) and soluble CD14 (sCD14), as well as C-reactive protein (CRP), interleukin 6 (IL-6) and tumor necrosis factor alpha (TNF-α) were used to assess inflammation. Particits with more hostile marital interactions were shown to have higher LBP than those who were less hostile. These results indicate that, among other things, a difficult marriage and a history of mood disorders may promote a pro-inflammatory environment through increased intestinal permeability, thus fueling inflammation-related disorders [111].

Research conducted in 2007 by Vaccarino et al. showed a strong relationship between depression and biomarkers of inflammation, and partly explains the link between depression and cardiovascular disease [112].

Cardiovascular health deteriorates with age, and age is one of the strongest risk factors for cardiovascular complications, including myocardial infarction, heart failure, arrhythmias, and heart-related death. An important risk factor for complications of cardiovascular diseases is age. The expression of pro-inflammatory cytokines increases throughout human life. Their increased concentrations are not only markers of chronic low-grade inflammation, but also affect the cardiovascular system. They promote autonomic and sympathetic nervous-system imbalance, increase myocardial electrical instability, stimulate remodeling and inhibit cardiac function, accelerate endothelial dysfunction, vasoconstriction, and atherosclerosis progression. Additionally, they impair kidney function. Through these mechanisms, the cardiovascular system ages faster and, consequently, increases its susceptibility to cardiovascular morbidity and death [113]. The findings of Zhou et al. suggest that systemic inflammation in patients with heart failure is causally related to the function of mitochondria in peripheral blood mononuclear cells [114]. Ridker et al. conducted a joint analysis of patients with or at high risk of atherosclerotic disease who were receiving modern statins and were participants in international trials. It was shown that among patients receiving modern statins, inflammation assessed by high-sensitivity CRP was a stronger predictor of the risk of future cardiovascular events and death than cholesterol assessed via LDLC. These data influence the choice of adjuvant therapy in addition to statin therapy and suggest that the combination of aggressive lipid-lowering and anti-inflammatory therapies may be necessary to further reduce the risk of atherosclerosis [115]. Koenig et al. used a sensitive immunoradiometric assay to investigate the association of serum C-reactive protein (CRP) with the rate of first major ischemic heart event (CHD). There was a positive and statistically significant unadjusted relationship between CRP values and the incidence of CHD events. These results confirm the prognostic importance of CRP for CVD risk. They suggest that low-grade inflammation, and especially its thrombo-occlusive complications, are involved in the pathogenesis of atherosclerosis [116]. Gusev et al. reviewed research on the underlying cause of atherosclerosis, noting that atherosclerosis was not initially thought of as an inflammatory disease. Many authors subsequently believed it to be a chronic, low-grade inflammatory condition. There is now ample evidence that the formation of atherosclerosis more closely resembles classical variants of productive inflammation involving various immune-response vectors [117]. Garcia-Arellano et al. used the Dietary Inflammatory Index (DII) in their research to assess the inflammatory potential of nutrients and foods in the context of dietary pattern. In their study, they prospectively investigated the relationship between DII and CVD. The results provide direct prospective evidence that a pro-inflammatory diet is associated with a higher risk of clinical cardiovascular events [118]. Sandoo et al. showed in their studies that classic CVD risk may affect endothelial function more than disease-related inflammatory markers in rheumatoid arthritis. Classic CVD risk factors and anti-TNF-α drugs have different effects on microvascular and macrovascular endothelial function, suggesting that combined CVD prevention strategies may be necessary [119].

Microglia are specialized immune cells that make up 5–10% of all brain cells and perform functions similar to macrophages and other specialized cells [120]. It consists of macrophage cells that reside in the central nervous system. They have the ability to migrate to all areas of the central nervous system through the brain parenchyma. They develop a specific, branched morphological phenotype known as "resting microglia". A large number of signaling pathways allow it to communicate with macroglia as well as neurons and cells of the immune system. Microglial cells are the most sensitive sensors of brain pathology. They activate when signs of brain damage or nervous system dysfunction are detected. The "activated microglial cell" has the ability to release a large number of substances that can be harmful or beneficial to surrounding cells. They are also able to migrate to the site of damage, proliferation and phagocytosis of cells and cell compartments [121]. These processes ultimately lead to the production of pro-inflammatory cytokines by microglial cells. This event requires two events with different timing: the activation of a fast afferent neural pathway and the slower propagation of the cytokine message in the brain. This is likely to sensitize target brain structures to the production and action of cytokines that spread from the periventricular organs and choroid plexus to the brain. The peripheral innate immune response of the brain is similar in many respects to the peripheral response. The difference is that this brain response does not involve the invasion of immune cells into the parenchyma and is not distorted by tissue damage at the site of infection [122]. Macrophages play a key functional role in the pathogenesis of various cardiovascular diseases, such as atherosclerosis and aortic aneurysms. Their accumulation in the vascular wall leads to a persistent local inflammatory response characterized by the secretion of chemokines, cytokines, and enzymes that degrade matrix proteins [123].

Minocycline, which inhibits microglial activation, represents a promising diversion candidate for the treatment of treatment-resistant depression. Therefore, this theory was tested by Hellmann-Regen et al. Interestingly, minocycline 200 mg/d was added to antidepressant treatment for 6 weeks. Minocycline was well tolerated but no better than a placebo in reducing depressive symptoms. The results of this work highlight the unmet need for therapeutic approaches and predictive biomarkers in drug-resistant depressive disorders [124]. Additionally, a study conducted by Hasebe et al. aimed to investigate the effect of minocycline adjuvant treatment on inflammatory and neurogenesis markers in major depressive disorder (MDD). Serum samples were collected from a randomized, placebo-controlled 12-week clinical trial of minocycline (200 mg/day, added as usual to treatment) in adults experiencing MDD to determine changes in interleukin-6 (IL-6), lipopolysaccharide binding protein (LBP) and brain-derived neurotrophic factor (BDNF). There was no difference between the adjuvant minocycline or placebo groups at baseline or week 12 in IL-6, LBP, or BDNF levels. Interestingly, higher levels of IL-6 at the start of the study were predictive of greater clinical improvement. Exploratory analyzes suggested that a change in IL-6 levels was significantly associated with anxiety symptoms and quality of life [125].

The blood–brain barrier (BBB) is a kind of link between the plasma and the brain. Its task is to prevent the entry of neurotoxic plasma components, blood cells and pathogens into the brain and to regulate the transport of molecules to and from the central nervous system (CNS), which maintains a strictly controlled chemical composition of the entire nervous system and an environment that is necessary for the proper functioning of neurons [126,127]. BBB transport is selective. Some of the transported substances are also some cytokines. These include interleukin (IL)-1α and IL-1β, IL-1 receptor antagonist (IL-1ra), IL-6, tumor necrosis factor-α (TNF), leukemia inhibitory factor (LIF) and ciliated neurotrophic factor, and many adipokines. They play an important role in the physiological response to inflammation and neuro-regeneration. Cytokines are known to be associated with autoimmune diseases, infections, trauma-related inflammation, ischemia, hemorrhage, neurodegeneration, and some genetic disorders. Not without significance is their impact on brain physiology, including eating behavior (Table 3), sleep, thermoregulation, emotions, and memory [128]. Cytokines such as IL-1, IL-6, IL-10, and TNF-alpha also play a major role in the inflammatory processes underlying cardiovascular disease [129].

Table 3. The influence of selected cytokines on behavior.

Cytokine	Behavior
IL-1	Has a pivotal role in the occurrence of fatigue as assessed by a decreased resistance to forced exercise on a treadmill [129,130]
IL-1β i TNF-α	Flatten the diurnal rhythm of activity by decreasing the expression of steady-state mRNAs for clock genes that control the amplitude but not the period of activity rhythms [126]
IL-10 and insulin-like growth factor I (IGF-I)	Growth factor that behaves like an anti-inflammatory cytokine in the brain, attenuates behavioral signs of sickness induced by centrally injected LPS [126]
IL-6	Chronic mild stress showed anhedonia and increased levels of circulating pro-inflammatory cytokines, including IL-6 [131,132]

IL-1—Interleukin 1, pro-inflammatory cytokine. IL-1β—Interleukin 1-β, pro-inflammatory cytokine. TNF-α—tumor necrosis factor-α, pro-inflammatory cytokine. IL-10—Interleukin 10, pro-inflammatory cytokine. IGF-I—insulin-like growth factor I. IL-6—Interleukin 6, pro-inflammatory cytokine.

Kruse et al. attempted to test whether IL-8 predicts a depressive response to ketamine and whether it depends on participants' gender. Plasma IL-8 levels were assessed at baseline and post-treatment. The change in IL-8 levels from baseline to post-treatment differed significantly by response status (defined as a $\geq$50% decrease in the Hamilton Depression Rating Scale) by gender. Increasing IL-8 was associated with a decrease in HAM-D score in women, while the opposite was found in men [89]. In another study in 2022 by another team, Kruse et al. investigated whether higher levels of IL-8 attenuated increases in depressed mood in response to an experimental model of inflammation-induced depression. Given the epidemiological associations identified between IL-6, tumor necrosis factor (TNF)-α, and subsequent depression, the levels of these pro-inflammatory cytokines have also been studied as potential moderators of the depressed mood response to endotoxins. Their findings suggest that IL-8 may be a biological agent that reduces the risk of inflammation-related depression [133]. The aim of Yang et al. was to check whether the level of pro-inflammatory cytokines in the serum is correlated with the development of post-stroke depression. The concentration of pro-inflammatory cytokines (IL-6, IL-18 and TNF-alpha) in the serum of all patients was determined on the 1st and 7th days after admission. Serum IL-18 concentration on day 7 was significantly higher in patients with post-stroke depression than in patients without post-stroke depression. This may suggest that serum IL-18 determination on day 7 after admission may predict the risk of post-stroke depression both in the acute stage of stroke and 6 months after stroke [134]. Depressed people are prone to sleep disturbances, which in turn can perpetuate depression. The aim of the study conducted by Siu-Man et al. was to evaluate the effect of these two mind–body therapies on people with depressive symptoms and sleep disorders. The outcome measures were plasma IL-6 and IL-1β concentrations and a questionnaire including the Pittsburgh Sleep Quality Index, the Center for Epidemiology Research Depression Scale, the Somatic Symptoms Inventory, the Perceived Stress Scale, and the Holistic Body–Mind–Spirit Well-Being Scale. The study showed a bidirectional relationship between depression and sleep disorders, and a significant effect of depression and sleep disorders on IL-6 and IL-1β [135].

Increased inflammation alerts organisms to danger. The immune system produces cytokines by affecting the CNS, a complex mediated by pro-inflammatory cytokines.

(Figure 1). Common immune-inflammatory pathways underlie the physiology of sickness behavior and the clinical pathophysiology of depression. This relationship is two-way [136]. The main cause of cardiovascular disease is atherosclerosis. It is a chronic inflammatory disease of blood vessels. Various inflammatory cells and inflammatory factors are believed to play a significant role in its pathogenesis. The pathological response to various vascular wall lesions induces classical inflammation that leads to degeneration, exudation, and hypertrophy. The detection of inflammatory biomarkers, such as CRP or IL-6 adhesion molecules, may be a good way of diagnosing atherosclerosis and cardiovascular disease [137]. Scientists are still looking for the causes of civilization diseases, such as depression and atherosclerosis. Many cytokines and their levels have been studied in patients suffering from the diseases mentioned above. Elevated levels of the same cytokines in these disease entities may suggest links between depression and atherosclerosis. A brief summary of examples of cytokines associated with both depression and atherosclerosis is provided in Table 4.

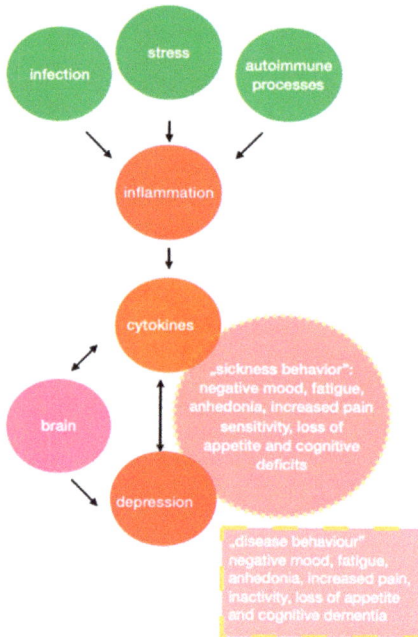

Figure 1. The common mechanism of inflammation and depression.

Table 4. Selected cytokines and their relationships with atherosclerosis and depression.

Cytokine	Atherosclerosis	Depression
IL-1	Changes the functions of cardiac myocytes and cells in the blood vessel wall, impairing systolic function, and may intensify ischemia-reperfusion injury and expansive cardiac remodeling [138]	Can cause mood disorders, a key mediator in various behavioral effects of stress [139]

Table 4. Cont.

Cytokine	Atherosclerosis	Depression
IL-6	Impaired function of vascular mitochondria accelerates the development of atherosclerosis. In mouse studies, it caused dysfunction associated with increased levels of the inflammatory cytokine IL-6 in the aorta. Human and mouse studies—aging leads to the deterioration of vascular mitochondrial function and the impairment of mitophagy. The aging of blood vessels and bone marrow cells is associated with IL-6 signaling [140]	was tested on animals and in clinical trials. Increased IL-6 activity is a factor contributing to the development of depression by activating the hypothalamic-pituitary-adrenal axis or by affecting the metabolism of neurotransmitters [141]
TNF-α	The development of atherosclerosis is closely related to the activation of TNF-α, and promotes various inflammatory reactions associated with atherosclerosis, induces vascular adhesion molecules and the recruitment and proliferation of monocytes/macrophages, participates in lipid metabolism, inhibits the activity of 7α-hydroxylase and lipoprotein lipase, and enhances the production of triglycerides in the liver [142]	Elevated plasma concentrations of tumor necrosis factor (TNF)-α in patients with mood disorders, disturbances in TNF-α levels and mental deterioration, including suicidal thoughts and response to treatment, collide [143]
IL-17	T helper-17 lymphocytes produce interleukin-17, which are important in the defense of the host mucosa against pathogenic microorganisms and fungi, constituting the anti-atherosclerotic effect of IL-17, but also the pro-atherogenic effect of IL-17 [144,145]	In depression, the number of Th17 cells increase. Th17 cells produce interleukin-17A (IL-17A), through which they promote inflammation of the nerves and activation of microglia and astrocytes. In this mechanism, they can contribute to neuronal damage, which is secondary to depression [146]

IL-1—Interleukin 1, pro-inflammatory cytokine. IL-6—Interleukin 6, pro-inflammatory cytokine. TNF-α—tumor necrosis factor-α, pro-inflammatory cytokine. IL-17—Interleukin 17, pro-inflammatory cytokine.

In the above paragraphs, the authors have focused on possible factors, including obesity, inflammation, diabetes and physical activity constituting links between depression and CVS. A detailed review of each has been presented along with a possible linking pathway between depression and CVDs.

7. Discussion

As we can see, many authors and researchers have been looking for answers to questions about the relationship between depression and CVD for a very long time. Inflammation seems to be the strongest variable influencing these relationships. Further research in this area should be considered. There are a number of factors to consider when interpreting scientific publications and research results. First, depression and cardiovascular disease are very complex issues in terms of medical knowledge and their social consequences. Many studies do not control for potential confounders, and most of the literature is cross-sectional. A growing body of the literature is focusing on the interaction between depression and inflammatory diseases, which include most CVDs. The number of patients visiting a doctor with a complex set of overlapping symptoms, including emotional and physical ailments, including stenocardia, is growing. Physical ailments usually do not indicate the cause of the physical condition of the patient. Factors linking depression and cardiovascular disease has been researched worldwide for many years. In our narrative review, we looked for evidence of comorbidity between depression and CVD. For many years, factors linking depression and cardiovascular disease have been studied all over the world. We found many studies that showed a positive correlation between depression and CVD. The results showed that people with CVD are more likely to suffer from depression than the general population. Common risk factors for these diseases are also evident, such as obesity, physical inactivity, diabetes, and inflammation. The scheduled state seems to be the most widely studied issue here. Reports have indicated a significant association between CVD and depression. Depression is a mental health disorder characterized by persistent feelings of sadness, loss of interest, and other emotional and physical symptoms. CVD refers to a range of conditions affecting the heart and blood vessels, including coronary artery disease, heart failure, and stroke. Studies have consistently shown that individuals with depression have a higher risk of developing CVD. The relationship between the two conditions is bidirectional, meaning that depression can contribute to the development of CVD, and having CVD can increase the risk of developing depression. Depression can lead to unhealthy behaviors such as poor diet, sedentary lifestyle, smoking, and non-adherence to medication, which are risk factors for CVD. Additionally, depression is associated with physiological changes in the body, including inflammation, hormonal imbalances, and increased sympathetic nervous system activity, all of which can contribute to the development and progression of CVD. Conversely, individuals with CVD are more prone to developing depression due to the psychological and emotional impact of dealing with a chronic illness. The physical limitations imposed by CVD, the fear of future cardiac events, and the disruption of daily life can lead to feelings of hopelessness, sadness, and anxiety. Both depression and CVD share common underlying mechanisms, such as dysregulation of the hypothalamic-pituitary-adrenal axis, increased oxidative stress, and endothelial dysfunction. These shared pathways may help explain the strong association between the two conditions. Recognition of the link between depression and CVD is crucial for healthcare providers. Identifying and treating depression in individuals with CVD can improve their quality of life and potentially reduce the risk of further cardiovascular events. Similarly, addressing cardiovascular risk factors in individuals with depression can help prevent the development of CVD. Integrative approaches that combine pharmacological interventions, psychotherapy, lifestyle modifications, and social support have shown promise in managing both depression and CVD. Collaborative care models, where primary care physicians, cardiologists, and mental health professionals work together, have been effective in improving outcomes for patients with comorbid depression and CVD. Depression and cardiovascular disease are closely linked, with each condition increasing the risk of the other. Recognizing and addressing this association is important for providing comprehensive care to individuals affected by these conditions. Further research is needed to better understand the mechanisms underlying the relationship and to develop more targeted interventions. Research suggests a strong link between depression and obesity. People with depression are more likely to be obese, and individuals who are obese have a higher risk of developing depression. The exact nature of this association is still under investigation. Factors such as emotional eating, sedentary behavior, and hormonal imbalances may contribute to the development of obesity in individuals with depression. Similarly, the psychosocial consequences of obesity, such as body image dissatisfaction and social stigma, may increase the risk of depression. Obesity is a well-established risk factor for cardiovascular disease. Excess body weight, particularly abdominal obesity, is associated with an increased likelihood of developing conditions such as hypertension, dyslipidemia, and type 2 diabetes, all of which contribute to the development of cardiovascular disease. Obesity-induced inflammation, insulin resistance, and adverse metabolic changes play significant roles in the progression of CVD. Lifestyle modifications, including weight loss, are crucial in reducing the risk of cardiovascular events in obese individuals. Overall, the reports highlight the interconnectedness of depression, cardiovascular disease, and obesity. There is substantial evidence indicating a link between depression and inflammation. Depressed individuals often exhibit elevated levels of pro-inflammatory markers, such as C-reactive protein (CRP), interleukin-6 (IL-6), and tumor necrosis factor-alpha (TNF-alpha). The relationship between depression and inflammation is thought to be bidirectional. Chronic inflammation can contribute to the development of depression, while depression-related alterations in the stress-response system and neurotransmitter imbalances can promote inflammation. Inflammatory processes may impair the functioning of neurotransmitters such as serotonin, which plays a crucial role in mood regulation. This disruption can contribute to the development and maintenance of depressive symptoms. Inflammation is recognized as a significant contributor to the development and progression of CVD. Conditions such as atherosclerosis, which underlies many CVDs, involve an inflammatory response within arterial walls. Inflammatory markers, including CRP, IL-6, and TNF-alpha, have been associated with an increased risk of CVD. These markers can predict the likelihood of future cardiovascular events and help assess the effectiveness of treatment. Chronic inflammation can contribute to the formation of arterial plaques, increase blood clot formation, and impair endothelial function, all of which are important factors in CVD pathogenesis. Depression, CVD, and inflammation are interconnected, with each influencing the other. Depression can contribute to the development of CVD through behavioral and physiological mechanisms, while inflammation plays a significant role in both depression and CVD. Recognizing and addressing the links between these conditions is essential for effective prevention and treatment strategies.

Depression and cardiovascular disease are two prevalent health conditions that can significantly impact an individual's well-being. Research has indicated a complex and bidirectional relationship between these two conditions, suggesting that they can influence each other's development and progression. Several studies have established a link between depression and an increased risk of developing cardiovascular disease. Similarly, a meta-analysis performed by Nicholson et al. demonstrated a 64% increased risk of cardiac events in depressed individuals [147]. A systematic review and meta-analysis performed by van Melle et al. analyzed 20 studies and found that depression was associated with a two-fold increased risk of mortality in patients with coronary artery disease. Another meta-analysis performed by Thombs et al. involving 22 studies [148]. concluded that depression was associated with a 31% increased risk of adverse cardiovascular events in patients with heart disease [149]. Meng et al. conducted a prospective study of 512,712 adults (302,509 women and 210,203 men) aged 30–79 to assess depression as a risk factor for all-cause and cardiovascular mortality. The results showed that depression was associated with an increased risk of all-cause and cardiovascular mortality in Chinese adults, especially males [150]. On the other hand, cardiovascular disease can also contribute to the development of depression. Patients with cardiovascular disease often experience physical limitations, chronic pain, and reduced quality of life, which can lead to depressive symptoms. A longitudinal study conducted by Lett et al. observed that individuals with heart disease had a two-fold increased risk of developing depression compared to those without heart disease [151]. The underlying mechanisms linking depression and cardiovascular disease are still being investigated. One proposed pathway is the dysregulation of the autonomic nervous system, characterized by increased sympathetic activity and decreased parasympathetic activity, which can contribute to both depression and cardiovascular dysfunction [152]. Depression can negatively affect cardiovascular disease outcomes through various mechanisms. Behavioral factors such as poor medication adherence, unhealthy lifestyle choices, and increased rates of smoking and alcohol consumption have been associated with depression, which can further exacerbate cardiovascular disease [153]. Additionally, depression is associated with physiological alterations, including increased inflammation, platelet activation, and autonomic dysregulation, which can contribute to adverse cardiovascular outcomes [154,155]. Effective management of depression in patients with cardiovascular disease is essential for improving outcomes. Collaborative care interventions, which involve integrating mental health care into the cardiovascular disease management process, have shown promise in reducing depressive symptoms and improving cardiovascular outcomes [156]. Bucciarelii et al. in their work concluded that the presence of depression may worsen cardiovascular morbidity and mortality. They suggest that awareness among cardiologists should be promoted. They pay attention to and emphasize gender issues in order to provide specific answers to male and female patients with CVD due to the different etiology and course of these diseases [157]. Recent studies have begun to address gender and individual differences in susceptibility to both disorders. It is generally believed that the predominance of women in depression is widespread and significant. Parker and Brotchie decided to test these theories in their review. They concluded that while external factors play a role, it is concluded that there is a higher order biological factor (variably defined neuroticism, "stress response" or "limbic overactivity") that fundamentally contributes to sex differentiation in some manifestations both depression and anxiety, and reflects the impact of steroid changes in the gonads during puberty. Instead of concluding that "anatomy is destiny", a model of blemish stress, taking into account varied epidemiological outcomes, will emphasize the importance. Ref. [158] Salk et al. found in their meta-analysis that the gender difference in depression is a health disparity, especially during adolescence; however, the magnitude of this difference indicates that depression in men should not be underestimated, as the gender gap peaked during adolescence but then declined and remained stable in adulthood. International analyzes found that greater gender differences were found in countries with greater gender equality for major depression, but not for depressive symptoms [159]. There is much talk about CVD risk factors such as hypertension, dyslipidemia, diabetes, obesity, and smoking. However, despite differences in CVD risk between men and women, most studies evaluating the magnitude of the effect of each risk factor have traditionally focused on men [160]. For many years, female participation in clinical trials was minimal, resulting in a lack of gender-specific analysis of clinical trial data, and, therefore, no specific assessment of risk factors among women. However, scientific advances in the last decade have identified a spectrum of risk factors for cardiovascular disease that may be specific to women. These risk factors, which may include menopause, hypertension, pregnancy disease, and depression, pose additional risks to women beyond traditional risk factors. The current state of knowledge and awareness about these risk factors is currently suboptimal [161]. It is still not known whether the same mechanisms affect sensitivity and immunity in women as in men. Obtaining more information on gender and individual differences in susceptibility to depression and CVD would contribute to both better prevention and treatment [162]. Depression and cardiovascular disease are two prevalent health conditions that can have a significant impact on an individual's well-being. While they differ in their manifestations, there are several common risk factors that contribute to the development of both conditions. Hare et al. in their clinical review also emphasize the importance of the co-occurrence of systemic disease and depression. It is a common comorbidity that is associated with higher rates of mortality and morbidity. They note that there is sufficient evidence to support the introduction of exercise, talk therapies, and antidepressants to reduce depression in patients with CVD [163]. Meanwhile, lifestyle recommendations in the form of sufficient physical activity and dietary modification can be an invaluable, safe, and useful tool in the treatment of depression, cardiovascular disease and many related immunometabolic disorders [164]. Engaging in regular exercise has been shown to have positive effects on mental health and cardiovascular health. Exercise is efficacious in treating depression and depressive symptoms and should be offered as an evidence-based treatment option focusing on supervised and group exercise with moderate intensity and aerobic exercise regimes [165,166]. Unhealthy eating patterns, such as consuming a diet high in processed foods, added sugars, and saturated fats, are linked to an increased risk of depression and cardiovascular disease [167,168]. Conversely, a diet rich in fruits, vegetables, whole grains, and lean proteins has been associated with a lower risk of both conditions. Obesity is a significant risk factor for both depression and cardiovascular disease. Studies have demonstrated a bidirectional relationship between obesity and depression, with each condition increasing the risk of the other [169,170]. Moreover, obesity is strongly linked to an elevated risk of developing cardiovascular diseases [171]. Chronic stress plays a crucial role in the development of both depression and cardiovascular disease. Prolonged exposure to stress can lead to the dysregulation of various physiological systems, including the immune and cardiovascular systems, and can contribute to the onset and progression of these conditions [172,173]. Joynt et al., in the conclusions of their work, gave theories that stress may be the primary trigger that leads to the development of both depression and cardiovascular disease [174]. However, not every stressed person becomes depressed or suffers from CVD. Dudek et al. emphasize the need to identify not only the biological determinants of susceptibility to stress, but also resilience. Based on the reverse translation approach, rodent depression models were developed to investigate the mechanisms underlying susceptibility and resistance. Both innate and adaptive hormonal and immune responses are enhanced in depressed individuals and in mice exhibiting depressive-like behavior. Neurovascular health is receiving increasing attention as patients with depressive disorders are more likely to have cardiovascular disease, and inflammation is associated with depression, treatment resistance, and relapse [162]. It is important to note that while these risk factors are associated with an increased likelihood of developing depression or cardiovascular disease, they do not guarantee the onset of these conditions. Other factors, such as individual susceptibility and environmental influences, also contribute to the overall risk. Glassman et al. in their work present studies that clearly showed that depression is a risk factor for both incident and recurrence of ischemic heart disease diseases. They also drew attention to the fact that biological factors modifiable health behaviors, especially physical ones, among which inactivity, smoking, and non-compliance seem to be the most critical mediators. This outcome may occur because once a person develops depression, especially if it is recurrent, the illness triggers a series of health behaviors that will undoubtedly increase the risk of vascular disease. It has been repeatedly shown that people with depression take less care of their health, exercise less often, are more likely to be obese and have difficulty quitting smoking [175]. The prospect of integrating the treatment of depression and CVD on the basis of their common pathophysiological elements brings hope. However, there is still not enough research on them. Halaris, in his article, summarizes the evidence showing that the aforementioned co-morbidity is well established, though the relationship between these two serious conditions is complex and multi-faceted. Based on the available literature, inflammation has become a dominant theme and is considered a major mechanism contributing to co-morbidity. An active inflammatory process is present during the active stages of either disease, possibly preceding the onset of debilitating symptoms, and possibly extending beyond mood normalization and symptom remission [176].

Our narrative review reveals how many papers present correlations between depression and CVD. Scientific studies recognize that there is a strong link between the two conditions. Although correlation does not imply causation, the relationship between depression and CVD is complex and involves various factors. Here are some correlations and factors related to depression and CVD (Table 5).

Table 5. Correlations between factors related to depression and CVD.

Increased risk of cardiovascular disease	Depression is associated with an increased risk of developing cardiovascular disease. Many studies show that people with depression are more likely to develop cardiovascular conditions, such as coronary artery disease, heart attacks, heart failure, and strokes.
Common Risk Factors	Depression and CVD share several common risk factors, such as a sedentary lifestyle, poor eating habits, smoking, excessive alcohol consumption, and obesity. These risk factors can contribute to both depression and cardiovascular problems.

Table 5. *Cont.*

Biological mechanisms	There are a wide range of biological mechanisms that may help explain the relationship between depression and CVD. Chronic stress, which is often associated with depression, can lead to increased inflammation and oxidative stress within the human body. These processes may contribute to the development and progression of cardiovascular diseases.
Behavioral factors	Depression can also affect an individual's behavior and lifestyle choices in ways that increase the risk of developing CVD. For example, people with depression may engage in less physical activity, have difficulty complying with medical advice, or use unhealthy coping mechanisms, such as overeating or substance abuse.
Poor adherence to treatment	People with depression may have poor adherence to treatment required for cardiovascular disease. This lack of commitmernt can lead to inadequate treatment of risk factors, exacerbation of CVD symptoms, and increased complications.

Our review of common risk factors for depression and cardiovascular disease provides valuable insights into the relationship between the two conditions and could potentially aid in the development of prevention strategies and interventions. This study could improve our understanding of common risk factors between depression and cardiovascular disease. Identifying common factors can help scientists and healthcare professionals develop a more comprehensive approach to prevention and treatment. By identifying common risk factors, the study has the potential to facilitate early intervention strategies targeting both depression and cardiovascular disease. This multifaceted approach could lead to better health outcomes and improved quality of life for those at risk. Depression and cardiovascular disease are often treated separately in healthcare systems. Studying common risk factors can promote a more integrated and holistic approach to healthcare by recognizing the link between mental and physical health. It can also inform the development of public health campaigns, policies, and interventions to reduce the incidence and burden of both depression and cardiovascular disease.

However, there are also limitations to this study. For example, establishing causality in observational studies can be difficult. The study may find correlations between some risk factors and depression and cardiovascular disease; however, determining whether these risk factors directly contribute to the development of these conditions requires further research.

Moreover, findings from a particular study may not be universally applicable. Factors such as population demographics, cultural differences, and regional differences in healthcare systems may limit the generalizability of results in other populations. Numerous confounding variables may influence the associations between risk factors, depression, and cardiovascular disease. Factors such as socioeconomic status, genetics, and lifestyle can complicate the interpretation of results. Conducting a mental and physical health examination may also raise ethical concerns. Researchers need to protect participants' confidentiality, provide adequate support to people with mental health issues, and address any potential stigma associated with depression. Overall, while research into common risk factors for depression and cardiovascular disease has the potential to provide valuable insights, researchers must overcome limitations and challenges to obtain meaningful and reliable results.

Civilization diseases are closely related through common risk factors. It is easy to see that this relationship is bidirectional (Figure 2). Many studies present similar results leading to the conclusion that the relationship between somatic diseases and mood disorders is close.

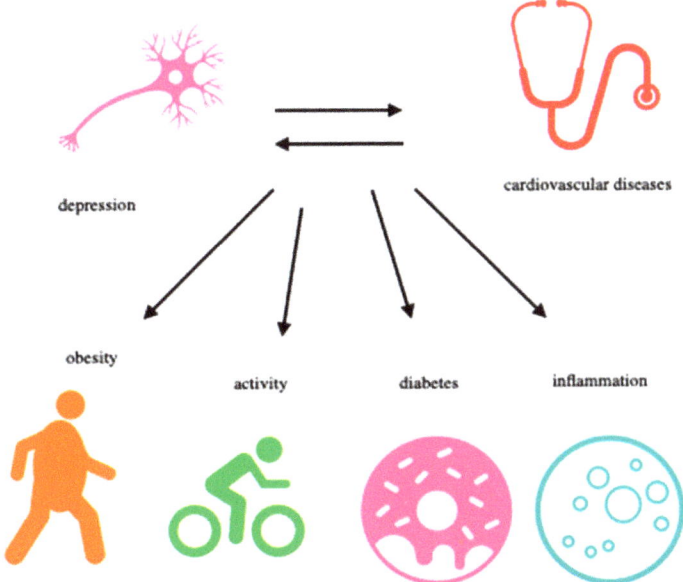

Figure 2. Two-way relationship between depression and cardiovascular disease.

Being overweight or obese is associated with an increased risk of both depression and cardiovascular disease, and physical activity is a protective factor against the development of these disorders. The morbidity of mood disorders and CVD in diabetics is higher than in the general population (Table 6). Underlying both of these disorders, the inflammatory process heals [93].

It is important for a healthy society to prevent, identify, and treat health problems. The World Health Organization warns us of an increase in both cardiovascular disease and depressive disorders. These measures will probably continue to increase due to, among others, lifestyle and an increase in life expectancy in highly developed countries. The co-occurrence of mental and physical disorders is a major challenge in healthcare around the world. There are two ways to fight civilization diseases, treat or prevent them. This issue seems to be very important and requires further research. Based on our review, there is no doubt that there is a well-established link between cardiovascular disease (CVD) and depression. Studies have consistently shown that people with depression have a higher risk of developing cardiovascular disease, and people with cardiovascular disease have a higher risk of developing depression. Depression is a common mental health condition that can lead to behavioral changes such as reduced physical activity, poor diet, and increased smoking or alcohol consumption. These behavioral changes can increase the risk of developing further disorders, such as obesity and diabetes, and cardiovascular diseases, such as heart attack, stroke, and heart failure. In addition to these behavioral changes, depression has also been linked to biological changes in the body that may contribute to CVD. For example, depression can cause inflammation, which is a key factor in the development of atherosclerosis (a buildup of plaque in the arteries) [158]. Depression can also cause changes in the autonomic nervous system, which can lead to increased heart rate and blood pressure. An interesting direction for further research could be the issue of perceived stress and anxiety related to CVD and their condition, which in turn may lead to the development of depression. Patients may also feel isolated or restricted in their activities, which can contribute to feelings of depression. Treatment is mainly based on pharmacotherapy and interestingly, many authors focus on anti-inflammatory potential of antidepressants [159,160]. Worth clinical attention is also potential treatment targets in CVD [161–163]. Prevention should consist of appropriate social education on physical activity and proper diet, preventive programs and screening tests. It is important for healthcare professionals to remember to educate patients about the consequences of leading a harmful lifestyle at each visit [175]. Also, worth attention is the fact that observed associations are present worldwide [144] and probably somehow associated with genetics [176]. Interestingly, depression, CVDs, and systemic blood hypertension are also linked, which seems to be a promising line of future clinical consideration [176] and highlights even more strongly the importance of early detection and diagnosis [162].

Table 6. Results related to obesity, physical activity, and diabetes.

	Depression	Cardiovascular Disease	Depression and Cardiovascular Disease
Obesity	The prevalence of depression was 17.83% in patients with central obesity and 12.6% in non-obese patients [39]	That reducing BMI reduces the risk of CVD, at least in overweight or moderately obese patients [31]	Behavioral weight control resulted in short-term improvements in weight, mood, and CVD risk, comparable to a combination treatment of cognitive-behavioral therapy for depression [45]
	That depression and anxiety were associated with more severe obesity among adolescents seeking treatment [40]		
Physical activity	A strong antidepressant effect of exercise [52]	The impact of physical fitness and physical activity on the risk, management, and prognosis of heart failure [49]	The online cognitive-behavioral therapy group, a significant correlation was found between changes in depressive symptoms and changes in physical activity [54]
	Behavioral activation (BA) and physical activity (PA) can reduce the severity of depressive symptoms in adults [52]		Physical activity of ≥ 336 kcal/week had significantly lower rates of cardiovascular morbidity and mortality at 12 months [55]
	Physical exercise in a physiotherapeutic setting seems to have an effect on depressive severity and performance in major depression. Their findings suggest that physical therapy may be a viable clinical strategy that inspires and guides people with major depression to exercise [50]		Patients with coronary heart disease, exercise programs were well attended, safe, and beneficial in terms of improving physical and mental health [53]
Diabetes			The dysregulation of the hypothalamic-pituitary-adrenal HPA axis is a critical link in the high incidence of depression and comorbid diabetes [48]

It is considered appropriate to conduct further research in this area. It would be worthwhile for further research to focus, among other things, on screening for depression in people with CVD and vice versa. Conducting a study on the relationship between depression and cardiovascular disease can provide valuable insights into the potential link between these two conditions. However, it is important to consider the pros and limitations associated with such studies (Table 7). It is important to acknowledge these pros and limitations when designing and interpreting studies on depression and cardiovascular disease. By addressing methodological challenges and ethical considerations, researchers

73. Thorp, A.A.; Owen, N.; Neuhaus, M.; Dunstan, D.W. Sedentary Behaviors and Subsequent Health Outcomes in Adults: A Systematic Review of Longitudinal Studies, 1996–2011. *Am. J. Prev. Med.* **2011**, *41*, 207–215. [CrossRef]
74. Reed, J.L.; Terada, T.; Cotie, L.M.; Tulloch, H.E.; Leenen, F.H.; Mistura, M.; Hans, H.; Wang, H.-W.; Vidal-Almela, S.; Reid, R.D.; et al. The effects of high-intensity interval training, Nordic walking and moderate-to-vigorous intensity continuous training in functional capacity, depression and quality of life in patients with coronary artery disease enrolled in cardiac rehabilitation: A randomized controlled trial (CRX study). *Prog. Cardiovasc. Dis.* **2021**, *70*, 73–83. [CrossRef] [PubMed]
75. Johansson, P.; Svensson, E.; Andersson, G.; Lundgren, J. Trajectories and associations between depression and physical activity in patients with cardiovascular disease during participation in an internet-based cognitive behavioural therapy programme. *Eur. J. Cardiovasc. Nurs.* **2020**, *20*, 124–131. [CrossRef] [PubMed]
76. Peterson, J.C.; Charlson, M.E.; Wells, M.T.; Altemus, M. Depression, Coronary Artery Disease, and Physical Activity: How Much Exercise Is Enough? *Clin. Ther.* **2014**, *36*, 1518–1530. [CrossRef]
77. World Health Organization. Available online: https://www.who.int/health-topics/diabetes#tab=tab_1 (accessed on 16 September 2022).
78. Roy, T.; Lloyd, C.E. Epidemiology of depression and diabetes: A systematic review. *J. Affect. Disord.* **2012**, *142*, S8–S21. [CrossRef]
79. Strain, W.D.; Paldanius, P.M. Diabetes, cardiovascular disease and the microcirculation. *Cardiovasc. Diabetol.* **2018**, *17*, 57. [CrossRef]
80. Vos, T.; Allen, C.; Arora, M.; Barber, R.M.; Bhutta, Z.A.; Brown, A.; Carter, A.; Casey, D.C.; Charlson, F.J.; Chen, A.Z.; et al. Global, regional, and national incidence, prevalence, and years lived with disability for 310 diseases and injuries, 1990–2015: A systematic analysis for the Global Burden of Disease Study 2015. *Lancet* **2016**, *388*, 1545–1602. [CrossRef]
81. Sartorius, N. Depression and diabetes. *Dialog-Clin. Neurosci.* **2018**, *20*, 47–52. [CrossRef]
82. Ali, S.; Stone, M.A.; Peters, J.L.; Davies, M.J.; Khunti, K. The prevalence of co-morbid depression in adults with Type 2 diabetes: A systematic review and meta-analysis. *Diabet. Med.* **2006**, *23*, 1165–1173. [CrossRef] [PubMed]
83. Nouwen, A.; Winkley, K.; Twisk, J.; Lloyd, C.E.; Peyrot, M.; Ismail, K.; Pouwer, F. Type 2 diabetes mellitus as a risk factor for the onset of depression: A systematic review and meta-analysis. *Diabetologia* **2010**, *53*, 2480–2486. [CrossRef] [PubMed]
84. Black, C.N.; Bot, M.; Scheffer, P.G.; Cuijpers, P.; Penninx, B.W. Is depression associated with increased oxidative stress? A systematic review and meta-analysis. *Psychoneuroendocrinology* **2015**, *51*, 164–175. [CrossRef]
85. Fisher, L.; Skaff, M.M.; Mullan, J.T.; Arean, P.; Mohr, D.; Masharani, U.; Glasgow, R.; Laurencin, G. Clinical depression versus distress among patients with type 2 diabetes: Not just a question of semantics. *Diabetes Care* **2007**, *30*, 542–548. [CrossRef] [PubMed]
86. Gonzalez, J.S.; Peyrot, M.; McCarl, L.A.; Collins, E.M.; Serpa, L.; Mimiaga, M.J.; Safren, S.A. Depression and Diabetes Treatment Nonadherence: A Meta-Analysis. *Diabetes Care* **2008**, *31*, 2398–2403. [CrossRef] [PubMed]
87. Fisher, L.; Gonzalez, J.S.; Polonsky, W.H. The confusing tale of depression and distress in patients with diabetes: A call for greater clarity and precision. *Diabet. Med.* **2014**, *31*, 764–772. [CrossRef]
88. Lustman, P.J.; Clouse, R.E.; Nix, B.D.; Freedland, K.E.; Rubin, E.H.; McGill, J.B.; Williams, M.M.; Gelenberg, A.J.; Ciechanowski, P.S.; Hirsch, I.B. Sertraline for prevention of depression recurrence in diabetes mellitus: A randomized, double-blind, placebo-controlled trial. *Arch. Gen. Psychiatry* **2006**, *63*, 521–529. [CrossRef]
89. Lustman, P.J.; Anderson, R.J.; Freedland, K.E.; de Groot, M.; Carney, R.M.; Clouse, R.E. Depression and poor glycemic control: A meta-analytic review of the literature. *Diabetes Care* **2000**, *23*, 934–942. [CrossRef]
90. Knol, M.J.; Twisk, J.W.R.; Beekman, A.T.F.; Heine, R.J.; Snoek, F.J.; Pouwer, F. Depression as a risk factor for the onset of type 2 diabetes mellitus. A meta-analysis. *Diabetologia* **2006**, *49*, 837–845. [CrossRef]
91. Joseph, J.J.; Golden, S.H. Cortisol dysregulation: The bidirectional link between stress, depression, and type 2 diabetes mellitus. *Ann. N. Y. Acad. Sci.* **2017**, *1391*, 20–34. [CrossRef] [PubMed]
92. The Emerging Risk Factors Collaboration; Sarwar, N.; Gao, P.; Seshasai, S.R.; Gobin, R.; Kaptoge, S.; Di Angelantonio, E.; Ingelsson, E.; Lawlor, D.A.; Selvin, E.; et al. Diabetes mellitus, fasting blood glucose concentration, and risk of vascular disease: A collaborative meta-analysis of 102 prospective studies. *Lancet* **2010**, *375*, 2215–2222. [CrossRef] [PubMed]
93. Haffner, S.M.; Lehto, S.; Rönnemaa, T.; Pyörälä, K.; Laakso, M. Mortality from Coronary Heart Disease in Subjects with Type 2 Diabetes and in Nondiabetic Subjects with and without Prior Myocardial Infarction. *N. Engl. J. Med.* **1998**, *339*, 229–234. [CrossRef]
94. Brownlee, M. The Pathobiology of Diabetic Complications: A unifying mechanism. *Diabetes* **2005**, *54*, 1615–1625. [CrossRef]
95. Beckman, J.A.; Creager, M.A.; Libby, P. Diabetes and atherosclerosis: Epidemiology, pathophysiology, and management. *JAMA* **2002**, *287*, 2570–2581. [CrossRef]
96. Rutter, M.K.; Meigs, J.B.; Sullivan, L.M.; D'agostino, R.B.; Wilson, P.W. Insulin Resistance, the Metabolic Syndrome, and Incident Cardiovascular Events in the Framingham Offspring Study. *Diabetes* **2005**, *54*, 3252–3257. [CrossRef]
97. Laakso, M. Cardiovascular disease in type 2 diabetes: Challenge for treatment and prevention. *J. Intern. Med.* **2001**, *249*, 225–235. [CrossRef]
98. Jia, G.; Hill, M.A.; Sowers, J.R. Diabetic Cardiomyopathy: An Update of Mechanisms Contributing to This Clinical Entity. *Circ. Res.* **2018**, *122*, 624–638. [CrossRef] [PubMed]
99. Patti, G.; Cavallari, I.; Andreotti, F.; Calabrò, P.; Cirillo, P.; Denas, G.; Galli, M.; Golia, E.; Maddaloni, E.; Marcucci, R.; et al. Prevention of atherothrombotic events in patients with diabetes mellitus: From antithrombotic therapies to new-generation glucose-lowering drugs. *Nat. Rev. Cardiol.* **2018**, *16*, 113–130. [CrossRef]

100. Morrish, N.J.; Wang, S.-L.; Stevens, L.K.; Fuller, J.H.; Keen, H. Mortality and causes of death in the WHO multinational study of vascular disease in diabetes. *Diabetologia* **2001**, *44* (Suppl. 2), S14–S21. [CrossRef]
101. American Diabetes Association. 5. Facilitating Behavior Change and Well-being to Improve Health Outcomes: Standards of Medical Care in Diabetes—2021. *Diabetes Care* **2021**, *44* (Suppl. 1), S53–S72. [CrossRef] [PubMed]
102. Grundy, S.M.; Benjamin, I.J.; Burke, G.L.; Chait, A.; Eckel, R.H.; Howard, B.V.; Mitch, W.; Smith, S.C.; Sowers, J.R. Diabetes and Cardiovascular Disease: A statement for healthcare professionals from the American Heart Association. *Circulation* **1999**, *100*, 1134–1146. [CrossRef] [PubMed]
103. Harvard Health Publishing. Available online: https://www.health.harvard.edu/heart-disease/ask-the-doctor-what-is-inflammation (accessed on 12 April 2021).
104. Beurel, E.; Toups, M.; Nemeroff, C.B. The Bidirectional Relationship of Depression and Inflammation: Double Trouble. *Neuron* **2020**, *107*, 234–256. [CrossRef] [PubMed]
105. Soysal, P.; Arik, F.; Smith, L.; Jackson, S.E.; Isik, A.T. Inflammation, Frailty and Cardiovascular Disease. *Adv. Exp. Med. Biol.* **2020**, *1216*, 55–64. [CrossRef] [PubMed]
106. Singh, N.; Baby, D.; Rajguru, J.P.; Patil, P.B.; Thakkannavar, S.S.; Pujari, V.B. Inflammation and cancer. *Ann. Afr. Med.* **2019**, *18*, 121–126. [CrossRef] [PubMed]
107. Scott, L., Jr.; Li, N.; Dobrev, D. Role of inflammatory signaling in atrial fibrillation. *Int. J. Cardiol.* **2019**, *287*, 195–200. [CrossRef] [PubMed]
108. Liu, C.S.; Adibfar, A.; Herrmann, N.; Gallagher, D.; Lanctôt, K.L. Evidence for Inflammation-Associated Depression. *Curr. Top. Behav. Neurosci.* **2017**, *31*, 3–30. [CrossRef]
109. Gałecki, P. Teoria zapalna depresji—Podstawowe fakty. *Psychiatria* **2012**, *9*, 68–75.
110. Moludi, J.; Khedmatgozar, H.; Nachvak, S.M.; Abdollahzad, H.; Moradinazar, M.; Tabaei, A.S. The effects of co-administration of probiotics and prebiotics on chronic inflammation, and depression symptoms in patients with coronary artery diseases: A randomized clinical trial. *Nutr. Neurosci.* **2022**, *25*, 1659–1668. [CrossRef]
111. Kiecolt-Glaser, J.K.; Wilson, S.J.; Bailey, M.L.; Andridge, R.; Peng, J.; Jaremka, L.M.; Fagundes, C.P.; Malarkey, W.B.; Laskowski, B.; Belury, M.A. Marital distress, depression, and a leaky gut: Translocation of bacterial endotoxin as a pathway to inflammation. *Psychoneuroendocrinology* **2018**, *98*, 52–60. [CrossRef]
112. Vaccarino, V.; Johnson, B.D.; Sheps, D.S.; Reis, S.E.; Kelsey, S.F.; Bittner, V.; Rutledge, T.; Shaw, L.J.; Sopko, G.; Merz, C.N.B. National Heart, Lung, and Blood Institute. Depression, inflammation, and incident cardiovascular disease in women with suspected coronary ischemia: The National Heart, Lung, and Blood Institute-sponsored WISE study. *J. Am. Coll. Cardiol.* **2007**, *50*, 2044–2050. [CrossRef] [PubMed]
113. Smykiewicz, P.; Segiet, A.; Keag, M.; Żera, T. Proinflammatory cytokines and ageing of the cardiovascular-renal system. *Mech. Ageing Dev.* **2018**, *175*, 35–45. [CrossRef] [PubMed]
114. Zhou, B.; Wang, D.D.-H.; Qiu, Y.; Airhart, S.; Liu, Y.; Stempien-Otero, A.; O'brien, K.D.; Tian, R. Boosting NAD level suppresses inflammatory activation of PBMCs in heart failure. *J. Clin. Investig.* **2020**, *130*, 6054–6063. [CrossRef] [PubMed]
115. Ridker, P.M.; Bhatt, D.L.; Pradhan, A.D.; Glynn, R.J.; MacFadyen, J.G.; Nissen, S.E. PROMINENT, REDUCE-IT, and STRENGTH Investigators. Inflammation and cholesterol as predictors of cardiovascular events among patients receiving statin therapy: A collaborative analysis of three randomised trials. *Lancet* **2023**, *401*, 1293–1301. [CrossRef]
116. Koenig, W.; Sund, M.; Fröhlich, M.; Fischer, H.-G.; Löwel, H.; Döring, A.; Hutchinson, W.L.; Pepys, M.B. C-Reactive protein, a sensitive marker of inflammation, predicts future risk of coronary heart disease in initially healthy middle-aged men: Results from the MONICA (Monitoring Trends and Determinants in Cardiovascular Disease) Augsburg Cohort Study, 1984 to 1992. *Circulation* **1999**, *99*, 237–242. [CrossRef]
117. Gusev, E.; Sarapultsev, A. Atherosclerosis and Inflammation: Insights from the Theory of General Pathological Processes. *Int. J. Mol. Sci.* **2023**, *24*, 7910. [CrossRef]
118. Garcia-Arellano, A.; Ramallal, R.; Ruiz-Canela, M.; Salas-Salvadó, J.; Corella, D.; Shivappa, N.; Schröder, H.; Hébert, J.R.; Ros, E.; Gómez-Garcia, E.; et al. Dietary Inflammatory Index and Incidence of Cardiovascular Disease in the PREDIMED Study. *Nutrients* **2015**, *7*, 4124–4138. [CrossRef]
119. Sandoo, A.; Kitas, G.D.; Carroll, D.; van Zanten, J.J.V. The role of inflammation and cardiovascular disease risk on microvascular and macrovascular endothelial function in patients with rheumatoid arthritis: A cross-sectional and longitudinal study. *Arthritis. Res. Ther.* **2012**, *14*, R117. [CrossRef]
120. Maes, M.; Galecki, P.; Chang, Y.S.; Berk, M. A review on the oxidative and nitrosative stress (O&NS) pathways in major depression and their possible contribution to the (neuro)degenerative processes in that illness. *Prog. Neuro-Psychopharmacol. Biol. Psychiatry* **2011**, *35*, 676–692. [CrossRef]
121. Gałecki, P.; Gałecka, E.; Maes, M.; Chamielec, M.; Orzechowska, A.; Bobińska, K.; Lewiński, A.; Szemraj, J. The expression of genes encoding for COX-2, MPO, iNOS, and sPLA2-IIA in patients with recurrent depressive disorder. *J. Affect. Disord.* **2012**, *138*, 360–366. [CrossRef]

122. Kim, S.U.; de Vellis, J. Microglia in health and disease. *J. Neurosci. Res.* **2005**, *81*, 302–313. [CrossRef]
123. Khoury, M.K.; Yang, H.; Liu, B. Macrophage Biology in Cardiovascular Diseases. *Arter. Thromb. Vasc. Biol.* **2021**, *41*, e77–e81. [CrossRef]
124. Hellmann-Regen, J.; Clemens, V.; Grözinger, M.; Kornhuber, J.; Reif, A.; Prvulovic, D.; Goya-Maldonado, R.; Wiltfang, J.; Gruber, O.; Schüle, C.; et al. Effect of Minocycline on Depressive Symptoms in Patients with Treatment-Resistant Depression: A Randomized Clinical Trial. *JAMA Netw. Open* **2022**, *5*, e2230367. [CrossRef] [PubMed]
125. Hasebe, K.; Mohebbi, M.; Gray, L.; Walker, A.J.; Bortolasci, C.C.; Turner, A.; Berk, M.; Walder, K.; Maes, M.; Kanchanatawan, B.; et al. Exploring interleukin-6, lipopolysaccharide-binding protein and brain-derived neurotrophic factor following 12 weeks of adjunctive minocycline treatment for depression. *Acta Neuropsychiatr.* **2021**, *34*, 220–227. [CrossRef] [PubMed]
126. Dantzer, R.; O'Connor, J.C.; Freund, G.G.; Johnson, R.W.; Kelley, K.W. From inflammation to sickness and depression: When the immune system subjugates the brain. *Nat. Rev. Neurosci.* **2008**, *9*, 46–56. [CrossRef] [PubMed]
127. Sweeney, M.D.; Zhao, Z.; Montagne, A.; Nelson, A.R.; Zlokovic, B.V. Blood-Brain Barrier: From Physiology to Disease and Back. *Physiol. Rev.* **2019**, *99*, 21–78. [CrossRef] [PubMed]
128. Bliźniewska-Kowalska, K.; Szewczyk, B.; Gałecka, M.; Su, K.-P.; Maes, M.; Szemraj, J.; Gałecki, P. Is Interleukin 17 (IL-17) Expression A Common Point in the Pathogenesis of Depression and Obesity? *J. Clin. Med.* **2020**, *9*, 4018. [CrossRef] [PubMed]
129. Liberale, L.; Ministrini, S.; Carbone, F.; Camici, G.G.; Montecucco, F. Cytokines as therapeutic targets for cardio- and cerebrovascular diseases. *Basic Res. Cardiol.* **2021**, *116*, 23. [CrossRef]
130. Pan, W.; Stone, K.P.; Hsuchou, H.; Manda, V.K.; Zhang, Y.; Kastin, A.J. Cytokine Signaling Modulates Blood-Brain Barrier Function. *Curr. Pharm. Des.* **2011**, *17*, 3729–3740. [CrossRef]
131. Gałecka, M.; Bliźniewska-Kowalska, K.; Maes, M.; Su, K.-P.; Gałecki, P. Update on the neurodevelopmental theory of depression: Is there any 'unconscious code'? *Pharmacol. Rep.* **2020**, *73*, 346–356. [CrossRef]
132. Roohi, E.; Jaafari, N.; Hashemian, F. On inflammatory hypothesis of depression: What is the role of IL-6 in the middle of the chaos? *J. Neuroinflamm.* **2021**, *18*, 45. [CrossRef]
133. Kruse, J.L.; Vasavada, M.M.; Olmstead, R.; Hellemann, G.; Wade, B.; Breen, E.C.; Brooks, J.O.; Congdon, E.; Espinoza, R.; Narr, K.L.; et al. Depression treatment response to ketamine: Sex-specific role of interleukin-8, but not other inflammatory markers. *Transl. Psychiatry* **2021**, *11*, 167. [CrossRef] [PubMed]
134. Yang, L.; Zhang, Z.; Sun, D.; Xu, Z.; Zhang, X.; Li, L. The serum interleukin-18 is a potential marker for development of post-stroke depression. *Neurol. Res.* **2010**, *32*, 340–346. [CrossRef] [PubMed]
135. Ng, S.-M.; Yin, M.X.C.; Chan, J.S.M.; Chan, C.H.Y.; Fong, T.C.T.; Li, A.; So, K.-F.; Yuen, L.-P.; Chen, J.-P.; Chung, K.-F.; et al. Impact of mind–body intervention on proinflammatory cytokines interleukin 6 and 1β: A three-arm randomized controlled trial for persons with sleep disturbance and depression. *Brain Behav. Immun.* **2021**, *99*, 166–176. [CrossRef]
136. Maes, M.; Berk, M.; Goehler, L.; Song, C.; Anderson, G.; Gałecki, P.; Leonard, B. Depression and sickness behavior are Janus-faced responses to shared inflammatory pathways. *BMC Med.* **2012**, *10*, 66. [CrossRef]
137. Zhu, Y.; Xian, X.; Wang, Z.; Bi, Y.; Chen, Q.; Han, X.; Tang, D.; Chen, R. Research Progress on the Relationship between Atherosclerosis and Inflammation. *Biomolecules* **2018**, *8*, 80. [CrossRef]
138. Libby, P. Interleukin-1 Beta as a Target for Atherosclerosis Therapy: Biological Basis of CANTOS and Beyond. *J. Am. Coll. Cardiol.* **2017**, *70*, 2278–2289. [CrossRef]
139. Koo, J.W.; Duman, R.S. Evidence for IL-1 receptor blockade as a therapeutic strategy for the treatment of depression. *Curr. Opin. Investig. Drugs* **2009**, *10*, 664–671. [PubMed]
140. Tyrrell, D.J.; Goldstein, D.R. Ageing and atherosclerosis: Vascular intrinsic and extrinsic factors and potential role of IL-6. *Nat. Rev. Cardiol.* **2020**, *18*, 58–68. [CrossRef]
141. Ting, E.Y.-C.; Yang, A.C.; Tsai, S.-J. Role of Interleukin-6 in Depressive Disorder. *Int. J. Mol. Sci.* **2020**, *21*, 2194. [CrossRef]
142. Kim, C.W.; Oh, E.; Park, H.J. A strategy to prevent atherosclerosis via TNF receptor regulation. *FASEB J.* **2021**, *35*, e21391. [CrossRef]
143. Uzzan, S.; Azab, A.N. Anti-TNF-α Compounds as a Treatment for Depression. *Molecules* **2021**, *26*, 2368. [CrossRef] [PubMed]
144. Chen, S.; Crother, T.R.; Arditi, M. Emerging Role of IL-17 in Atherosclerosis. *J. Innate Immun.* **2010**, *2*, 325–333. [CrossRef] [PubMed]
145. Taleb, S.; Tedgui, A.; Mallat, Z. IL-17 and Th17 Cells in Atherosclerosis: Subtle and contextual roles. *Arter. Thromb. Vasc. Biol.* **2015**, *35*, 258–264. [CrossRef]
146. Beurel, E.; Lowell, J.A. Th17 cells in depression. *Brain, Behav. Immun.* **2018**, *69*, 28–34. [CrossRef]
147. Nicholson, A.; Kuper, H.; Hemingway, H.; Adrie, C.; Cariou, A.; Mourvillier, B.; Laurent, I.; Dabbane, H.; Hantala, F.; Rhaoui, A.; et al. Depression as an aetiologic and prognostic factor in coronary heart disease: A meta-analysis of 6362 events among 146 538 participants in 54 observational studies. *Eur. Heart J.* **2006**, *27*, 2763–2774. [CrossRef]
148. van Melle, J.P.; de Jonge, P.; Spijkerman, T.A.; Tijssen, J.G.P.; Ormel, J.; van Veldhuisen, D.J.; van den Brink, R.H.S.; van den Berg, M.P. Prognostic Association of Depression Following Myocardial Infarction with Mortality and Cardiovascular Events: A Meta-analysis. *Psychosom. Med.* **2004**, *66*, 814–822. [CrossRef]

149. Thombs, B.D.; de Jonge, P.; Coyne, J.C.; Whooley, M.A.; Frasure-Smith, N.; Mitchell, A.J.; Zuidersma, M.; Eze-Nliam, C.; Lima, B.B.; Smith, C.G.; et al. Depression Screening and Patient Outcomes in Cardiovascular Care. *JAMA* **2008**, *300*, 2161–2171. [CrossRef] [PubMed]
150. Meng, R.; Yu, C.; Liu, N.; He, M.; Lv, J.; Guo, Y.; Bian, Z.; Yang, L.; Chen, Y.; Zhang, X.; et al. Association of Depression with All-Cause and Cardiovascular Disease Mortality Among Adults in China. *JAMA Netw. Open* **2020**, *3*, e1921043. [CrossRef]
151. Lett, H.S.; Blumenthal, J.A.; Babyak, M.A.; Sherwood, A.; Strauman, T.; Robins, C.; Newman, M.F. Depression as a Risk Factor for Coronary Artery Disease: Evidence, Mechanisms, and Treatment. *Psychosom. Med.* **2004**, *66*, 305–315. [CrossRef]
152. Carney, R.M.; Freedland, K.E.; Miller, G.E.; Jaffe, A.S. Depression as a risk factor for cardiac mortality and morbidity. *J. Psychosom. Res.* **2002**, *53*, 897–902. [CrossRef] [PubMed]
153. Berkman, L.F.; Blumenthal, J.; Burg, M.; Carney, R.M.; Catellier, D.; Cowan, M.J.; Czajkowski, S.M.; DeBusk, R.; Hosking, J.; Jaffe, A.; et al. Effects of Treating Depression and Low Perceived Social Support on Clinical Events After Myocardial Infarction: The Enhancing Re-covery in Coronary Heart Disease Patients (ENRICHD) randomized trial. *JAMA* **2003**, *289*, 3106–3116. [CrossRef] [PubMed]
154. Barth, J.; Schumacher, M.; Herrmann-Lingen, C. Depression as a Risk Factor for Mortality in Patients with Coronary Heart Disease: A Meta-analysis. *Psychosom. Med.* **2004**, *66*, 802–813. [CrossRef]
155. Whooley, M.A.; de Jonge, P.; Vittinghoff, E.; Otte, C.; Moos, R.; Carney, R.M.; Ali, S.; Dowray, S.; Na, B.; Feldman, M.D.; et al. Depressive Symptoms, Health Behaviors, and Risk of Cardiovascular Events in Patients with Coronary Heart Disease. *JAMA* **2008**, *300*, 2379–2388. [CrossRef] [PubMed]
156. Katon, W.J.; Lin, E.H.; Von Korff, M.; Ciechanowski, P.; Ludman, E.J.; Young, B.; Peterson, D.; Rutter, C.M.; McGregor, M.; McCulloch, D. Collaborative Care for Patients with Depression and Chronic Illnesses. *N. Engl. J. Med.* **2010**, *363*, 2611–2620. [CrossRef] [PubMed]
157. Bucciarelli, V.; Caterino, A.L.; Bianco, F.; Caputi, C.G.; Salerni, S.; Sciomer, S.; Maffei, S.; Gallina, S. Depression and cardiovascular disease: The deep blue sea of women's heart. *Trends Cardiovasc. Med.* **2020**, *30*, 170–176. [CrossRef]
158. Parker, G.; Brotchie, H. Gender differences in depression. *Int. Rev. Psychiatry* **2010**, *22*, 429–436. [CrossRef]
159. Salk, R.H.; Hyde, J.S.; Abramson, L.Y. Gender differences in depression in representative national samples: Meta-analyses of diagnoses and symptoms. *Psychol. Bull.* **2017**, *143*, 783–822. [CrossRef]
160. Connelly, P.J.; Azizi, Z.; Alipour, P.; Delles, C.; Pilote, L.; Raparelli, V. The Importance of Gender to Understand Sex Differences in Cardiovascular Disease. *Can. J. Cardiol.* **2021**, *37*, 699–710. [CrossRef]
161. Saeed, A.; Kampangkaew, J.; Nambi, V. Prevention of Cardiovascular Disease in Women. *Methodist DeBakey Cardiovasc. J.* **2017**, *13*, 185–192. [CrossRef]
162. Dudek, K.A.; Dion-Albert, L.; Kaufmann, F.N.; Tuck, E.; Lebel, M.; Menard, C. Neurobiology of resilience in depression: Immune and vascular insights from human and animal studies. *Eur. J. Neurosci.* **2021**, *53*, 183–221. [CrossRef]
163. Hare, D.L.; Toukhsati, S.R.; Johansson, P.; Jaarsma, T. Depression and cardiovascular disease: A clinical review. *Eur. Heart J.* **2014**, *35*, 1365–1372. [CrossRef]
164. Chávez-Castillo, M.; Nava, M.; Ortega, Á.; Rojas, M.; Núñez, V.; Salazar, J.; Bermúdez, V.; Rojas-Quintero, J. Depression as an Immunometabolic Disorder: Exploring Shared Pharmacotherapeutics with Cardiovascular Disease. *Curr. Neuropharmacol.* **2020**, *18*, 1138–1153. [CrossRef]
165. Heissel, A.; Heinen, D.; Brokmeier, L.L.; Skarabis, N.; Kangas, M.; Vancampfort, D.; Stubbs, B.; Firth, J.; Ward, P.B.; Rosenbaum, S.; et al. Exercise as medicine for depressive symptoms? A systematic review and meta-analysis with meta-regression. *Br. J. Sports Med.* **2023**. [CrossRef]
166. Warburton, D.E.R.; Nicol, C.W.; Bredin, S.S.D. Health benefits of physical activity: The evidence. *Can. Med. Assoc. J.* **2006**, *174*, 801–809. [CrossRef]
167. Akbaraly, T.N.; Brunner, E.J.; Ferrie, J.E.; Marmot, M.G.; Kivimaki, M.; Singh-Manoux, A. Dietary pattern and depressive symptoms in middle age. *Br. J. Psychiatry* **2009**, *195*, 408–413. [CrossRef] [PubMed]
168. Hu, F.B. Dietary pattern analysis: A new direction in nutritional epidemiology. *Curr. Opin. Lipidol.* **2002**, *13*, 3–9. [CrossRef] [PubMed]
169. Luppino, F.S.; de Wit, L.M.; Bouvy, P.F.; Stijnen, T.; Cuijpers, P.; Penninx, B.W.J.H.; Zitman, F.G. Overweight, Obesity, and Depression: A systematic review and meta-analysis of longitudinal studies. *Arch. Gen. Psychiatry* **2010**, *67*, 220–229. [CrossRef] [PubMed]
170. Pan, A.; Sun, Q.; Czernichow, S.; Kivimaki, M.; Okereke, O.I.; Lucas, M.; Manson, J.E.; Ascherio, A.; Hu, F.B. Bidirectional association between depression and obesity in middle-aged and older women. *Int. J. Obes.* **2011**, *36*, 595–602. [CrossRef]
171. Lavie, C.J.; McAuley, P.A.; Church, T.S.; Milani, R.V.; Blair, S.N. Obesity and cardiovascular diseases: Implications regarding fitness, fatness, and severity in the obesity paradox. *J. Am. Coll. Cardiol.* **2014**, *63*, 1345–1354. [CrossRef] [PubMed]
172. Pariante, C.M. Risk Factors for Development of Depression and Psychosis. *Ann. N. Y. Acad. Sci.* **2009**, *1179*, 144–152. [CrossRef]
173. Rozanski, A.; Blumenthal, J.A.; Kaplan, J. Impact of Psychological Factors on the Pathogenesis of Cardiovascular Disease and Implications for Therapy. *Circulation* **1999**, *99*, 2192–2217. [CrossRef] [PubMed]
174. Joynt, K.E.; Whellan, D.J.; O'Connor, C.M. Depression and cardiovascular disease: Mechanisms of interaction. *Biol. Psychiatry* **2003**, *54*, 248–261. [CrossRef] [PubMed]

175. Glassman, A.H. Depression and cardiovascular comorbidity. *Dialog. Clin. Neurosci.* **2007**, *9*, 9–17. [CrossRef] [PubMed]
176. Halaris, A. Inflammation-associated co-morbidity between depression and cardiovascular disease. *Curr. Top. Behav. Neurosci.* **2017**, *31*, 45–70. [CrossRef]

Disclaimer/Publisher's Note: The statements, opinions and data contained in all publications are solely those of the individual author(s) and contributor(s) and not of MDPI and/or the editor(s). MDPI and/or the editor(s) disclaim responsibility for any injury to people or property resulting from any ideas, methods, instructions or products referred to in the content.

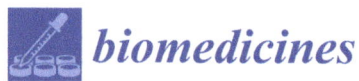

Review

Move Your Body, Boost Your Brain: The Positive Impact of Physical Activity on Cognition across All Age Groups

Felice Festa, Silvia Medori and Monica Macrì *

Department of Innovative Technologies in Medicine & Dentistry, University "G. D'Annunzio" of Chieti-Pescara, 66100 Chieti, Italy
* Correspondence: m.macri@unich.it

Abstract: While the physical improvements from exercise have been well documented over the years, the impact of physical activity on mental health has recently become an object of interest. Physical exercise improves cognition, particularly attention, memory, and executive functions. However, the mechanisms underlying these effects have yet to be fully understood. Consequently, we conducted a narrative literature review concerning the association between acute and chronic physical activity and cognition to provide an overview of exercise-induced benefits during the lifetime of a person. Most previous papers mainly reported exercise-related greater expression of neurotransmitter and neurotrophic factors. Recently, structural and functional magnetic resonance imaging techniques allowed for the detection of increased grey matter volumes for specific brain regions and substantial modifications in the default mode, frontoparietal, and dorsal attention networks following exercise. Here, we highlighted that physical activity induced significant changes in functional brain activation and cognitive performance in every age group and could counteract psychological disorders and neural decline. No particular age group gained better benefits from exercise, and a specific exercise type could generate better cognitive improvements for a selected target subject. Further research should develop appropriate intervention programs concerning age and comorbidity to achieve the most significant cognitive outcomes.

Keywords: age groups; attention; brain; cognition; default mode network; executive function; exercise; magnetic resonance imaging; memory; mental health

Citation: Festa, F.; Medori, S.; Macrì, M. Move Your Body, Boost Your Brain: The Positive Impact of Physical Activity on Cognition across All Age Groups. *Biomedicines* 2023, 11, 1765. https://doi.org/10.3390/biomedicines11061765

Academic Editors: Masaru Tanaka and Eleonóra Spekker

Received: 23 April 2023
Revised: 11 June 2023
Accepted: 16 June 2023
Published: 20 June 2023

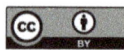

Copyright: © 2023 by the authors. Licensee MDPI, Basel, Switzerland. This article is an open access article distributed under the terms and conditions of the Creative Commons Attribution (CC BY) license (https://creativecommons.org/licenses/by/4.0/).

1. Introduction

Physical activity (PA) is defined as "any bodily movement produced by skeletal muscles that requires energy expenditure" [1] (p. 126) and can encompass several activities, such as housework, sports, and active recreation [2]. Limitations to or, often, a complete absence of exercise cause various health problems, including postural and somatic disorders, diabetes, overweight, obesity, cardiovascular disease, and even premature death [3–5]. Existing literature suggests that regular PA, particularly aerobic activity, promotes physical and mental improvements in healthy and impaired people [6].

While several papers have dealt with exercise-induced benefits on body health, only in recent years has the study of the relationship between PA and cognition received considerable attention. This relationship directly influences cognitive functioning associated with structural and functional changes in the brain and improves psychophysical well-being [7]. Although a definition of cognition has yet to be standardized [8], the term cognition includes a series of mental abilities that enable us to perceive, process, and store valuable information in daily life. It has been widely demonstrated that PA can positively influence different cognitive functions (e.g., attention, memory, and executive functions) and has more generic effects on the mechanisms involved in learning. Pioneering research on rodents demonstrated how PA could induce growth factor production and changes in the hippocampus, improving memory [9]. These favourable outcomes on mice have spurred research on humans.

The first human studies indicated that these benefits are mediated by complex neurophysiological and biochemical systems, such as the brain-derived neurotrophic factor (BDNF), which over time, leads to a more efficient, adaptive, and plastic brain [10]. In humans, circulating BDNF and vascular endothelial growth factors are acutely and chronically enhanced after aerobic exercise, leading to brain structure and function changes and neurogenesis [11]. Considering recent mouse studies, the expression of BDNF and cytokines following a systemic administration of myokines released during muscular contraction, such as irisin, could have an anti-depressant effect [12]. However, these neurobiological mechanisms have yet to be understood entirely [13], primarily due to a need for suitable procedures for evaluating brain function in vivo during a dynamic motor task.

Cognitive functioning is commonly assessed through mental status examinations, which evaluate the level of consciousness, orientation, constructional ability, and cognitive abilities. Nowadays, neuroimaging methods detail the link between exercise and cognitive function, provide the physical-exercise-induced changes in the neural correlates of cognition in both short-term and long-term practice, and assess brain health [14]. Among the methods available to investigate the impact on functional brain activation, functional near-infrared spectroscopy (fNIRS), electroencephalography (EEG), and structural and functional magnetic resonance imaging (MRI) have been used in previous research [15,16]. fNIRS and EEG have a limited spatial resolution and may only allow for the evaluation of brain activation patterns in superficial cerebral areas. However, functional magnetic resonance imaging (fMRI) has recently overcome these shortcomings.

fMRI is a fundamental non-invasive instrument of investigation to acquire high-definition images of whole brain activity during different motor tasks and to estimate the brain activation changes in cortical and subcortical areas (cerebral networks) via the blood oxygenation level-dependent (BOLD) signal [17–19]. The human brain comprises anatomical regions (nodes or hubs) and synaptic connections among the various regions (edges) [20]. The cerebral networks may change after PA and usually encompasses all body muscles, or after jaw-related therapeutic interventions that involve especially masticatory muscles [21]. Task-based fMRI and resting-state fMRI examine BOLD changes obtained during a cognitive task and while performing no straightforward task, respectively. These two methods are suitable for exploring the modification in neural correlates driving cognitive improvements and measuring brain functional connectivity after exercise or other environmental factors, such as thermal stress [22]. Functional connectivity relates to areas of the brain that are spatially separated but temporally connected in their signalling [23]. A good use of fMRI is in the preclinical models [24]. Indeed, fMRI may even detect abnormal mitochondrial functions, especially in severe inheritable metabolic diseases with neurological manifestations [25].

Previous reviews have investigated the current literature concerning the link between chronic exercise and cognition, mainly among older adults [26–28]. These reviews generally encompassed studies evaluating exercise-induced changes at the molecular and cellular levels and in cognitive functions. Moreover, most papers analysed the impact of PA in patients with mild cognitive impairment [29]. Few fMRI reviews dealt with older people and reported better functional connectivity, especially after light-intensity aerobic exercise [30,31]. Recent studies pointed out the positive impact of exercise since PA could counteract the loss of brain white and grey matter and promote the efficiency of brain circuits and neuronal plasticity, especially in adults [32,33]. Regarding children, most papers evaluated the impact of PA through standardised tests of academic and cognitive outcomes. Few reviews included neuroimaging effects following exercise [34,35]. A 2019 review examined cognitive improvements among elders, adults, and children through neuropsychological tests but had only two fMRI studies concerning children [36]. Therefore, the authors did not provide a complete analysis of functional changes during the lifetime of a person.

To provide a more up-to-date and in-depth analysis, we described the relationship between PA and brain health using standardised tests, and structural and functional MRI in this review. **We reviewed recent, peer-reviewed studies with original data and published in English that concerned the effects of exercise and the cognitive benefits across all age groups. We investigated the effect of acute and chronic PA.** Acute PA indicates a single bout of physical exercise, while chronic PA indicates PA that is repeated and persists longer than a single session or episode. Acute PA studies showed the transitory response to a single session of PA, whereas chronic PA illustrated a long shift in an individual's life. Due to heterogeneity among the studies, the studies selected were divided into "acute exercise" and "chronic exercise" to provide readily comprehensible data. We used PA or exercise to refer to coordinative activities (e.g., yoga, Tai Chi exercise, and dance) and aerobic fitness (e.g., walking, cycling, and treadmill running).

The present narrative review aimed to understand what mechanisms and brain changes were involved following acute and chronic PA in older people, adults, and children; whether a specific age showed the most significant cognitive improvements following PA; and lastly, whether a particular exercise type could provide better cognitive performances in a selected age group.

2. Acute Exercise

Previous studies have targeted cognitive abilities as evidence suggests that a single exercise session may temporarily alter them [37]. A 2001 study observed that older patients with chronic obstructive pulmonary disease (COPD) showed better verbal fluency following 35 min of acute aerobic exercise (20 min cycling and 15 min recovery period) [38]. **Therefore, acute exercise positively impacts both healthy and impaired people.** Although previous papers recommended acute physical exercise [39], the relationship between acute PA and cognition remains to be determined. **Consequently, we investigated the cognitive improvements** in subjects of different ages via fMRI and the cognitive test for attention, cognitive control, or memory, especially following a single cycling or treadmill running session (Table 1).

Table 1. Summary of studies investigating acute exercise.

Study	Sample	Physical Activity	Methods	Main Findings
Coelho et al., 2014 [40]	21 AD * patients (76.3 ± 6.2 yrs) 18 healthy controls (74.6 ± 4.7 yrs)	Treadmill	Treadmill grade, time to exhaustion, VO2, maximal lactate, Baecke Questionnaire	Increase in BDNF * plasma levels
Won et al., 2019 [41]	26 healthy older adults (65.9 ± 7.2 yrs)	30 min of cycling	fMRI * scan	Activation of semantic memory
Won et al., 2019 [42]	32 healthy older adults (66.2 ± 7.3 yrs)	30 min cycling	fMRI scan	Activation in the left inferior frontal gyrus and inferior parietal lobule
Voss et al., 2020 [43]	34 healthy older adults (67.1 ± 4.3 yrs)	20 min of light and moderate cycling	fMRI scan	Improvements in hippocampal–cortical connections and working memory
Suwabe et al., 2018 [44]	36 healthy young adults (20.9 ± 1.8 yrs)	10 min of light exercise	fMRI scan	Increase in connectivity between dentate gyrus and cortical regions
Li et al., 2014 [45]	15 female students (19–22 yrs)	20 min of moderate exercise	fMRI scan	Activation in the right middle prefrontal gyrus, right lingual gyrus, and left fusiform gyrus; deactivations in anterior cingulate cortex: left inferior frontal gyrus and right paracentral lobule

Table 1. Cont.

Study	Sample	Physical Activity	Methods	Main Findings
Marian Bosch et al., 2020 [46]	15 healthy male young adults (23.7 ± 4.02 yrs)	30 min of moderate exercise/15 min of vigorous exercise	fMRI scan	Significant improvements in motor sequence memory (high intensity)/improvements tending towards significance (moderate intensity)
Perini et al., 2016 [47]	84 healthy male young adults: 44 (23.0 ± 2.2 yrs) in the orientation discrimination task group and 40 (22.9 ± 2.2 yrs) in the motor task group	30 min of exercise	Physiological and behavioural tests	Gradual up-regulation of a functional network
Mehren et al., 2019 [48]	20 ADHD * patients (29.9 ± 9.5 yrs) 20 healthy controls (29.0 ± 7.4 yrs)	30 min of moderate cycling	fMRI scan	Improvements in reaction times and attention in ADHD patients; activation in frontal and sensorimotor regions in patients and controls
Mehren et al., 2019 [49]	64 healthy young adults: 32 participants (29.3 ± 8.5 yrs) in the moderate-intensity group; 32 participants (28.6 ± 7.7 yrs) in the high-intensity group	Moderate- and high-intensity cycling	fMRI scan	Activation in the insula, superior frontal gyrus, precentral gyrus, and supplementary motor area in the moderate-intensity group
Schmitt et al., 2019 [50]	21 male athletes (27.2 ± 4.2 yrs)	30 min of low- and high-intensity exercise	fMRI scan	Reduced activation in posterior cingulate cortex/precuneus for low intensity; reduced activation in the caudate nucleus and ventral anterior putamen for high intensity
Li et al., 2019 [51]	12 healthy high-fit and 12 healthy low-fit female students	30 min of aerobic exercise	fMRI scan	Activation in the right cerebellum and subcortical regions
Choi et al., 2016 [52]	37 ADHD children; 18 healthy controls (12.8 ± 0.79 yrs)	13 min of aerobic stretching and moderate exercise	EEG *	Increased alpha activity; decreased theta activity
Chen et al., 2016 [53]	9 healthy children (10 yrs)	30 min of moderate cycling	fMRI scan	Activation in bilateral parietal cortex: left hippocampus and bilateral cerebellum
Chen et al., 2017 [54]	9 healthy children (10 yrs)	30 min of moderate cycling	fMRI scan	Connectivity between left cerebellum and right inferior frontal gyrus
Metcalfe et al., 2016 [55]	30 BD * adolescents (16.8 ± 1.4 yrs); 20 healthy controls (16.1 ± 1.5 yrs)	20 min of recumbent cycling	fMRI scan	Deactivation in the left inferior frontal gyrus, right frontal pole, temporal pole, hippocampus, and right amygdala

* AD: Alzheimer's disease; ADHD: attention deficit hyperactivity disorder; BD: bipolar disorder; BDNF: brain-derived neurotrophic factor; EEG: electroencephalography; fMRI: functional magnetic resonance imaging.

Regarding older adults, a low level of PA is considered a risk factor for dementia. Acute aerobic exercise increased the BDNF plasma levels in patients with Alzheimer's disease and healthy controls. In addition, the BDNF levels had an association with the level of PA [40]. Following 30 min of moderate-intensity exercise in healthy older adults, higher activation was observed in the middle frontal, inferior temporal, middle temporal, and fusiform gyri during a semantic memory task and in the bilateral hippocampus after exercise compared with at rest [41]. Moreover, 30 min moderate-intensity bicycling generated greater activation in the left inferior frontal gyrus and left inferior parietal lobule and deactivation in the right anterior cingulate gyrus [42]. Functional connectivity did not differ significantly between acute light- and moderate-intensity training in cognitively normal older adults. A correlation between the right postcentral/parietal cortex, the right ventral lateral prefrontal cortex, the right posterior superior temporal gyrus, and the right dorsolateral prefrontal cortex was detected after acute exercise [43]. In older adults, 20 min cycling, especially at moderate intensity, improved working memory [43], while 30 min moderate-intensity cycling enhanced executive function and functional processing [42].

Regarding younger adults, we reported some studies concerning the influence of different duration and intensities of PA. Recent papers have reported that a single session of PA increased functional connectivity in specific brain networks. These findings are essential for cognitive and motor functions, often the primary goal of neurorehabilitation strategies [56]. Suwabe et al. observed that young adults showed a higher hippocampal memory function thanks to better functional connectivity between dentate gyrus and cortical networks following a 10 min, very light-intensity PA bout [44]. According to Li et al., in younger adults, a 20 min moderate-intensity physical session slightly improved working memory; however, this single bout generated a greater activation in the right middle prefrontal gyrus, the right lingual gyrus, and the left fusiform gyrus [45]. The improvement in executive control processes after acute exercise was related to activation of the prefrontal and occipital cortexes and deactivation of the anterior cingulate cortexes and left frontal hemisphere. Moreover, motor sequence memory in connection with the hippocampus increased significantly for high-intensity PA while tending towards significance for moderate PA in healthy young males; the bilateral precuneus activity improved for both moderate- and high-intensity PA [46]. The mnemonic discrimination task, working memory, and executive function were enhanced in younger adults after 20 min moderate-intensity cycling, while executive function improved in younger adults with attention-deficit/hyperactivity disorder (ADHD) after 30 min moderate-intensity cycling. A single bout of aerobic exercise significantly improved learning mechanisms in young male adults' visual and motor domains. These benefits could last for at least 30 min after exercise. Moreover, moderate-intensity acute PA could allow for a gradual up-regulation of a functional network due to a constant rise in synapse strength, which could encourage brain plasticity in motor and non-motor areas [47]. Mehren et al. analysed the impact of a 30 min single session of aerobic exercise on attention and executive functions in adult patients with and without ADHD. Moderate-intensity PA significantly improved reaction times in patients with ADHD compared with healthy adults [48]. Although the authors noticed no changes in brain activation between the two groups, they supported the importance of acute exercise for patients with ADHD. In another study, Mehren et al. compared moderate-intensity exercise with high-intensity exercise in healthy younger adults [49]. A better behavioural performance (sensitivity index) and greater activation in areas related to executive function, attention, and motor processes (insula, superior frontal gyrus, precentral gyrus, and supplementary motor area) was noticed following moderate PA. Higher cardiorespiratory fitness was also linked to increased brain activation of the right insult and left rolandic operculum after moderate exercise and decreased brain activation of the right postcentral gyrus after high-intensity exercise. Thirty minutes of low-intensity acute exercise in healthy male athletes led to reduced brain activation in the posterior cingulate cortex/precuneus. In contrast, a 30 min high-intensity acute workout reduced the caudate nucleus and ventral anterior putamen [50]. Schmitt et al. also described a positive interference of intense acute PA in emotion-processing brain regions during fearful face elaboration [50]. The authors concluded that single acute exercise sessions are usually beneficial for mood. Moreover, after 30 min acute aerobic exercise, Li et al. noticed that the right cerebellum played a decisive role in processing simple executive tasks [51]. At the same time, the subcortical regions were involved in the processing of relatively complex executive tasks.

A few papers dealt with acute PA's impact on adolescents and children. Acute aerobic stretching and moderate-intensity exercise affected the theta and alpha waves of the EEG and, thus, had beneficial effects on brain maturation and development of children aged 12 to 14 years, especially those with ADHD [52]. Executive function and working memory performance improved in healthy children after 30 min moderate-intensity cycling [53,54]. During a working memory task, a more significant change in functional brain haemodynamics was also detected in the bilateral parietal cortexes, the left hippocampus, and the bilateral cerebellum. A 30 min cycling session also led to higher brain connectivity between the right dorsolateral prefrontal and left cerebellum, inversely associated with improved cognitive performance. Metcalfe et al. observed no significant modifications in the attentional task after 20 min moderate-intensity cycling in adolescents with and without bipolar disorder [55]. In adolescents with bipolar problems, the authors noticed a reduced functional activation in the orbital part of the left inferior frontal gyrus, the right frontal pole extending to the temporal pole, the bilateral hippocampus, and the right amygdala.

Regardless of age, brain changes following acute exercise were mainly found in the frontal and temporal lobes, the cerebellum, and the hippocampal regions. Moreover, executive functions associated with the frontal lobe and hippocampus could be selectively maintained or enhanced in humans with higher fitness levels. Herold et al. underlined that different acute exercise protocols (cycling or treadmill running) and various intensities (light, moderate, and high), as well as the cardiorespiratory fitness level and sex of the participants, affect PA-related shifts in functional brain haemodynamics [57].

3. Chronic Exercise

A more significant number of studies dealt with the benefits of PA on cognition following a period longer than a single bout. Therefore, descriptions of the positive impact of regular exercise have been divided according to the age of the subjects analysed in the reviewed studies. **Figures 1–3 summarise the main PA-induced effects on cognition among older adults, adults, adolescents, and children. These benefits are described in detail in the following subsections.**

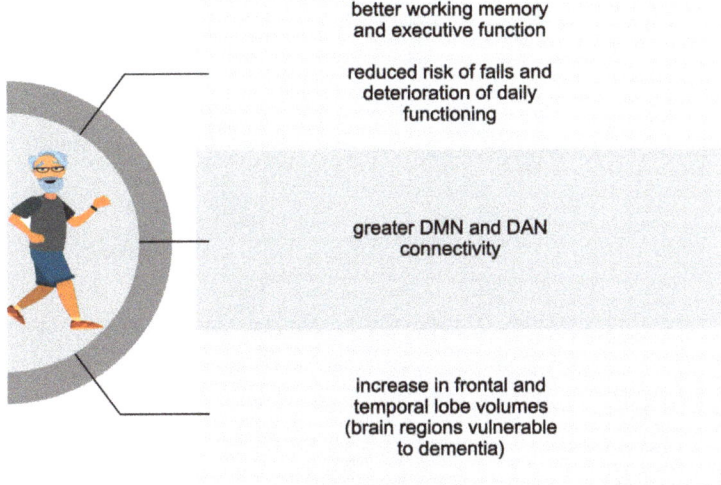

Figure 1. The main cognitive effects of chronic exercise among older adults.

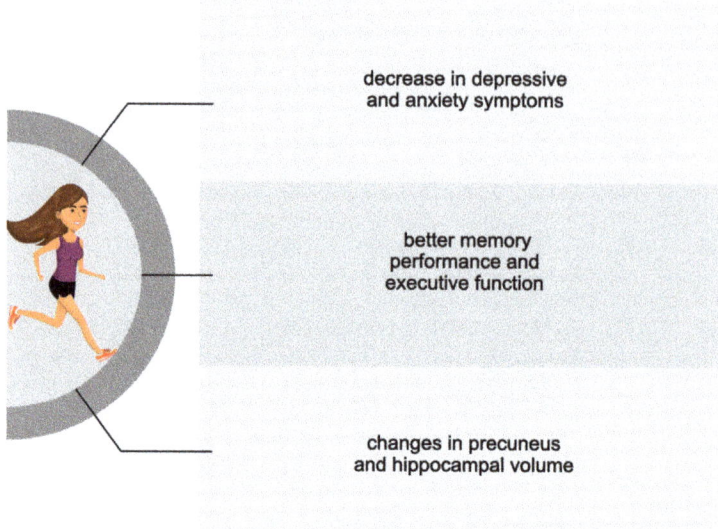

Figure 2. The main cognitive effects of chronic exercise among adults.

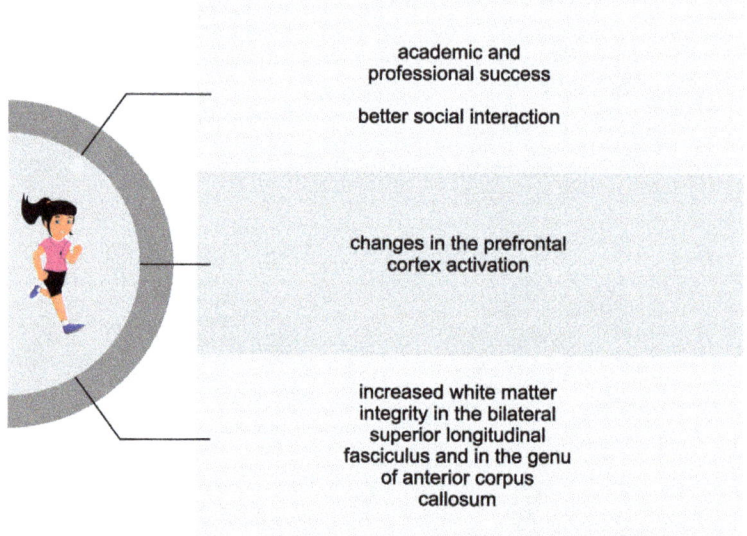

Figure 3. The main cognitive effects of chronic exercise among adolescents and children.

3.1. Older Adults

The elderly population is increasing worldwide; according to the World Health Organization (WHO), by 2030, one in six people will be 60 years or over [58]. This leads to an increasing interest on the part of the scientific research community in ageing and the quality of life of the elderly population. With age, cognitive impairments, such as dementia and Alzheimer's disease, may occur in addition to physical conditions. Therefore, older people should implement preventive strategies and lead healthy lifestyles. Several risk factors, for instance, smoking, physical inactivity, being overweight, and high blood pressure, may contribute to the onset of dementia and related diseases. Most people need to be fully aware of the relationship between lifestyle and brain health, especially in subgroups with low socioeconomic statuses or low levels of social health literacy. It, therefore, appears essential to raise awareness in the general population on modifiable risk and protective factors for dementia, as was the goal in an awareness campaign in the Netherlands, "my brain coach" [59]. Numerous studies pointed out a compatible correlation between regular physical exercise and a lower incidence of dementia and cognitive impairment [60–62].

However, the underlying mechanism by which PA may improve cognition is still unknown. Some studies found that the level of training intensity influenced the increase in cognitive ability in older adults [63,64]. In contrast, others stated that simple daily movement was significantly linked to cognition [65,66]. An improved cognition reduces the risks of falls, cognitive complaints, and deterioration of everyday functioning. The duration of PA sessions varied from 60 to 90 min. On the contrary, Langhammer et al. proposed an activity time of 150 min weekly for at least six months [67]. Taylor et al. recommended 30 daily aerobic exercises five days a week and two days of strength-based training [68]. In addition, a systematic review suggested that moderate-intensity exercise programs with aerobic and resistance training, lasting at least 45 min per session on as many days of the week as possible, could benefit older healthy adults' cognition [62]. Pietrelli et al. analysed the benefits of moderate-intensity aerobic exercise, performed regularly throughout life, on brain health and anxiety-related behaviour in old rats [69]. By studying cognitive response with the radial maze (RM) and anxiety-related behaviours with the open field (OF) and higher maze (EPM), the authors found improved cognitive function and protection from the deleterious effects of ageing and decreased anxiety. Thus, regular and chronic aerobic exercise generated time- and dose-dependent, neuroprotective, and reparative effects on physiological brain ageing, reducing anxiety-related behaviours. With regard to PA type, Klimova et al. reported that dance improved cognitive performance in healthy older people thanks to emotional involvement, balance control, memory, and coordination [70]. On the contrary, the effects of high-intensity interval training (HIIT) interventions on functional brain changes in the elderly remain unclear. A Korean preliminary study demonstrated that a HIIT program that included flexibility, endurance, and balance effectively improved cognitive function, physical fitness, and electroencephalographic markers in older Koreans; thus, HIIT interventions could help improve functional brain activity in this population [71]. Several studies described that exercise could activate different mechanisms at the brain level, promoting various physiologic phenomena, such as angiogenesis, neurogenesis, synaptogenesis, and stimulation of neurotrophic factors improving memory and brain plasticity. PA modulated Aβ turnover, inflammation, the synthesis and release of neurotrophins, and cerebral blood flow in older populations. Moreover, encouraging lifestyle changes in the pre-symptomatic and pre-dementia disease stages could potentially delay a third of dementia worldwide [72].

Table 2 summarises the findings of the following reviewed studies.

Table 2. Summary of studies investigating chronic exercise among older adults.

Study	Sample	Physical Activity	Methods	Main Findings
Engeroff et al., 2018 [73]	Healthy older adults (>65 yrs)	Moderate-to-vigorous exercise	MRS *-based marked	Increase in BDNF * and hippocampus volume
Wheeler et al., 2020 [74]	67 healthy older adults (67 ± 7 yrs)	6 days of moderate exercise	Cognitive testing	Increase in BDNF, working memory, and executive function
Gaitán et al., 2021 [75]	23 late middle-aged adults (mean age 65 yrs)	26 weeks of treadmill training	Cognitive function test and Enzyme-Linked Immunosorbent Assay (ELISA)	Increased plasma Cathepsin B; unchanged serum klotho

Table 2. Cont.

Study	Sample	Physical Activity	Methods	Main Findings
Neale et al., 2017 [76]	95 healthy older adults (65–92 yrs)	Light exercise	EEG *	Association between neural signature and environment
Gogniat et al., 2022 [77]	47 healthy older adults (>65 yrs)	7 days of exercise	Neuropsychological tests and fMRI * scan	Increased DMN * and DAN * functional connectivity
Gogniat et al., 2022 [78]	51 healthy older adults (>65 yrs)	Light exercise	Neuropsychological tests and fMRI scan	Relationship between low DMN/DAN anti-correlations levels and better executive function
Pieramico et al., 2012 [79]	30 healthy older adults (60–75 yrs): 15 participants; 15 controls	6 months of structured multimodal activities (cognitive, aerobic, and sensorial stimuli and fun recreational activities)	fMRI scan	Improvements in cognitive performance and reorganization of functional connectivity
Li et al., 2014 [80]	34 healthy male older adults: 17 (68.6 ± 5.7 yrs) participants; 17 (71.7 ± 4.0) controls	6 weeks of multimodal activities (Tai Chi and counselling group); lecture for the control group	Cognitive tests and fMRI scan	Improved functional connectivity between the medial prefrontal cortex and medial temporal lobe
Tao et al., 2016 [81]	62 older adults: 21 in the Tai Chin Chaun group; 16 in the Baduanjin group; 25 in the control group	12 weeks of Tai Chin Chuan or Baduanjin exercise	Memory function measurement and fMRI scan	Increased memory quotient; improved functional connectivity between the hippocampus and medial prefrontal cortex
Dorsman et al., 2020 [82]	212 older adults (73.3 ± 6.2 yrs)	7 days of exercise	fMRI scan	Greater frontal-subcortical and within-subcortical network synchrony
Ji et al., 2017 [83]	24 older adults: 12 (67.0 ± 6.40 yrs) participants; 12 (73.0 ± 8.0 yrs) controls	6 weeks of exercise	Cognitive tests, and MRI * and fMRI scans	Improved memory and executive function; increased posterior cingulate volume; higher connectivity between the striatum and cingulate, temporal, parietal, and occipital regions
Voss et al., 2010 [84]	65 older adults: 30 (67.3 ± 5.8 yrs) participants; 35 (65.4 ± 5.2 yrs) controls	6 and 12 months of moderate aerobic exercise	Cognitive tests and fMRI scan	Improved executive function; increased functional connectivity within DMN and FEN *
Flodin et al., 2017 [85]	47 older adults: 22 (68.4 ± 2.6 yrs) participants; 25 (69.16 ± 3.0 yrs) controls	6 months of aerobic exercise	fMRI scan	Decreased connectivity between left hippocampus and contralateral precentral gyrus; Better connectivity between right mid-temporal areas and frontal and parietal region
Voss et al., 2019 [86]	189 healthy older adults (65.4 ± 4.4 yrs)	6 months of aerobic exercise (dance and walk)	fMRI scan	Increased salience network connectivity via nutritional supplementation
Kimura et al., 2013 [87]	72 healthy older adults (70.3 ± 4.0)	3 months of short and long brisk walking	fMRI scan	Activation in left prefrontal and parietal regions and in dorsolateral prefrontal cortex
Bugg et al., 2011 [88]	52 healthy older adults (69.0 ± 6.7 yrs)	exercise (running or walking) practiced over the last 10 yrs	MRI scan	Larger frontal volume and medial temporal lobule

Table 2. Cont.

Study	Sample	Physical Activity	Methods	Main Findings
Papenberg et al., 2016 [89]	414 healthy older adults	exercise practiced in the last 12 months	MRI scan	Correlation between physical inactivity and small grey matter volume
Well et al., 2013 [90]	14 MCI patients: 9 participants; 5 controls	8 weeks of mindfulness	fMRI scan	Increased connectivity between posterior cingulate cortex, bilateral medial prefrontal cortex, and left hippocampus
Eyre et al., 2016 [91]	25 MCI * patients: 14 in the yoga group; 11 in the memory enhancement training group	12 weeks of yoga	fMRI scan	Greater connectivity between the DMN and medial frontal cortex, pregenual anterior cingulate cortex, right middle frontal cortex, posterior cingulate cortex, and left lateral occipital cortex
Tao et al., 2019 [92]	47 MCI patients: 20 (66.17 ± 4.17 yrs) in the Baduanjin group; 17 (64.32 ± 2.60 yrs) in the brisk walking group; 20 (65.97 ± 5.66 yrs) in the control group	24 weeks of exercise (Baduanjin and brisk walking)	Montreal cognitive test, and MRI and fMRI scans	Improved cognitive function; greater hippocampus grey matter volume; higher connectivity between the hippocampus and right angular gyrus
Suo et al., 2016 [93]	100 MCI older adults (70.1 ± 6.7 yrs)	6 months of resistance training	Neuropsychological tests, and MRI and fMRI scans	Better global cognition; greater cortical thickness in the posterior cingulate; improved connectivity between the hippocampus and superior frontal cortex
Hsu et al., 2017 [94]	21 SIVCI * older adults	6 months of aerobic exercise	fMRI scan	FPN * linked to better mobility performance
Veldsman et al., 2017 [95]	62 stroke patients (67 ± 12.6 yrs) 27 healthy controls (68.0 ± 5.94 yrs)	3 months of exercise	fMRI scan	Increased connectivity of superior parietal lobule in DAN

* BDNF: brain-derived neurotrophic factor; DMN: default mode network; DAN: dorsal attention network; EEG: electroencephalography; FEN: frontal executive network; FPN: frontoparietal network; fMRI: functional magnetic resonance imaging; MCI: mild cognitive impairment; MRI: magnetic resonance imaging; MRS: magnetic resonance spectroscopy; SIVCI: subcortical ischemic vascular cognitive impairment.

Engeroff et al. described the associations of objectively assessed habitual PA and physical performance with brain plasticity in cognitively healthy older adults [73]. The brain plasticity was analysed using magnetic resonance spectroscopy (MRS)-based markers and BDNF serum levels. Overall, PA and exceeding current recommendations for moderate-to-vigorous PA were positively related to BDNF. On the contrary, sedentary behaviour was negatively correlated with the bioavailability of neurotrophic factors in the elderly. Moderate-intensity morning exercise improved serum BDNF and working memory or executive function in older adults, depending on whether the next session was interrupted with light-intensity intermittent walking [74]. A recent study evaluated systemic biomarkers in learning and memory in 23 asymptomatic late middle-aged adults with familiar and genetic AD risk after 26 weeks of supervised treadmill training [75]. Systemic biomarkers included myokine cathepsin B (CTSB), BDNF, and Klotho. The authors observed a modification in the metabolic regulation of exercise-induced plasma BDNF. They concluded that CTSB is a marker of cognitive changes in late middle-aged adults with a risk for dementia.

A study proposed another aspect: the evaluation of older people's neural activation via electroencephalography (EEG) in response to the environment in which walking was carried out [76]. Levels of 'engagement' (related to immersion) were higher in urban green spaces than in crowded or quiet residential areas, while levels of 'excitement' (linked to classic arousal indicators such as increased heart rate and blood flow) were higher in busy urban streets than in green areas and quiet urban spaces. Therefore, green spaces in an urban setting could favour walking in older adults.

Some studies aimed to evaluate functional connectivity after PA in older adults. The default mode network (DMN) and the dorsal attention network (DAN) represent the most susceptible brain networks to ageing. The DMN is positioned in the ventromedial prefrontal and posterior cingulate cortex and is active at rest [96]. At the same time, the DAN is located in the intraparietal sulcus and frontal eye fields and is active during tasks that require voluntary and sustained attention [97]. The posterior cingulate cortex controls memory functioning, whereas the left frontal eye field controls attention.

In older adults without significant neurological (e.g., Alzheimer's and Parkinson's) or psychiatric diseases, the DMN and DAN were strongly positively correlated with PA. The DMN plays a crucial role in high-level cognitive and self-referential processes; abnormal functioning of the DMN is related to psychological diseases, such as depression, anxiety, and attention deficit. The DAN is involved in top-down control of attention and sensory–motor information integration. The relation between PA and DMN varied depending on the levels of executive function: this association was only significant for high executive function. Moreover, PA was not significantly related to whole brain global or local efficiency [77]. In elders with the lowest DMN/DAN anti-correlation levels, higher PA and fitness were associated with improved executive function [78]. As reported in other studies, better executive function performance would be related to greater DMN and DAN connectivity.

Walking or dancing together with sensorial stimuli (musical stimulation) and fun-recreational activities (for example, book reading, crossword, and sudoku) led to significant changes in DMN, especially the precuneus, the right angular gyrus, and the posterior cingulate cortex, and in DAN, particularly the left frontal eye field [79]. The prefrontal cortex and medial temporal lobe are susceptible to ageing consequences. These areas showed resting-state functional connectivity following Tai Chi exercise, mainly if associated with cognitive training and group counselling [80]. Regarding memory processes, the hippocampus and medial prefrontal cortex communication play a key role [98,99]. Resting-state functional magnetic resonance imaging showed increased functional connectivity between the hippocampus and medial prefrontal cortex after Tai Chi Chuan and Baduanjin practices [81]. Moreover, frontal and subcortical networks also improved after exercise [82].

As concerns duration of PA, 6 weeks of PA produced significant changes in the right striatum (including both the putamen and the globus pallidus) and the posterior cingulate cortex/precuneus area, and no volume reduction in the right striatum [83]. On the contrary, an improvement in functional connectivity between the frontal, posterior, and temporal cortexes within the DMN and the frontal executive network was only found after one year of walking. Voss et al. noticed a non-significant but trending effect on the connectivity of the DMN following 6 months of training [84], which was confirmed by Flodin et al., who reported modulation of mid-temporal brain regions and hippocampus [85]. Voss et al. also suggested a boost in exercise-induced effects on functional connectivity thanks to nutritional supplements, including beta-alanine [86].

As for the intensity of daily PA, easy-paced walking (light activity) generated a greater BOLD in the left prefrontal and parietal regions. At the same time, brisk walking (moderate exercise) induced a greater BOLD response in the dorsolateral prefrontal cortex. Therefore, Kimura et al. concluded that moderate activity could counteract neurocognitive degradations [87].

PA has been positively associated with grey matter integrity. In structural MRI papers, the frontal and temporal lobes, including the hippocampus, were the areas with the most significant benefits from exercise. Higher levels of PA produced an augmentation and preservation of grey matter in the frontal cortex. An increase in medial temporal lobe volume was described in fit older adults [88]; moreover, this effect could be desirable in subjects with a genetic risk of Alzheimer's disease [100]. Thus, PA-induced modifications seem to limit the ageing effect of temporal lobes. The pro-inflammatory cytokines affect brain ageing negatively and have been linked to dementia. Indeed, Papenberg et al. reported that grey matter volume could be preserved thanks to an active lifestyle [89]. On the contrary, inflammation related to inactivity could lead to a cognitive decline across 6 years.

In cognitively impaired older people, neural regions associated with language, superior-parietal regions, and frontoparietal regions are the most common brain networks involved after exercise. In older adults with mild cognitive impairment, improvements in functional connectivity between the posterior cingulate cortex and bilateral medial prefrontal cortex and between the posterior cingulate cortex and left hippocampus, as well as a trend of reduced bilateral hippocampal volume atrophy, were noticed after 8 weeks of mindfulness (non-judgmental moment-to-moment awareness obtained through sitting and walking meditation, body scan, and yoga) [90]. The elders who underwent a 12-week yoga intervention showed an enhancement of memory functions and functional connectivity related to verbal, attentional, and self-regulatory performance [91]. Yoga also improved connectivity between the DMN and lingual network, which is positively related to better memory performance. Moreover, Baduanjin training increased grey matter volume in the hippocampus, functional connectivity between the hippocampus and angular gyrus, and the amplitude of low-frequency fluctuations in the anterior cingulate cortex, compared with brisk walking and non-exercise. Tao et al. suggested the potential of Baduanjin in preventing the progression of mild cognitive impairment [92]. Progressive resistance training decreased posterior cingulate–anterior cingulate cortex functional connectivity. Suo et al. also described a greater cortical thickness in the posterior cingulate after 6 months of progressive resistance training [93]. The authors concluded that this mechanism might benefit long-term protection against further cognitive decline, as posterior cingulate grey matter loss is a biomarker of Alzheimer's disease [101].

Stroke survivors frequently show cognitive impairments; hence, a selected PA intervention could improve post-stroke recovery. Aerobic exercise provides cognitive benefits, enhancing memory and attention after stroke [102]. The positive exercise-induced effects on cognition are often present even in the chronic stroke phase [103]. Moreover, combined interventions substantially impacted cognition improvement, especially regarding executive function [104]. However, the mechanisms underpinning these positive effects have yet to be fully understood. The following studies described functional brain changes following PA. Hsu et al. investigated the effect of 6 months of progressive aerobic exercise training in subjects with mild subcortical ischemic vascular cognitive impairment [94]. Six months of walking outdoors with progressive intensity did not significantly increase frontoparietal network (FPN) connectivity; that, however, was especially linked to improved mobility performance. Older people stroke survivors showed a positive correlation between daily exercise and DAN [95]. Stroke patients also improved attention performance thanks to PA.

3.2. Adults

The studies concerning the impact of chronic PA in adults encompassed a wide range of ages, from young adults to middle-aged people (Table 3). They mainly described the cognitive improvement to counteract psychological disorders and brain ageing. Moreover, the papers concerning adults embraced patients with psychological disorders and healthy people.

Table 3. Summary of studies investigating chronic exercise among adults.

Study	Sample	Physical Activity	Methods	Main Findings
Goldin et al., 2012 [105]	42 adults with SAD * (32.88 ± 7.97 yrs): 24 in the MBSR group; 18 in the aerobic group	8 sessions of weekly MBSR; 8 weeks of aerobic exercise	fMRI * scan	Greater brain responses in the posterior cingulate cortex in the MBSR group
Goldin et al., 2013 [106]	42 adults with SAD (32.88 ± 7.97 yrs): 24 in the MBSR * group; 18 in the aerobic group	8 sessions of weekly MBSR; 8 weeks of aerobic exercise	fMRI scan	Reduced negative emotions; increase in attention-related parietal cortical regions in the MBSR group
Gourgouvelis et al., 2017 [107]	16 adults: 8 patients with depression and anxiety (37.25 ± 8.0 yrs); 8 healthy controls (20.63 ± 1.19 yrs)	8 weeks of moderate intervention: resistance training, and mild to vigorous aerobic session	fMRI scan	Reduced hippocampal activity in patients
Huang et al., 2021 [108]	70 adults (18–50 yrs): 38 StD patients; 32 healthy controls	8 weeks of moderate aerobic exercise	fMRI scan	Reduced right inferior parietal lobule activity in StD * patients
Stern et al., 2019 [109]	132 healthy adults (20–67 yrs)	6 months of aerobic exercise/stretching and toning	MRI scan	Increased cortical thickness in the left caudal middle frontal cortex Brodmann area in the aerobic group
Bashir et al., 2021 [110]	45 healthy adults (19–27 yrs): 25 in the exercise group; 20 in the control group	6 months of aerobic and anaerobic exercise	MRI scan	Increased cortical thickness in left peri calcarine area, left superior parietal area, right rostral middle frontal, and right lateral occipital gyrus
Kaiser et al., 2022 [111]	45 healthy adults (18–30 yrs)	12 weeks of high- vs. low-intensity exercise	MRI scan	Increased left hippocampal and decreased right hippocampal volume after vigorous exercise
Fontes et al., 2013 [112]	7 healthy male adults (26.6 ± 4.0 yrs)	6 sessions of cycling	fMRI scan	Relation between posterior cingulate cortex and precuneus and higher levels of perceived exertion
Ishihara et al., 2020 [113]	1033 healthy adults (22–37 yrs)	Not specified	fMRI scan	Increased functional connectivity within DMN and FPN *
Nakagawa et al., 2020 [114]	58 healthy adults (22.4 ± 2.4)	Moderate-to-vigorous exercise vs. low-to-moderate exercise	Cognitive tests	Better cognitive performance in moderate-to-vigorous group
Bezzola et al., 2012 [115]	32 healthy middle-aged adults (51.2 ± 7.2 yrs): 11 in the golf group; 11 in the control group	40 h of golf training	fMRI scan	Reduction in neuronal recruitment in the right and left dorsal premotor cortex
Wadden et al., 2013 [116]	10 healthy middle-aged adults (64.7 ± 8.5 yrs)	7 days of exercise	fMRI scan	Bilateral cerebellar activation
Pensel et al., 2018 [117]	25 healthy middle-aged adults (52.21 ± 6.39 yrs)	6 months of aerobic exercise	fMRI scan	Bilateral frontal activation

* DMN: default mode network; fMRI: functional magnetic resonance imaging; FPN: frontoparietal network; MRI: magnetic resonance imaging; MBSR: mindfulness-based stress reduction; SAD: social anxiety disorder; StD: subthreshold depression.

Goldin et al. investigated the effects of mindfulness meditation associated with Hatha yoga and 8 weeks of aerobic exercise in patients with social anxiety disorder [105]. Both mindfulness and aerobic training significantly reduced social symptoms and increased mindfulness skills. Nevertheless, mindfulness meditation generated excellent functional connectivity in the posterior cingulate and dorsomedial prefrontal cortex and improved attention-related parietal cortical regions [106]. Eight weeks of exercise in adults with major depressive disorder led to a marginal reduction in hippocampal activations; therefore, exercise reduced the level of depressive disorder from severe to mild [107]. Huang et al. investigated the changes in brain activity in adults aged between 18 and 50 years with and without subthreshold depression/subsyndromal depression before and after 8 weeks of moderate-intensity aerobic exercise [108]. All individuals showed changes in the right precuneus, right fusiform gyrus, right middle cingulate, and right superior parietal lobule and an augmentation of precuneal activity. The right inferior parietal lobule activity was enhanced only in subjects with subthreshold depression. The authors reported a decrease in depressive and anxiety symptoms and underlined the importance of PA in preventing the development of major depression.

Regarding healthy adults, Stern et al. compared the effects of 6 months of aerobic PA with that of stretching/toning exercises on the cognition and brain structure of healthy adults aged 20 to 67 years [109]. Executive function improved significantly after aerobic PA and increased with the subject's age. Increased cortical thickness in the left caudal middle frontal cortex Brodmann area was observed after aerobic PA. Another recent MRI study reported significantly increased cortical thickness following 6 months of aerobic and anaerobic exercise [110].

Kaiser et al. evaluated the changes in hippocampal volume, vasculature, neuro metabolites, and peripheral growth factors after a 12-week low- (toning) or high-intensity (aerobic) exercise program [111]. The concentrations of N-acetyl aspartate in the dorsal anterior cingulate cortex and BDNF, and peripheral insulin-like growth factor-1 (IGF-1), as markers for neuronal development, were positively linked to cardiorespiratory fitness changes. Moreover, the authors found an improvement in cardiorespiratory function, an increase in left hippocampal, and a decrease in right hippocampal volume, particularly after the high-intensity exercise condition.

Fontes et al. detected the associations of the precentral gyrus and cerebellar vermis with dynamic cycling activity using an fMRI-compatible cycling ergometer [112]. The authors found that the posterior cingulate cortex and precuneus were linked with higher levels of perceived exertion in healthy male young adults. Hence, the primary motor cortex and cerebellum regulate motor activity during cycling. In another study, Ishihara et al. described the cognitive impact of exercise in a broad sample of healthy young adults aged 22–37 years, focusing on the concomitant and independent relations between PA and working memory domains [113]. Superior working memory was linked to higher cardiorespiratory fitness and hand dexterity, mediated by task-evoked functional activity in parts of the FPN and DMN; instead, gait speed and muscular strength did not affect working memory.

As concerns exercise intensity, compared with low-to-moderate-intensity PA (for instance, walking), regular moderate-to-vigorous-intensity PA was associated with better cognitive and mental health measures in young people aged between 20 and 39 years [114].

Regarding healthy middle-aged adults, light- or moderate-intensity PA could lead to functional neuroplastic changes. After short-duration training, Bezzola et al. noticed a significant reduction in neuronal recruitment in the right and left dorsal premotor cortex [115]. Seven days of PA led to a bilateral cerebellar activation. Moreover, better sequence-specific temporal performance generated greater activation in the precentral gyrus, middle occipital gyrus, and putamen of the right hemisphere and the thalamus, cuneus, and cerebellum of the left hemisphere, which was linked to speed rather than the precision of movements [116]. Six months of moderate exercise in sedentary males produced brain activity in bilateral frontal regions that depended on individual fitness gains [117].

As reported above, the studies concerning cognitively normal adults mainly focused on the link between PA, and memory performance and executive function since both cognitive domains are affected by ageing and may change according to age.

3.3. Adolescents and Children

Several papers emphasised the importance of chronic PA during childhood and adolescence to prevent cardiac, muscular, and metabolic diseases and to improve cognitive function and scholastic performance [118]. A previous meta-analysis evaluated the correlation between regular physical exercise lasting at least one month and children's executive functions and noticed a small and measurable improvement in neuropsychological tests of executive functions, mainly inhibitory control. Some studies examined whether specific biomarkers (e.g., BDNF, cathepsin B (CTSB), and fibroblast growth factor 21) were involved in brain health after PA. According to Rodriguez-Ayllon et al., no biomarkers mediated the effects of exercise on brain health [119]. On the contrary, a systematic review reported that adolescent athletes show lower serum but higher plasma BDNF concentrations than sedentary individuals [120]. Moreover, exercise could increase serum BDNF concentrations in inactive adolescents to a small extent.

In children, a sedentary life may negatively affect the development of the growing brain. Therefore, promoting PA and reducing sedentary behaviour may preserve mental health in children and adolescents. PA is a simple and important method for improving children's mental functioning, such as executive function, which is critical to cognitive development [121]. Regular PA may contribute to academic and professional success, as well as success in social interaction [122].

Most of the following reviewed studies evaluated PA's impact on cognition by neuroimaging (Table 4).

Table 4. Summary of studies investigating chronic exercise among adolescents and children.

Study	Sample	Physical Activity	Methods	Main Findings
Kjellenberg et al., 2022 [123]	1139 adolescent (13.4 ± 0.3 yrs)	7 days of moderate-to-vigorous exercise	Cognitive tests	Better cognitive function
Kamijo et al., 2011 [124]	43 children (7–9 yrs): 22 in the exercise group; 21 in the control group	9 months of aerobic exercise	Cognitive tests	Improved working memory
Quinzi et al., 2022 [125]	64 children	Racket sport, martial arts, and indoor climbing	Cognitive tests	Improved specific domains related to exercise type
Hillmann et al., 2014 [126]	221 children (7–9 yrs): 109 in the exercise group; 112 in the control group	9 months of aerobic exercise	fMRI * scan	Improved executive control and brain activity
Chaddock-Heyman et al., 2013 [127]	23 children (8.9 ± 5.8)	9 months of moderate-to-vigorous aerobic exercise	fMRI scan	Reduced activation in the right anterior prefrontal cortex
Chaddock-Heyman et al., 2013 [128]	143 children (8.7 ± 0.55)	9 months of aerobic exercise	MRI * scan	Improved white matter microstructure in the genu of the anterior corpus callosum
Logan et al., 2021 [129]	206 children (8–10 yrs): 103 normal weight; 103 obese	9 months of aerobic exercise	EEG *	Reduced neuroleptic indices in obese
Ortega et al., 2022 [130]	90 overweight children (8–10 yrs)	20 weeks of high-intensity aerobic exercise	Standardised tests and MRI scan	Improved intelligence and cognitive flexibility; unidentified structural changes

Table 4. *Cont.*

Study	Sample	Physical Activity	Methods	Main Findings
Davis et al., 2011 [121]	19 overweight children (9.8 ± 1.0 yrs)	3 months of regular aerobic exercise	fMRI scan	Increased bilateral prefrontal cortex activity. Reduced bilateral posterior parietal cortex activity
Kraff et al., 2014 [131]	43 overweight children (9.8 ± 0.8 yrs)	8 months of aerobic exercise	fMRI scan	Reduced activation in prefrontal and parietal areas; increased activation in the frontal gyrus and anterior cingulate
Kraff et al., 2014 [132]	22 overweight children (9.5 ± 0.7 yrs): 13 in the exercise group; 9 in the control group	8 months of aerobic exercise	fMRI scan	Reduced synchrony in motor, default mode, and cognitive control networks; increased synchrony only between the motor network and frontal regions
Kraff et al., 2014 [133]	18 overweight children (9.7 ± 0.7 yrs): 10 in the exercise group; 8 in the control group	8 months of aerobic exercise	DTI *	Increased white matter integrity in the bilateral superior longitudinal fasciculus
Schaeffer et al., 2014 [134]	18 overweight children (9.7 ± 0.7 yrs): 10 in the exercise group; 8 in the control group	8 months of aerobic exercise	DTI	Positive change in bilateral uncinate fasciculus

* DTI: diffusion tensor imaging; EEG: electroencephalography; fMRI: functional magnetic resonance imaging; MRI: magnetic resonance imaging.

A Swedish study investigated the effects of moderate-to-vigorous PA and screen time on mental health in 1139 Swedish adolescents (mean age 13.4 years). After seven consecutive days, moderate-to-vigorous PA was associated with better mental health, while the opposite was observed following screen time [123]. These associations were inconsistent across time domains, genders, and mental health outcomes. Kamijo et al. detected increased cardiorespiratory fitness associated with improved cognitive control of working memory in preadolescent children following 9 months of randomised control PA compared with that in a waitlist control group [124]. Quinzi et al. analysed the effects of different disciplines on electrophysiological levels and behaviours in children [125]. The racket players showed the most consistent response time and greater attentional control, and the climbers were characterised by more intense top-down anticipatory attention. The martial arts practitioners had the fastest response time and a more speed-oriented response. Nine months of PA in preadolescent children determined changes in physical fitness (maximum oxygen consumption) and brain electrical activity and, significantly, an enhancement in executive control; therefore, exercise could improve infant cognition and brain health [126].

MRI and fMRI papers mainly analysed the impact of moderate-to-vigorous PA on cognition. After 9 months of moderate-to-vigorous aerobic PA, 8- to 9-year-old children showed a reduction in brain activation in the right anterior prefrontal cortex, which was consistent with patterns of young adults [127]. Following exercise, no changes were detected in the anterior cingulate cortex, insula, and occipital cortex. Moreover, white matter microstructure in the genu of the anterior corpus callosum was enhanced: in 7- to 9-year-old children, the fractional anisotropy increased and the radial diffusivity decreased, whereas no changes in axonal fibre diameter were found following 9 months of aerobic exercise [128]. In addition, the children not subjected to aerobic PA showed typical development without any modification of white matter microstructure. The anterior prefrontal cortex and the corpus callosum were involved in cognitive control. A specific corpus callosum development could prevent cognitive and behaviour deficits, e.g., attention-deficit hyperactivity disorder, autism, and schizophrenia.

A more significant number of studies have been carried out on the impact of PA in overweight children. Youth obesity is rising; according to the WHO European Regional Obesity Report 2022, approximately one-third of European children are overweight or obese [135]. A Mexican study reported a reduction in the hippocampal volume and a lower executive cognitive performance on neuropsychological evaluations in overweight/obese 6- to 8-year-old children, positively correlated with the increase in body mass index (BMI) [136]. Therefore, regular PA could reduce BMI and benefit cognitive performance, as described in the following reviewed papers (Table 4).

Nine months of PA led to many cognitive and brain health benefits in both standard and overweight children [129]. Obese children showed a reduction in neuroleptic indices compared with normal-weight children. In addition, normal-weight children exhibited a decrease in visceral adipose tissue associated with faster task performance. A recent study investigated the positive effects of PA on intelligence, executive function, academic performance, and brain outcomes in overweight or obese children [130]. Brain health indicators, including intelligence, executive function (cognitive flexibility, inhibition, and working memory), and academic performance, were assessed using standardised tests, whereas MRI measured hippocampal volume. In total, 109 obese or overweight participants, aged between 8 and 11 years, underwent 90 min of exercise three times a week. Training positively affects intelligence and cognitive flexibility during development among children with overweight or obesity. However, structural and functional brain changes were not identified. Overweight Black and White 7- to 11-year-old children showed improved bilateral prefrontal cortex activity and reduced bilateral posterior parietal cortex activity following 3 months of regular aerobic exercise [121]. As for executive function, an enhancement in mathematics was detected. No dose–response correlation between PA and cognition, and no changes in motor regions (frontal and supplementary eye fields) were observed. The outcomes concerning prefrontal and parietal cortexes are consistent with those observed in older people. The activation of several regions supporting antisaccade performance, i.e., bilateral precentral gyrus, medial frontal gyrus, paracentral lobule, postcentral gyrus, superior parietal lobule, inferior parietal lobule, anterior cingulate cortex, right inferior frontal gyrus, insula, and left precuneus, decreased in overweight, predominantly Black 8- to 11-year-old children after 8 months of aerobic exercise [131]. In contrast, the activation of other areas supporting flanker performance, i.e., left medial frontal gyrus, superior frontal gyrus, middle frontal gyrus, superior temporal gyrus, cingulate gyrus, and insula, was enhanced. Hence, differences in task strategies could modify different neural circuitries in children with higher BMI. Still, whether the functional connectivity changes depended on increased fitness or decreased body fat was determined. Eight months of aerobic exercise was also associated with reduced synchrony with three resting state networks (motor, default mode, and cognitive control networks) and increased synchrony only between the motor network and frontal regions (right medial frontal, middle frontal, and superior frontal gyri) [132]. A decrease in synchrony becomes more focal and refined synchrony in those regions.

The following papers described the effects of PA on white matter integrity in overweight young people via diffusion tensor MRI. Overweight, predominantly Black 8- to 11-year-old children showed changes in white matter integrity after approximately 8 months of aerobic exercise [133]. PA increased white matter integrity in the bilateral superior longitudinal fasciculus due to increased fractional anisotropy and reduced radial diffusivity. The enhancement of white matter integrity in the right superior longitudinal fasciculus indicated greater selective attention. In contrast, the improvement in white matter integrity in the left superior longitudinal fasciculus showed higher teacher ratings of classroom behaviour [133]. In addition, 8 months of PA generated significantly positive change in bilateral uncinate fasciculus, a white matter fibre tract connecting frontal and temporal lobes [134]. These outcomes indicated an enhancement of white matter structural coherence and myelination.

4. Discussion

The current review focused on the association between exercise and cognition in every age group. We found a positive correlation between PA and cognition in humans, which was widely supported by MRI and fMRI studies. **Indeed, PA generated substantial changes in functional brain activation and cognitive performance across all age groups. No particular age group showed more advantage from PA. Still, a specific exercise type could improve cognition in selected subjects.**

The papers reviewed here mainly investigated the effect of chronic PA rather than acute PA. Studies concerning acute PA differed in intensity and duration of exercise, whereas they were similar regarding the type of exercise, i.e., treadmill running or stationary cycling. However, acute aerobic exercise would provide more favourable cognitive improvements. It could create a healthy environment by facilitating cortical activity, haemodynamics, and metabolism, especially at moderate intensity [137].

In line with previous studies [36,138], we noted the exercise-induced mechanisms on cognition at multiple levels of analysis in every age group. Regarding molecular and cellular levels, PA induces the expression of neurotransmitter and neurotrophic factors involved in changes in brain structure and neurogenesis [139]. Indeed, BDNF underpins neuron growth, survival, synaptic plasticity, axonal pruning, and regeneration. Decreased BDNF levels represent a lack of trophic support and may contribute to cognitive impairment in Alzheimer's disease. In children and older adults, moderate-intensity resistance training was more effective in maintaining or increasing BDNF levels than other exercise types [140]. **Moreover, BDNF seems to mediate the link between exercise and functional connectivity** [141].

Regarding structural and functional brain changes, MRI studies reported increased grey matter volume in brain regions, especially in the hippocampus, prefrontal regions, and caudate nucleus. Exercise is crucial in preventing brain volume loss, a phenomenon linked to brain ageing. Consistent with previous papers [142], we found a positive impact of PA on frontal and temporal lobes; in particular, exercise may reduce the risk of temporal lobe atrophy [143]. PA was also associated with greater white matter integrity. The increase in white matter integrity in bilateral superior longitudinal fasciculus found in children was linked to a reduction in radial diffusivity, in accordance with studies concerning adults [144]. The frontotemporal white matter integrity increased in unfit children and older adults [145], although the extent of integrity could vary in the age group.

Regarding functional brain connectivity, through fMRI, children, adults, and older adults showed significant changes in brain functional connectivity, especially in the frontal lobe, the cerebellum, and the hippocampus after acute PA. These outcomes are consistent with those detected by other functional neuroimaging techniques (i.e., fNIRS) [15]. In older adults, PA led to more excellent DMN connectivity: in older adults without major neurological diseases, the association between PA and DMN was higher for higher executive function and more extended training periods. Moreover, PA generated changes, especially in frontal, temporal, and parietal regions, i.e., areas sensitive to neurodegeneration [100]. FPN and DAN modifications usually occur in young adults and older people. In adults, the changes were detected in the left parietal regions, especially in the precuneus. The precuneus manages highly integrated mental processes and is often involved in the early stages of Alzheimer's disease and mild cognitive impairments [146]. PA seems to counteract cognitive decline by improving functional integration of the frontoparietal control network via effects on the precuneus [147,148]. PA increased prefrontal cortex activity and reduced posterior parietal cortex activity in children. There was also better functional connectivity in DMN. **Different study designs can explain these results.**

PA improved attention, working memory, and executive function in all ages. Exercise improved performance on various cognitive task categories, including attention, visuospatial functions, information processing, memory, and executive function. Moreover, the benefits of acute exercise could help prepare for situations demanding high executive control (e.g., complex daily tasks or necessary examinations in educational settings) [149]. Increased functional connectivity in DMN and DAN was associated with more significant enhancement in executive function. An improvement in working memory was noticed in several studies after chronic PA [150]: working memory is involved in daily activities, such as performing mathematical calculations, recognising to-do lists, and turning instructions into action plans. Longer PA interventions in young people improved mental health and cognition outcomes, especially neurobiological alterations [151,152]. However, **most papers focused on working memory and executive function, neglecting other cognitive domains.**

When we analysed whether a particular age or population gained the most significant advantages from PA, we noticed no big differences among different ages. Since most studies dealt with older adults and children, available data are insufficient to state which age exhibited the greatest cognitive improvements from PA. However, overweight children and subjects with subthreshold depression or subsyndromal depression seemed to benefit from exercise, which could prevent worsening clinical status. Consequently, future research should investigate whether exercise-induced benefits are more significant in a specific age or population than others.

Lastly, we evaluated whether a selected age or population achieved better cognitive performance for a specific exercise type. The studies focusing on older adults with cognitive impairment and adults with depression comprised participants who underwent light or moderate PA. These subjects were generally involved in coordinated exercise, for instance, yoga, which has beneficial effects on mood, cognitive function, and neural structure and function via lowering stress, reducing inflammation, and improving neuroplasticity processes. Quinzi et al. demonstrated how different sports (racket sport, martial arts, and indoor climbing) could promote specific changes in cognitive functions [125]. Practising specific sports could lead to differential benefits on cognitive processing. Therefore, selecting the most appropriate PA depending on individual demands would be helpful.

fMRI represents the best available neuroimaging method in neurological fields. However, some studies preferred resting-state fMRI in subjects unable to perform tasks accurately because of physical or cognitive impairment, eliminating the confounding effects due to differences in task performance [153,154]. Children showed resting-state networks more defined by anatomical proximity, whereas adults showed patterns more related to functional relationships [155]. However, fMRI reproducibility can be compromised by experimental factors, e.g., length of scan, cognitive task design, and motion artefacts. In addition, total sleep duration and sleepiness could affect the measures of the cortical hemodynamic response; cognitive performance is linked to some biopsychosocial factors, such as circadian rhythms [156–158], tiredness [159], and level of arousal.

The current review was subjected to the following limitations. We did not include behavioural mechanisms since only some studies dealt with this aspect. Exercise-induced positive benefits on sleep and mood could enhance cognitive function [160]. In addition, motivation, fatigue, and perception of pain could affect training compliance and, thus, brain health [161]. Individuals with serious psychological disorders, with a potential lack of motivation were usually excluded from the studies. Future studies should investigate how behavioural mechanisms could regulate the effects of PA on cognition. Our research was conducted in a single database. Therefore, it could be possible that potentially eligible papers were omitted.

Overall, the results tended to need more generalisability; brain changes did not manifest equally or uniformly throughout the brain, probably because the studies differed in terms of their study samples, imaging methods, and type of exercises. Several study limitations should be noted. The fMRI studies generally encompassed a small sample size with a homogeneous population. Moreover, including participants with higher educational levels could be a confounding variable. Most fMRI studies limited their sample to right-handed people and did not investigate the potential different brain activations between right- and left-handed individuals. Few papers dealt with the effects of chronic physical exercise in adults [161]. Moreover, these studies included a large range of ages, from young adults to middle-aged people, without considering the hormonal changes that occur in the passage from young to middle-aged adulthood [161,162]. The duration of the studies was limited to a maximum of one year. Hence, assessing whether the PA-induced results remain stable over time following PA cessation would be interesting.

Given the differences in study design, cognitive tests, neuroimaging methods, and study samples in the reviewed studies, future studies should be drawn to overcome these limitations and to better understand the mechanisms underpinning the impact of PA on cognition. **More well-designed randomised controlled trials with appropriate sample sizes and post-PA follow-up assessments should be conducted to increase the findings' reliability.**

However, despite the heterogeneity among the research, **our findings provide a further and current understanding of PA-induced mechanisms** and highlight the strength of exercise-related effects on both the brain and cognition across all age groups. PA may be considered a powerful tool to preserve and foster neurocognitive functioning throughout a person's lifetime. **Furthermore, our review supports the importance of practising a specific type of PA in selected people, for instance, in patients with psychological disorders, to gain better cognitive performance.**

Regular PA could be an essential and decisive protective factor against cognitive decline and dementia in the elderly. It should be recommended during childhood and adolescence, characterised by rapid growth and development. **Thus, public health initiatives should be implemented to raise awareness among people of different ages regarding the impact of PA on mental health.**

5. Conclusions

Regular PA leads to positive effects in multiple cognitive domains at every stage of life, and neurological tests and neuroimaging widely support this evidence. A healthy lifestyle and proper PA reduce inflammatory states; increase the presence of synaptogenic, angiogenic, and neurotrophic factors; and improve cognitive functions (e.g., memory and executive function) and functional connectivity. It can be suggested that a particular exercise type could provide better cognitive improvements for a selected target of subjects, for instance, light-intensity exercise in patients with depression or neural diseases. However, our findings are inconclusive because of the heterogeneity among the papers reviewed here. Future well-designed studies should select the most suitable type of PA for every age group and to detail the impact of PA in adults. Therefore, correct and constant PA is fundamental for adolescents' and children's physical, psychophysical, and mental well-being and should be promoted and implemented in educational and recreational places. In addition, regular PA may prevent the onset of diseases related to cognitive decline with age.

Author Contributions: Conceptualisation, M.M. and F.F.; methodology, M.M.; validation, M.M.; formal analysis, S.M.; investigation, M.M.; resources, M.M.; data curation, M.M.; writing—original draft preparation, F.F.; writing—review and editing, M.M.; visualisation, S.M. and M.M.; supervision, M.M.; project administration, M.M.; funding acquisition, F.F. All authors have read and agreed to the published version of the manuscript.

Funding: This research received no external funding.

Institutional Review Board Statement: Not applicable.

Informed Consent Statement: Not applicable.

Data Availability Statement: Not applicable.

Conflicts of Interest: The authors declare no conflict of interest.

References

1. Caspersen, C.J.; Powell, K.E.; Christenson, G.M. Physical activity, exercise, and physical fitness: Definitions and distinctions for health-related research. *Public Health Rep.* **1985**, *100*, 126–131. [PubMed]
2. World Health Organization. Global Status Report on Physical Activity. 2022. Available online: https://www.who.int/publications/i/item/9789240059153 (accessed on 19 October 2022).
3. Hillman, C.H.; Erickson, K.I.; Kramer, A.F. Be smart, exercise your heart: Exercise effects on brain and cognition. *Nat. Rev. Neurosci.* **2008**, *9*, 58–65. [CrossRef] [PubMed]
4. Lipowski, M.; Zaleski, Z. Inventory of Physical Activity Objectives—A new method of measuring motives for physical activity and sport. *Health Psychol. Rep.* **2015**, *3*, 47–58. [CrossRef]
5. Lee, I.M.; Shiroma, E.J.; Lobelo, F.; Puska, P.; Blair, S.N.; Katzmarzyk, P.T. Lancet Physical Activity Series Working Group. Effect of physical inactivity on major non-communicable diseases worldwide: An analysis of disease burden and life expectancy. *Lancet* **2012**, *380*, 219–229. [CrossRef]
6. Sanad, E.A.; El-Shinnawy, H.A.E.H.; Hebah, H.A.; Farrag, D.A.; Soliman, E.R.A.; Abdelgawad, M.A. Effect of intra-dialytic physical exercise on depression in prevalent hemodialysis patients. *Egypt. J. Neurol. Psychiatry Neurosurg.* **2022**, *58*, 124. [CrossRef]
7. Colcombe, S.; Kramer, A.F. Fitness effects on the cognitive function of older adults: A meta-analytic study. *Psychol. Sci.* **2003**, *14*, 125–130. [CrossRef]
8. Allen, C. On (not) defining cognition. *Synthese* **2017**, *194*, 4233–4249. [CrossRef]
9. van Praag, H.; Kempermann, G.; Gage, F.H. Neural consequences of environmental enrichment. *Nat. Rev. Neurosci.* **2000**, *1*, 191–198. [CrossRef]
10. Colcombe, S.J.; Kramer, A.F.; Erickson, K.I.; Scalf, P.; McAuley, E.; Cohen, N.J.; Webb, A.; Jerome, G.J.; Marquez, D.X.; Elavsky, S. Cardiovascular fitness, cortical plasticity, and aging. *Proc. Natl. Acad. Sci. USA* **2004**, *101*, 3316–3321. [CrossRef]
11. Szuhany, K.L.; Bugatti, M.; Otto, M.W. A meta-analytic review of the effects of exercise on brain-derived neurotrophic factor. *J. Psychiatr. Res.* **2015**, *60*, 56–64. [CrossRef]
12. Pignataro, P.; Dicarlo, M.; Zerlotin, R.; Storlino, G.; Oranger, A.; Sanesi, L.; Lovero, R.; Buccoliero, C.; Mori, G.; Colaianni, G.; et al. Antidepressant Effect of Intermittent Long-Term Systemic Administration of Irisin in Mice. *Int. J. Mol. Sci.* **2022**, *23*, 7596. [CrossRef] [PubMed]
13. Noakes, T.D. Time to move beyond a brainless exercise physiology: The evidence for complex regulation of human exercise performance. *Appl. Physiol. Nutr. Metab.* **2011**, *36*, 23–35. [CrossRef] [PubMed]
14. Törpel, A.; Herold, F.; Hamacher, D.; Müller, N.G.; Schega, L. Strengthening the Brain—Is Resistance Training with Blood Flow Restriction an Effective Strategy for Cognitive Improvement? *J. Clin. Med.* **2018**, *7*, 377. [CrossRef]
15. Herold, F.; Wiegel, P.; Scholkmann, F.; Müller, N.G. Applications of Functional Near-Infrared Spectroscopy (fNIRS) Neuroimaging in Exercise—Cognition Science: A Systematic, Methodology-Focused Review. *J. Clin. Med.* **2018**, *7*, 466. [CrossRef]
16. Boecker, H.; Hillman, C.H.; Scheef, L.; Strüder, H.K. *Functional Neuroimaging in Exercise and Sport Sciences*; Springer: New York, NY, USA, 2012; pp. 419–446, ISBN 978-1-4614-3292-0.
17. Ciccarelli, O.; Toosy, A.T.; Marsden, J.F.; Wheeler-Kingshott, C.M.; Sahyoun, C.; Matthews, P.M.; Miller, D.H.; Thompson, A.J. Identifying brain regions for integrative sensorimotor processing with ankle movements. *Exp. Brain Res.* **2005**, *166*, 31–42. [CrossRef] [PubMed]
18. Glover, G.H. Overview of functional magnetic resonance imaging. *Neurosurg. Clin. N. Am.* **2011**, *22*, 133–139. [CrossRef] [PubMed]
19. Ogawa, S.; Lee, T.M.; Kay, A.R.; Tank, D.W. Brain magnetic resonance imaging with contrast dependent on blood oxygenation. *Proc. Natl. Acad. Sci. USA* **1990**, *87*, 9868–9872. [CrossRef]
20. Hahn, A.; Lanzenberger, R.; Kasper, S. Making Sense of Connectivity. *Int. J. Neuropsychopharmacol.* **2019**, *22*, 194–207. [CrossRef]
21. Festa, F.; Rotelli, C.; Scarano, A.; Navarra, R.; Caulo, M.; Macrì, M. Functional Magnetic Resonance Connectivity in Patients with Temporomadibular Joint Disorders. *Front. Neurol.* **2021**, *12*, 629211. [CrossRef]
22. Kawata, K.H.D.S.; Hirano, K.; Hamamoto, Y.; Oi, H.; Kanno, A.; Kawashima, R.; Sugiura, M. Motivational decline and proactive response under thermal environmental stress are related to emotion- and problem-focused coping, respectively: Questionnaire construction and fMRI study. *Front. Behav. Neurosci.* **2023**, *17*, 1143450. [CrossRef]
23. Damoiseaux, J.S.; Beckmann, C.F.; Arigita, E.J.; Barkhof, F.; Scheltens, P.; Stam, C.J.; Smith, S.M.; Rombouts, S.A. Reduced resting-state brain activity in the "default network" in normal aging. *Cereb. Cortex* **2008**, *18*, 1856–1864. [CrossRef] [PubMed]
24. Tanaka, M.; Szabó, Á.; Vécsei, L. Preclinical modelling in depression and anxiety: Current challenges and future research directions. *Adv. Clin. Exp. Med.* **2023**, *32*, 505–509. [CrossRef] [PubMed]
25. Tanaka, M.; Szabó, Á.; Spekker, E.; Polyák, H.; Tóth, F.; Vécsei, L. Mitochondrial Impairment: A Common Motif in Neuropsychiatric Presentation? The Link to the Tryptophan—Kynurenine Metabolic System. *Cells* **2022**, *11*, 2607. [CrossRef] [PubMed]
26. Stillman, C.M.; Donofry, S.D.; Erickson, K.I. Exercise, fitness and the aging brain: A Review of functional connectivity in aging. *Arch. Psychol.* **2019**, *3*. [CrossRef]
27. Eckstrom, E.; Neukam, S.; Kalin, L.; Wright, J. Physical Activity and Healthy Aging. *Clin. Geriatr. Med.* **2020**, *36*, 671–683. [CrossRef]
28. Won, J.; Callow, D.D.; Pena, G.S.; Gogniat, M.A.; Kommula, Y.; Arnold-Nedimala, N.A.; Jordan, L.S.; Smith, J.C. Evidence for exercise-related plasticity in functional and structural neural network connectivity. *Neurosci. Biobehav. Rev.* **2021**, *131*, 923–940. [CrossRef]

29. Haeger, A.; Costa, A.S.; Schulz, J.B.; Reetz, K. Cerebral changes improved by physical activity during cognitive decline: A systematic review on MRI studies. *Neuroimage Clin.* **2019**, *23*, 101933. [CrossRef]
30. Li, M.Y.; Huang, M.M.; Li, S.Z.; Tao, J.; Zheng, G.H.; Chen, L.D. The effects of aerobic exercise on the structure and function of DMN-related brain regions: A systematic review. *Int. J. Neurosci.* **2017**, *127*, 634–649. [CrossRef]
31. Teixeira-Machado, L.; Arida, R.M.; de Jesus Mari, J. Dance for neuroplasticity: A descriptive systematic review. *Neurosci. Biobehav. Rev.* **2019**, *96*, 232–240. [CrossRef]
32. Sigmundsson, H.; Dybendal, B.H.; Grassini, S. Motion, Relation, and Passion in Brain Physiological and Cognitive Aging. *Brain Sci.* **2022**, *12*, 1122. [CrossRef]
33. Turrini, S.; Bevacqua, N.; Cataneo, A.; Chiappini, E.; Fiori, F.; Battaglia, S.; Romei, V.; Avenanti, A. Neurophysiological Markers of Premotor–Motor Network Plasticity Predict Motor Performance in Young and Older Adults. *Biomedicines* **2023**, *11*, 1464. [CrossRef] [PubMed]
34. Gunnell, K.E.; Poitras, V.J.; LeBlanc, A.; Schibli, K.; Barbeau, K.; Hedayati, N.; Ponitfex, M.B.; Goldfied, G.S.; Dunlap, C.; Lehan, E.; et al. Physical activity and brain structure, brain function, and cognition in children and youth: A systematic review of randomized controlled trials. *Ment. Health Phys. Act.* **2019**, *16*, 105–127. [CrossRef]
35. Valkenborghs, S.R.; Noetel, M.; Hillman, C.H.; Nilsson, M.; Smith, J.J.; Ortega, F.B.; Lubans, D.R. The Impact of Physical Activity on Brain Structure and Function in Youth: A Systematic Review. *Pediatrics* **2019**, *144*, e20184032. [CrossRef] [PubMed]
36. Erickson, K.I.; Hillman, C.; Stillman, C.M.; Ballard, R.M.; Bloodgood, B.; Conroy, D.E.; Macko, R.; Marquez, D.X.; Petruzzello, S.J.; Powell, K.E.; et al. Physical Activity, Cognition, and Brain Outcomes: A Review of the 2018 Physical Activity Guidelines. *Med. Sci. Sports Exerc.* **2019**, *51*, 1242–1251. [CrossRef] [PubMed]
37. Chang, Y.K.; Labban, J.D.; Gapin, J.I.; Etnier, J.L. The effects of acute exercise on cognitive performance: A meta-analysis. *Brain Res.* **2012**, *1453*, 87–101. [CrossRef]
38. Emery, C.F.; Honn, V.J.; Frid, D.J.; Lebowitz, K.R.; Diaz, P.T. Acute effects of exercise on cognition in patients with chronic obstructive pulmonary disease. *Am. J. Respir. Crit. Care Med.* **2001**, *164*, 1624–1627. [CrossRef] [PubMed]
39. Pontifex, M.B.; Hillman, C.H.; Fernhall, B.; Thompson, K.M.; Valentini, T.A. The effect of acute aerobic and resistance exercise on working memory. *Med. Sci. Sports Exerc.* **2009**, *41*, 927–934. [CrossRef]
40. Coelho, F.G.; Vital, T.M.; Stein, A.M.; Arantes, F.J.; Rueda, A.V.; Camarini, R.; Teodorov, E.; Santos-Galduróz, R.F. Acute aerobic exercise increases brain-derived neurotrophic factor levels in elderly with Alzheimer's disease. *J. Alzheimer's Dis.* **2014**, *39*, 401–408. [CrossRef]
41. Won, J.; Alfini, A.J.; Weiss, L.R.; Michelson, C.S.; Callow, D.D.; Ranadive, S.M.; Gentili, R.J.; Smith, J.C. Semantic Memory Activation After Acute Exercise in Healthy Older Adults. *J. Int. Neuropsychol. Soc.* **2019**, *25*, 557–568. [CrossRef]
42. Won, J.; Alfini, A.J.; Weiss, L.R.; Callow, D.D.; Smith, J.C. Brain activation during executive control after acute exercise in older adults. *Int. J. Psychophysiol.* **2019**, *146*, 240–248. [CrossRef]
43. Voss, M.W.; Wenig, T.B.; Narayana-Kumanan, K.; Cole, R.C.; Wharff, C.; Reist, L.; Dubose, L.; Sigurdsson, G.; Mills, J.A.; Long, J.D.; et al. Acute Exercise Effects Predict Training Change in Cognition and Connectivity. *Med. Sci. Sports Exerc.* **2020**, *52*, 131–140. [CrossRef] [PubMed]
44. Suwabe, K.; Byun, K.; Hyodo, K.; Reagh, Z.M.; Roberts, J.M.; Matsushita, A.; Saotome, K.; Ochi, G.; Fukuie, T.; Suzuki, K.; et al. Rapid stimulation of human dentate gyrus function with acute mild exercise. *Proc. Natl. Acad. Sci. USA* **2018**, *115*, 10487–10492. [CrossRef] [PubMed]
45. Li, L.; Men, W.W.; Chang, Y.K.; Fan, M.X.; Ji, L.; Wei, G.X. Acute aerobic exercise increases cortical activity during working memory: A functional MRI study in female college students. *PLoS ONE* **2014**, *9*, e99222. [CrossRef] [PubMed]
46. Marin Bosch, B.; Bringard, A.; Logrieco, M.G.; Lauer, E.; Imobersteg, N.; Thomas, A.; Ferretti, G.; Schwartz, S.; Igloi, K. Effect of acute physical exercise on motor sequence memory. *Sci. Rep.* **2020**, *10*, 15322. [CrossRef]
47. Perini, R.; Bortoletto, M.; Capogrosso, M.; Fertonani, A.; Miniussi, C. Acute effects of aerobic exercise promote learning. *Sci. Rep.* **2016**, *6*, 25440. [CrossRef]
48. Mehren, A.; Özyurt, J.; Lam, A.P.; Brandes, M.; Müller, H.H.O.; Thiel, C.M.; Philipsen, A. Acute Effects of Aerobic Exercise on Executive Function and Attention in Adult Patients with ADHD. *Front. Psychiatry* **2019**, *10*, 132. [CrossRef]
49. Mehren, A.; Diaz Luque, C.; Brandes, M.; Lam, A.P.; Thiel, C.M.; Philipsen, A.; Özyurt, J. Intensity-Dependent Effects of Acute Exercise on Executive Function. *Neural Plast.* **2019**, *2019*, 8608317. [CrossRef]
50. Schmitt, A.; Martin, J.A.; Rojas, S.; Vafa, R.; Scheef, L.; Strüder, H.K.; Boecker, H. Effects of low- and high-intensity exercise on emotional face processing: An fMRI face-matching study. *Soc. Cogn. Affect. Neurosci.* **2019**, *14*, 657–665. [CrossRef]
51. Li, L.; Zhang, S.; Cui, J.; Chen, L.Z.; Wang, X.; Fan, M.; Wei, G.X. Fitness-Dependent Effect of Acute Aerobic Exercise on Executive Function. *Front. Physiol.* **2019**, *10*, 902. [CrossRef] [PubMed]
52. Choi, H.; Park, S.; Kim, K.K.; Lee, K.; Rhyu, H.S. Acute effects of aerobic stretching, health and happiness improving movement exercise on cortical activity of children. *J. Exerc. Rehabil.* **2016**, *12*, 320–327. [CrossRef]
53. Chen, A.G.; Zhu, L.N.; Yan, J.; Yin, H.C. Neural Basis of Working Memory Enhancement after Acute Aerobic Exercise: fMRI Study of Preadolescent Children. *Front. Psychol.* **2016**, *7*, 1804. [CrossRef] [PubMed]
54. Chen, A.G.; Zhu, L.N.; Xiong, X.; Li, Y. Acute aerobic exercise alters executive control network in preadolescent children. *J. Sport Psychol.* **2017**, *26*, 132–137.

55. Metcalfe, A.W.; MacIntosh, B.J.; Scavone, A.; Ou, X.; Korczak, D.; Goldstein, B.I. Effects of acute aerobic exercise on neural correlates of attention and inhibition in adolescents with bipolar disorder. *Transl. Psychiatry* **2016**, *6*, e814. [CrossRef] [PubMed]
56. Singh, A.M.; Staines, W.R. The effects of acute aerobic exercise on the primary motor cortex. *J. Mot. Behav.* **2015**, *47*, 328–339. [CrossRef]
57. Herold, F.; Aye, N.; Lehmann, N.; Taubert, M.; Müller, N.G. The Contribution of Functional Magnetic Resonance Imaging to the Understanding of the Effects of Acute Physical Exercise on Cognition. *Brain Sci.* **2020**, *10*, 175. [CrossRef] [PubMed]
58. World Health Organization. Ageing and Health. Available online: https://www.who.int/news-room/fact-sheets/detail/ageing-and-health (accessed on 1 October 2022).
59. Heger, I.; Deckers, K.; van Boxtel, M.; de Vugt, M.; Hajema, K.; Verhey, F.; Köhler, S. Dementia awareness and risk perception in middle-aged and older individuals: Baseline results of the MijnBreincoach survey on the association between lifestyle and brain health. *BMC Public Health* **2019**, *19*, 678. [CrossRef]
60. Dedeyne, L.; Deschodt, M.; Verschueren, S.; Tournoy, J.; Gielen, E. Effects of multi-domain interventions in (pre)frail elderly on frailty, functional, and cognitive status: A systematic review. *Clin. Interv. Aging* **2017**, *12*, 873–896. [CrossRef]
61. Karssemeijer, E.G.A.; Aaronson, J.A.; Bossers, W.J.; Smits, T.; Olde Rikkert, M.G.M.; Kessels, R.P.C. Positive effects of combined cognitive and physical exercise training on cognitive function in older adults with mild cognitive impairment or dementia: A meta-analysis. *Ageing Res. Rev.* **2017**, *40*, 75–83. [CrossRef]
62. Northey, J.M.; Cherbuin, N.; Pumpa, K.L.; Smee, D.J.; Rattray, B. Exercise interventions for cognitive function in adults older than 50: A systematic review with meta-analysis. *Br. J. Sports Med.* **2018**, *52*, 154–160. [CrossRef]
63. Kerr, J.; Marshall, S.J.; Patterson, R.E.; Marinac, C.R.; Natarajan, L.; Rosenberg, D.; Wasilenko, K.; Crist, K. Objectively measured physical activity is related to cognitive function in older adults. *J. Am. Geriatr. Soc.* **2013**, *61*, 1927–1931. [CrossRef]
64. Zhu, W.; Howard, V.J.; Wadley, V.G.; Hutto, B.; Blair, S.N.; Vena, J.E.; Colabianchi, N.; Rhodes, D.; Hooker, S.P. Association Between Objectively Measured Physical Activity and Cognitive Function in Older Adults-The Reasons for Geographic and Racial Differences in Stroke Study. *J. Am. Geriatr. Soc.* **2015**, *63*, 2447–2454. [CrossRef] [PubMed]
65. Barnes, D.E.; Blackwell, T.; Stone, K.L.; Goldman, S.E.; Hillier, T.; Yaffe, K.; Study of Osteoporotic Fractures. Cognition in older women: The importance of daytime movement. *J. Am. Geriatr. Soc.* **2008**, *56*, 1658–1664. [CrossRef]
66. Buchman, A.S.; Wilson, R.S.; Bennett, D.A. Total daily activity is associated with cognition in older persons. *Am. J. Geriatr. Psychiatry* **2008**, *16*, 697–701. [CrossRef] [PubMed]
67. Langhammer, B.; Bergland, A.; Rydwik, E. The Importance of Physical Activity Exercise among Older People. *Biomed. Res. Int.* **2018**, *2018*, 7856823. [CrossRef] [PubMed]
68. Taylor, D. Physical activity is medicine for older adults. *Postgrad. Med. J.* **2014**, *90*, 26–32. [CrossRef] [PubMed]
69. Pietrelli, A.; Lopez-Costa, J.; Goñi, R.; Brusco, A.; Basso, N. Aerobic exercise prevents age-dependent cognitive decline and reduces anxiety-related behaviors in middle-aged and old rats. *Neuroscience* **2012**, *202*, 252–266. [CrossRef]
70. Klimova, B.; Dostalova, R. The Impact of Physical Activities on Cognitive Performance among Healthy Older Individuals. *Brain Sci.* **2020**, *10*, 377. [CrossRef] [PubMed]
71. Lee, S.M.; Choi, M.; Chun, B.O.; Sun, K.; Kim, K.S.; Kang, S.W.; Song, H.S.; Moon, S.Y. Effects of a High-Intensity Interval Physical Exercise Program on Cognition, Physical Performance, and Electroencephalogram Patterns in Korean Elderly People: A Pilot Study. *Dement. Neurocogn. Disord.* **2022**, *21*, 93–102. [CrossRef]
72. De la Rosa, A.; Olaso-Gonzalez, G.; Arc-Chagnaud, C.; Millan, F.; Salvador-Pascual, A.; García-Lucerga, C.; Blasco-Lafarga, C.; Garcia-Dominguez, E.; Carretero, A.; Correas, A.G.; et al. Physical exercise in the prevention and treatment of Alzheimer's disease. *J. Sport Health Sci.* **2020**, *9*, 394–404. [CrossRef]
73. Engeroff, T.; Füzéki, E.; Vogt, L.; Fleckenstein, J.; Schwarz, S.; Matura, S.; Pilatus, U.; Deichmann, R.; Hellweg, R.; Pantel, J.; et al. Is Objectively Assessed Sedentary Behavior, Physical Activity and Cardiorespiratory Fitness Linked to Brain Plasticity Outcomes in Old Age? *Neuroscience* **2018**, *388*, 384–392. [CrossRef]
74. Wheeler, M.J.; Green, D.J.; Ellis, K.A.; Cerin, E.; Heinonen, I.; Naylor, L.H.; Larsen, R.; Wennberg, P.; Boraxbekk, C.J.; Lewis, J.; et al. Distinct effects of acute exercise and breaks in sitting on working memory and executive function in older adults: A three-arm, randomised cross-over trial to evaluate the effects of exercise with and without breaks in sitting on cognition. *Br. J. Sports Med.* **2020**, *54*, 776–781. [CrossRef] [PubMed]
75. Gaitán, J.M.; Moon, H.Y.; Stremlau, M.; Dubal, D.B.; Cook, D.B.; Okonkwo, O.C.; van Praag, H. Effects of Aerobic Exercise Training on Systemic Biomarkers and Cognition in Late Middle-Aged Adults at Risk for Alzheimer's Disease. *Front. Endocrinol.* **2021**, *12*, 660181. [CrossRef]
76. Neale, C.; Aspinall, P.; Roe, J.; Tilley, S.; Mavros, P.; Cinderby, S.; Coyne, R.; Thin, N.; Bennett, G.; Thompson, C.W. The Aging Urban Brain: Analyzing Outdoor Physical Activity Using the Emotiv Affectiv Suite in Older People. *J. Urban Health* **2017**, *94*, 869–880. [CrossRef] [PubMed]
77. Gogniat, M.A.; Robison, T.L.; Jean, K.R.; Stephen Miller, L. Physical activity moderates the association between executive function and functional connectivity in older adults. *Aging Brain* **2022**, *2*, 100036. [CrossRef] [PubMed]
78. Gogniat, M.A.; Robison, T.L.; Jean, K.R.; Stephen Miller, L. Physical activity and fitness moderate the association between executive function and anti-correlated networks in the aging brain. *Sport Sci. Health* **2022**, *18*, 1021–1031. [CrossRef]

79. Pieramico, V.; Esposito, R.; Sensi, F.; Cilli, F.; Mantini, D.; Mattei, P.A.; Frazzini, V.; Ciavardelli, D.; Gatta, V.; Ferretti, A.; et al. Combination training in aging individuals modifies functional connectivity and cognition, and is potentially affected by dopamine-related genes. *PLoS ONE* **2012**, *7*, e43901. [CrossRef]
80. Li, R.; Zhu, X.; Yin, S.; Niu, Y.; Zheng, Z.; Huang, X.; Wang, B.; Li, J. Multimodal intervention in older adults improves resting-state functional connectivity between the medial prefrontal cortex and medial temporal lobe. *Front. Aging Neurosci.* **2014**, *6*, 39. [CrossRef]
81. Tao, J.; Liu, J.; Egorova, N.; Chen, X.; Sun, S.; Xue, X.; Huang, J.; Zheng, G.; Wang, Q.; Chen, L.; et al. Increased Hippocampus-Medial Prefrontal Cortex Resting-State Functional Connectivity and Memory Function after Tai Chi Chuan Practice in Elder Adults. *Front. Aging Neurosci.* **2016**, *8*, 25. [CrossRef] [PubMed]
82. Dorsman, K.A.; Weiner-Light, S.; Staffaroni, A.M.; Brown, J.A.; Wolf, A.; Cobigo, Y.; Walters, S.; Kramer, J.H.; Casaletto, K.B. Get Moving! Increases in Physical Activity Are Associated with Increasing Functional Connectivity Trajectories in Typically Aging Adults. *Front. Aging Neurosci.* **2020**, *12*, 104. [CrossRef] [PubMed]
83. Ji, L.; Zhang, H.; Potter, G.G.; Zang, Y.F.; Steffens, D.C.; Guo, H.; Wang, L. Multiple Neuroimaging Measures for Examining Exercise-induced Neuroplasticity in Older Adults: A Quasi-experimental Study. *Front. Aging Neurosci.* **2017**, *9*, 102. [CrossRef]
84. Voss, M.W.; Prakash, R.S.; Erickson, K.I.; Basak, C.; Chaddock, L.; Kim, J.S.; Alves, H.; Heo, S.; Szabo, A.N.; White, S.M.; et al. Plasticity of brain networks in a randomized intervention trial of exercise training in older adults. *Front. Aging Neurosci.* **2010**, *2*, 32. [CrossRef] [PubMed]
85. Flodin, P.; Jonasson, L.S.; Riklund, K.; Nyberg, L.; Boraxbekk, C.J. Does Aerobic Exercise Influence Intrinsic Brain Activity? An Aerobic Exercise Intervention among Healthy Old Adults. *Front. Aging Neurosci.* **2017**, *9*, 267. [CrossRef] [PubMed]
86. Voss, M.W.; Sutterer, M.; Weng, T.B.; Burzynska, A.Z.; Fanning, J.; Salerno, E.; Gothe, N.P.; Ehlers, D.K.; McAuley, E.; Kramer, A.F. Nutritional supplementation boosts aerobic exercise effects on functional brain systems. *J. Appl. Physiol.* **2019**, *126*, 77–87. [CrossRef] [PubMed]
87. Kimura, K.; Yasunaga, A.; Wang, L.Q. Correlation between moderate daily physical activity and neurocognitive variability in healthy elderly people. *Arch. Gerontol. Geriatr.* **2013**, *56*, 109–117. [CrossRef] [PubMed]
88. Bugg, J.M.; Head, D. Exercise moderates age-related atrophy of the medial temporal lobe. *Neurobiol. Aging* **2011**, *32*, 506–514. [CrossRef] [PubMed]
89. Papenberg, G.; Ferencz, B.; Mangialasche, F.; Mecocci, P.; Cecchetti, R.; Kalpouzos, G.; Fratiglioni, L.; Bäckman, L. Physical activity and inflammation: Effects on gray-matter volume and cognitive decline in aging. *Hum. Brain Mapp.* **2016**, *37*, 3462–3473. [CrossRef] [PubMed]
90. Wells, R.E.; Yeh, G.Y.; Kerr, C.E.; Wolkin, J.; Davis, R.B.; Tan, Y.; Spaeth, R.; Wall, R.B.; Walsh, J.; Kaptchuk, T.J.; et al. Meditation's impact on default mode network and hippocampus in mild cognitive impairment: A pilot study. *Neurosci. Lett.* **2013**, *556*, 15–19. [CrossRef]
91. Eyre, H.A.; Acevedo, B.; Yang, H.; Siddarth, P.; van Dyk, K.; Ercoli, L.; Leaver, A.M.; Cyr, N.S.; Narr, K.; Baune, B.T.; et al. Changes in Neural Connectivity and Memory Following a Yoga Intervention for Older Adults: A Pilot Study. *J. Alzheimers Dis.* **2016**, *52*, 673–684. [CrossRef]
92. Tao, J.; Liu, J.; Chen, X.; Xia, R.; Li, M.; Huang, M.; Li, S.; Park, J.; Wilson, G.; Lang, C.; et al. Mind-body exercise improves cognitive function and modulates the function and structure of the hippocampus and anterior cingulate cortex in patients with mild cognitive impairment. *Neuroimage Clin.* **2019**, *23*, 101834. [CrossRef]
93. Suo, C.; Singh, M.F.; Gates, N.; Wen, W.; Sachdev, P.; Brodaty, H.; Saigal, N.; Wilson, G.C.; Meiklejohn, J.; Singh, N.; et al. Therapeutically relevant structural and functional mechanisms triggered by physical and cognitive exercise. *Mol. Psychiatry* **2016**, *21*, 1633–1642. [CrossRef]
94. Hsu, C.L.; Best, J.R.; Wang, S.; Voss, M.W.; Hsiung, R.G.Y.; Munkacsy, M.; Cheung, W.; Handy, T.C.; Liu-Ambrose, T. The Impact of Aerobic Exercise on Fronto-Parietal Network Connectivity and Its Relation to Mobility: An Exploratory Analysis of a 6-Month Randomized Controlled Trial. *Front. Hum. Neurosci.* **2017**, *11*, 344. [CrossRef] [PubMed]
95. Veldsman, M.; Churilov, L.; Werden, E.; Li, Q.; Cumming, T.; Brodtmann, A. Physical activity after stroke is associated with increased interhemispheric connectivity of the dorsal attention network. *Neurorehabil. Neural Repair* **2017**, *31*, 157–167. [CrossRef] [PubMed]
96. Fox, M.D.; Corbetta, M.; Snyder, A.Z.; Vincent, J.L.; Raichle, M.E. Spontaneous neuronal activity distinguishes human dorsal and ventral attention systems. *Proc. Natl. Acad. Sci. USA* **2006**, *103*, 10046–10051. [CrossRef]
97. Uddin, L.Q.; Kelly, A.M.; Biswal, B.B.; Castellanos, F.X.; Milham, M.P. Functional connectivity of default mode network components: Correlation, anticorrelation, and causality. *Hum. Brain Mapp.* **2009**, *30*, 625–637. [CrossRef]
98. Churchwell, J.C.; Kesner, R.P. Hippocampal-prefrontal dynamics in spatial working memory: Interactions and independent parallel processing. *Behav. Brain Res.* **2011**, *225*, 389–395. [CrossRef] [PubMed]
99. Kaplan, R.; Bush, D.; Bonnefond, M.; Bandettini, P.A.; Barnes, G.R.; Doeller, C.F.; Burgess, N. Medial prefrontal theta phase coupling during spatial memory retrieval. *Hippocampus* **2014**, *24*, 656–665. [CrossRef]
100. Dougherty, R.J.; Ellingson, L.D.; Schultz, S.A.; Boots, E.A.; Meyer, J.D.; Lindheimer, J.B.; van Riper, S.; Stegner, A.J.; Edwards, D.F.; Oh, J.M.; et al. Meeting physical activity recommendations may be protective against temporal lobe atrophy in older adults at risk for Alzheimer's disease. *Alzheimers Dement.* **2016**, *4*, 14–17. [CrossRef]

101. Vogt, B.A.; Vogt, L.J.; Vrana, K.E.; Gioia, L.; Meadows, R.S.; Challa, V.R.; Hof, P.R.; van Hoesen, G.W. Multivariate analysis of laminar patterns of neurodegeneration in posterior cingulate cortex in Alzheimer's disease. *Exp. Neurol.* **1998**, *153*, 8–22. [CrossRef] [PubMed]
102. Zheng, G.; Zhou, W.; Xia, R.; Tao, J.; Chen, L. Aerobic Exercises for Cognition Rehabilitation following Stroke: A Systematic Review. *J. Stroke Cerebrovasc. Dis.* **2016**, *25*, 2780–2789. [CrossRef]
103. Oberlin, L.E.; Waiwood, A.M.; Cumming, T.B.; Marsland, A.L.; Bernhardt, J.; Erickson, K.I. Effects of Physical Activity on Poststroke Cognitive Function: A Meta-Analysis of Randomized Controlled Trials. *Stroke* **2017**, *48*, 3093–3100. [CrossRef] [PubMed]
104. Sun, R.; Li, X.; Zhu, Z.; Li, T.; Li, W.; Huang, P.; Gong, W. Effects of Combined Cognitive and Exercise Interventions on Poststroke Cognitive Function: A Systematic Review and Meta-Analysis. *Biomed. Res. Int.* **2021**, *2021*, 4558279. [CrossRef] [PubMed]
105. Goldin, P.; Ziv, M.; Jazaieri, H.; Gross, J.J. Randomized controlled trial of mindfulness-based stress reduction versus aerobic exercise: Effects on the self-referential brain network in social anxiety disorder. *Front. Hum. Neurosci.* **2012**, *6*, 295. [CrossRef]
106. Goldin, P.; Ziv, M.; Jazaieri, H.; Hahn, K.; Gross, J.J. MBSR vs aerobic exercise in social anxiety: fMRI of emotion regulation of negative self-beliefs. *Soc. Cogn. Affect. Neurosci.* **2013**, *8*, 65–72. [CrossRef] [PubMed]
107. Gourgouvelis, J.; Yielder, P.; Murphy, B. Exercise Promotes Neuroplasticity in Both Healthy and Depressed Brains: An fMRI Pilot Study. *Neural Plast.* **2017**, *2017*, 8305287. [CrossRef] [PubMed]
108. Huang, L.; Huang, G.; Ding, Q.; Liang, P.; Hu, C.; Zhang, H.; Zhan, L.; Wang, Q.; Cao, Y.; Zhang, J.; et al. Amplitude of low-frequency fluctuation (ALFF) alterations in adults with subthreshold depression after physical exercise: A resting-state fMRI study. *J. Affect. Disord.* **2021**, *295*, 1057–1065. [CrossRef] [PubMed]
109. Stern, Y.; MacKay-Brandt, A.; Lee, S.; McKinley, P.; McIntyre, K.; Razlighi, Q.; Agarunov, E.; Bartels, M.; Sloan, R.P. Effect of aerobic exercise on cognition in younger adults: A randomized clinical trial. *Neurology* **2019**, *92*, e905–e916. [CrossRef]
110. Bashir, S.; Al-Sultan, F.; Jamea, A.A.; Almousa, A.; Alzahrani, M.S.; Alhargan, F.A.; Abualait, T.; Yoo, W.K. Physical exercise and cortical thickness in healthy controls: A pilot study. *Eur. Rev. Med. Pharmacol. Sci.* **2021**, *25*, 7375–7379. [CrossRef]
111. Kaiser, A.; Reneman, L.; Solleveld, M.M.; Coolen, B.F.; Scherder, E.J.A.; Knutsson, L.; Bjørnerud, A.; van Osch, M.J.P.; Wijnen, J.P.; Lucassen, P.J.; et al. A Randomized Controlled Trial on the Effects of a 12-Week High- vs. Low-Intensity Exercise Intervention on Hippocampal Structure and Function in Healthy, Young Adults. *Front. Psychiatry* **2022**, *12*, 780095. [CrossRef]
112. Fontes, E.B.; Okano, A.H.; De Guio, F.; Schabort, E.J.; Min, L.L.; Basset, F.A.; Stein, D.J.; Noakes, T.D. Brain activity and perceived exertion during cycling exercise: An fMRI study. *Br. J. Sports Med.* **2015**, *49*, 556–560. [CrossRef]
113. Ishihara, T.; Miyazaki, A.; Tanaka, H.; Matsuda, T. Identification of the brain networks that contribute to the interaction between physical function and working memory: An fMRI investigation with over 1,000 healthy adults. *Neuroimage* **2020**, *221*, 117152. [CrossRef]
114. Nakagawa, T.; Koan, I.; Chen, C.; Matsubara, T.; Hagiwara, K.; Lei, H.; Hirotsu, M.; Yamagata, H.; Nakagawa, S. Regular Moderate- to Vigorous-Intensity Physical Activity Rather Than Walking Is Associated with Enhanced Cognitive Functions and Mental Health in Young Adults. *Int. J. Environ. Res. Public Health* **2020**, *17*, 614. [CrossRef] [PubMed]
115. Bezzola, L.; Mérillat, S.; Jäncke, L. The effect of leisure activity golf practice on motor imagery: An fMRI study in middle adulthood. *Front. Hum. Neurosci.* **2012**, *6*, 67. [CrossRef] [PubMed]
116. Wadden, K.; Brown, K.; Maletsky, R.; Boyd, L.A. Correlations between brain activity and components of motor learning in middle-aged adults: An fMRI study. *Front. Hum. Neurosci.* **2013**, *7*, 169. [CrossRef] [PubMed]
117. Pensel, M.C.; Daamen, M.; Scheef, L.; Knigge, H.U.; Rojas Vega, S.; Martin, J.A.; Schild, H.H.; Strüder, H.K.; Boecker, H. Executive control processes are associated with individual fitness outcomes following regular exercise training: Blood lactate profile curves and neuroimaging findings. *Sci. Rep.* **2018**, *8*, 4893. [CrossRef]
118. De Greeff, J.W.; Bosker, R.J.; Oosterlaan, J.; Visscher, C.; Hartman, E. Effects of physical activity on executive functions, attention and academic performance in preadolescent children: A meta-analysis. *J. Sci. Med. Sport* **2018**, *21*, 501–507. [CrossRef] [PubMed]
119. Rodriguez-Ayllon, M.; Plaza-Florido, A.; Mendez-Gutierrez, A.; Altmäe, S.; Solis-Urra, P.; Aguilera, C.M.; Catena, A.; Ortega, F.B.; Esteban-Cornejo, I. The effects of a 20-week exercise program on blood-circulating biomarkers related to brain health in overweight or obese children: The ActiveBrains project. *J. Sport Health Sci.* **2023**, *12*, 175–185. [CrossRef]
120. De Menezes-Junior, F.J.; Jesus, Í.C.; Brand, C.; Mota, J.; Leite, N. Physical Exercise and Brain-Derived Neurotrophic Factor Concentration in Children and Adolescents: A Systematic Review with Meta-Analysis. *Pediatr. Exerc. Sci.* **2022**, *34*, 44–53. [CrossRef]
121. Davis, C.L.; Tomporowski, P.D.; McDowell, J.E.; Austin, B.P.; Miller, P.H.; Yanasak, N.E.; Allison, J.D.; Naglieri, J.A. Exercise improves executive function and achievement and alters brain activation in overweight children: A randomized, controlled trial. *Health Psychol.* **2011**, *30*, 91–98. [CrossRef]
122. Jackson, W.M.; Davis, N.; Sands, S.A.; Whittington, R.A.; Sun, L.S. Physical Activity and Cognitive Development: A Meta-Analysis. *J. Neurosurg. Anesthesiol.* **2016**, *28*, 373–380. [CrossRef]
123. Kjellenberg, K.; Ekblom, O.; Ahlen, J.; Helgadóttir, B.; Nyberg, G. Cross-sectional associations between physical activity pattern, sports participation, screen time and mental health in Swedish adolescents. *BMJ Open* **2022**, *12*, e061929. [CrossRef]
124. Kamijo, K.; Pontifex, M.B.; O'Leary, K.C.; Scudder, M.R.; Wu, C.T.; Castelli, D.M.; Hillman, C.H. The effects of an afterschool physical activity program on working memory in preadolescent children. *Dev. Sci.* **2011**, *14*, 1046–1058. [CrossRef]
125. Quinzi, F.; Modica, M.; Berchicci, M.; Bianco, V.; Perri, R.L.; Di Russo, F. Does sport type matter? The effect of sport discipline on cognitive control strategies in preadolescents. *Int. J. Psychophysiol.* **2022**, *177*, 230–239. [CrossRef] [PubMed]

126. Hillman, C.H.; Pontifex, M.B.; Castelli, D.M.; Khan, N.A.; Raine, L.B.; Scudder, M.R.; Drollette, E.S.; Moore, R.D.; Wu, C.T.; Kamijo, K. Effects of the FITKids randomized controlled trial on executive control and brain function. *Pediatrics* **2014**, *134*, e1063–e1071. [CrossRef] [PubMed]
127. Chaddock-Heyman, L.; Erickson, K.I.; Voss, M.W.; Knecht, A.M.; Pontifex, M.B.; Castelli, D.M.; Hillman, C.H.; Kramer, A.F. The effects of physical activity on functional MRI activation associated with cognitive control in children: A randomized controlled intervention. *Front. Hum. Neurosci.* **2013**, *7*, 72. [CrossRef] [PubMed]
128. Chaddock-Heyman, L.; Erickson, K.I.; Kienzler, C.; Drollette, E.S.; Raine, L.B.; Kao, S.C.; Bensken, J.; Weisshappel, R.; Castelli, D.M.; Hillman, C.H.; et al. Physical Activity Increases White Matter Microstructure in Children. *Front. Neurosci.* **2018**, *12*, 950. [CrossRef] [PubMed]
129. Logan, N.E.; Raine, L.B.; Drollette, E.S.; Castelli, D.M.; Khan, N.A.; Kramer, A.F.; Hillman, C.H. The differential relationship of an afterschool physical activity intervention on brain function and cognition in children with obesity and their normal weight peers. *Pediatr. Obes.* **2021**, *16*, e12708. [CrossRef]
130. Ortega, F.B.; Mora-Gonzalez, J.; Cadenas-Sanchez, C.; Esteban-Cornejo, I.; Migueles, J.H.; Solis-Urra, P.; Verdejo-Román, J.; Rodriguez-Ayllon, M.; Molina-Garcia, P.; Ruiz, J.R.; et al. Effects of an Exercise Program on Brain Health Outcomes for Children with Overweight or Obesity: The ActiveBrains Randomized Clinical Trial. *JAMA Netw. Open* **2022**, *5*, e2227893. [CrossRef] [PubMed]
131. Krafft, C.E.; Schwarz, N.F.; Chi, L.; Weinberger, A.L.; Schaeffer, D.J.; Pierce, J.E.; Rodrigue, A.L.; Yanasak, N.E.; Miller, P.H.; Tomporowski, P.D.; et al. An 8-month randomized controlled exercise trial alters brain activation during cognitive tasks in overweight children. *Obesity* **2014**, *22*, 232–242. [CrossRef]
132. Krafft, C.E.; Pierce, J.E.; Schwarz, N.F.; Chi, L.; Weinberger, A.L.; Schaeffer, D.J.; Rodrigue, A.L.; Camchong, J.; Allison, J.D.; Yanasak, N.E.; et al. An eight month randomized controlled exercise intervention alters resting state synchrony in overweight children. *Neuroscience* **2014**, *256*, 445–455. [CrossRef]
133. Krafft, C.E.; Schaeffer, D.J.; Schwarz, N.F.; Chi, L.; Weinberger, A.L.; Pierce, J.E.; Rodrigue, A.L.; Allison, J.D.; Yanasak, N.E.; Liu, T.; et al. Improved frontoparietal white matter integrity in overweight children is associated with attendance at an after-school exercise program. *Dev. Neurosci.* **2014**, *36*, 1–9. [CrossRef]
134. Schaeffer, D.J.; Krafft, C.E.; Schwarz, N.F.; Chi, L.; Rodrigue, A.L.; Pierce, J.E.; Allison, J.D.; Yanasak, N.E.; Liu, T.; Davis, C.L.; et al. An 8-month exercise intervention alters frontotemporal white matter integrity in overweight children. *Psychophysiology* **2014**, *51*, 728–733. [CrossRef] [PubMed]
135. World Health Organization. Regional Office for Europe. WHO European Regional Obesity Report. 2022. Available online: https://apps.who.int/iris/handle/10665/353747 (accessed on 3 May 2022).
136. Bauer, C.C.; Moreno, B.; González-Santos, L.; Concha, L.; Barquera, S.; Barrios, F.A. Child overweight and obesity are associated with reduced executive cognitive performance and brain alterations: A magnetic resonance imaging study in Mexican children. *Pediatr. Obes.* **2015**, *10*, 196–204. [CrossRef] [PubMed]
137. Kashihara, K.; Maruyama, T.; Murota, M.; Nakahara, Y. Positive effects of acute and moderate physical exercise on cognitive function. *J. Physiol. Anthropol.* **2009**, *28*, 155–164. [CrossRef] [PubMed]
138. Stillman, C.M.; Cohen, J.; Lehman, M.E.; Erickson, K.I. Mediators of Physical Activity on Neurocognitive Function: A Review at Multiple Levels of Analysis. *Front. Hum. Neurosci.* **2016**, *10*, 626. [CrossRef] [PubMed]
139. Mottola, L.; Crisostomi, S.; Ferrari, M.; Quaresima, V. Relationship between handgrip sustained submaximal exercise and prefrontal cortex oxygenation. *Adv. Exp. Med. Biol.* **2006**, *578*, 305–309. [CrossRef]
140. Zhou, B.; Wang, Z.; Zhu, L.; Huang, G.; Li, B.; Chen, C.; Huang, J.; Ma, F.; Liu, T.C. Effects of different physical activities on brain-derived neurotrophic factor: A systematic review and bayesian network meta-analysis. *Front. Aging Neurosci.* **2022**, *14*, 981002. [CrossRef]
141. Moore, D.; Jung, M.; Hillman, C.H.; Kang, M.; Loprinzi, P.D. Interrelationships between exercise, functional connectivity, and cognition among healthy adults: A systematic review. *Psychophysiology* **2022**, *59*, e14014. [CrossRef]
142. Domingos, C.; Pêgo, J.M.; Santos, N.C. Effects of physical activity on brain function and structure in older adults: A systematic review. *Behav. Brain Res.* **2021**, *402*, 113061. [CrossRef]
143. Erickson, K.I.; Voss, M.W.; Prakash, R.S.; Basak, C.; Szabo, A.; Chaddock, L.; Kim, J.S.; Heo, S.; Alves, H.; White, S.M.; et al. Exercise training increases size of hippocampus and improves memory. *Proc. Natl. Acad. Sci. USA* **2011**, *108*, 3017–3022. [CrossRef] [PubMed]
144. Johnson, N.F.; Kim, C.; Clasey, J.L.; Bailey, A.; Gold, B.T. Cardiorespiratory fitness is positively correlated with cerebral white matter integrity in healthy seniors. *Neuroimage* **2012**, *59*, 1514–1523. [CrossRef]
145. Voss, M.W.; Heo, S.; Prakash, R.S.; Erickson, K.I.; Alves, H.; Chaddock, L.; Szabo, A.N.; Mailey, E.L.; Wójcicki, T.R.; White, S.M.; et al. The influence of aerobic fitness on cerebral white matter integrity and cognitive function in older adults: Results of a one-year exercise intervention. *Hum. Brain Mapp.* **2013**, *34*, 2972–2985. [CrossRef] [PubMed]
146. Jacobs, H.I.; van Boxtel, M.P.; Jolles, J.; Verhey, F.R.; Uylings, H.B. Parietal cortex matters in Alzheimer's disease: An overview of structural, functional and metabolic findings. *Neurosci. Biobehav. Rev.* **2012**, *36*, 297–309. [CrossRef] [PubMed]
147. Kivipelto, M.; Mangialasche, F.; Ngandu, T. Lifestyle interventions to prevent cognitive impairment, dementia and Alzheimer disease. *Nat. Rev. Neurol.* **2018**, *14*, 653–666. [CrossRef] [PubMed]
148. Alty, J.; Farrow, M.; Lawler, K. Exercise and dementia prevention. *Pract. Neurol.* **2020**, *20*, 234–240. [CrossRef] [PubMed]

149. Ludyga, S.; Gerber, M.; Brand, S.; Holsboer-Trachsler, E.; Pühse, U. Acute effects of moderate aerobic exercise on specific aspects of executive function in different age and fitness groups: A meta-analysis. *Psychophysiology* **2016**, *53*, 1611–1626. [CrossRef] [PubMed]
150. Diamond, A. Executive functions. *Annu. Rev. Psychol.* **2013**, *64*, 135–168. [CrossRef] [PubMed]
151. Heinze, K.; Cumming, J.; Dosanjh, A.; Palin, S.; Poulton, S.; Bagshaw, A.P.; Broome, M.R. Neurobiological evidence of longer-term physical activity interventions on mental health outcomes and cognition in young people: A systematic review of randomised controlled trials. *Neurosci. Biobehav. Rev.* **2021**, *120*, 431–441. [CrossRef]
152. Birren, J.E.; Schaie, K.W. *Handbook of the Psychology of Aging*, 4th ed.; Academic Press: San Diego, CA, USA, 1996; ISBN 0-121-01260-3.
153. Voss, M.W.; Weng, T.B.; Burzynska, A.Z.; Wong, C.N.; Cooke, G.E.; Clark, R.; Fanning, J.; Awick, E.; Gothe, N.P.; Olson, E.A.; et al. Fitness, but not physical activity, is related to functional integrity of brain networks associated with aging. *Neuroimage* **2016**, *131*, 113–125. [CrossRef]
154. Fox, M.D.; Greicius, M. Clinical applications of resting state functional connectivity. *Front. Syst. Neurosci.* **2010**, *4*, 19. [CrossRef]
155. Fair, D.A.; Cohen, A.L.; Power, J.D.; Dosenbach, N.U.; Church, J.A.; Miezin, F.M.; Schlaggar, B.L.; Petersen, S.E. Functional brain networks develop from a "local to distributed" organization. *PLoS Comput. Biol.* **2009**, *5*, e1000381. [CrossRef]
156. Bruke, T.M.; Scheer, F.A.J.L.; Ronda, J.M.; Czeisler, C.A.; Wright, K.P. Sleep inertia, sleep homeostatic and circadian influences on higher-order cognitive functions. *J. Sleep Res.* **2015**, *24*, 364–371. [CrossRef]
157. Anderson, J.A.E.; Campbell, K.L.; Amer, T.; Grady, C.L.; Hasher, L. Timing is everything: Age differences in the cognitive control network are modulated by time of day. *Psychol. Aging* **2014**, *29*, 648–657. [CrossRef] [PubMed]
158. Hodyl, N.A.; Schneider, L.; Vallence, A.M.; Clow, A.; Ridding, M.C.; Pitcher, J.B. The cortisol awakening response is associated with performance of a serial sequence reaction time task. *Int. J. Psychophysiol.* **2016**, *100*, 12–18. [CrossRef] [PubMed]
159. Kojima, S.; Abe, T.; Morishita, S.; Inagaki, Y.; Qin, W.; Hotta, K.; Tsubaki, A. Acute moderate-intensity exercise improves 24-h sleep deprivation-induced cognitive decline and cerebral oxygenation: A near-infrared spectroscopy study. *Respir. Physiol. Neurobiol.* **2019**, *274*, 103354. [CrossRef]
160. Wilckens, K.A.; Erickson, K.I.; Wheeler, M.E. Physical Activity and Cognition: A Mediating Role of Efficient Sleep. *Behav. Sleep Med.* **2018**, *16*, 569–586. [CrossRef] [PubMed]
161. Macrì, M.; Flores, N.V.G.; Stefanelli, R.; Pegreffi, F.; Festa, F. Interpreting the prevalence of musculoskeletal pain impacting Italian and Peruvian dentists likewise: A cross-sectional study. *Front. Public Health* **2023**, *11*, 1090683. [CrossRef] [PubMed]
162. Macrì, M.; Murmura, G.; Scarano, A.; Festa, F. Prevalence of temporomandibular disorders and its association with malocclusion in children: A transversal study. *Front. Public Health* **2022**, *10*, 860833. [CrossRef] [PubMed]

Disclaimer/Publisher's Note: The statements, opinions and data contained in all publications are solely those of the individual author(s) and contributor(s) and not of MDPI and/or the editor(s). MDPI and/or the editor(s) disclaim responsibility for any injury to people or property resulting from any ideas, methods, instructions or products referred to in the content.

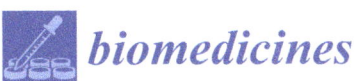 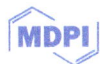

Article

Physical Health and Transition to Psychosis in People at Clinical High Risk

Andrea De Micheli [1,2,†], Umberto Provenzani [3,†], Kamil Krakowski [1,3,4], Dominic Oliver [1,5,6,7], Stefano Damiani [3], Natascia Brondino [3], Philip McGuire [5,6,7] and Paolo Fusar-Poli [1,2,3,8,*]

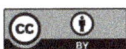

Citation: De Micheli, A.; Provenzani, U.; Krakowski, K.; Oliver, D.; Damiani, S.; Brondino, N.; McGuire, P.; Fusar-Poli, P. Physical Health and Transition to Psychosis in People at Clinical High Risk. *Biomedicines* **2024**, *12*, 523. https://doi.org/10.3390/biomedicines12030523

Academic Editor: Raul López Antón

Received: 31 October 2023
Revised: 9 January 2024
Accepted: 29 January 2024
Published: 26 February 2024

Copyright: © 2024 by the authors. Licensee MDPI, Basel, Switzerland. This article is an open access article distributed under the terms and conditions of the Creative Commons Attribution (CC BY) license (https://creativecommons.org/licenses/by/4.0/).

[1] Early Psychosis: Interventions and Clinical-Detection (EPIC) Lab, Department of Psychosis Studies, Institute of Psychiatry, Psychology & Neuroscience, King's College London, London SE5 8AB, UK; andrea.de_micheli@kcl.ac.uk (A.D.M.); kamil.krakowski@kcl.ac.uk (K.K.); dominic.a.oliver@kcl.ac.uk (D.O.)
[2] OASIS Service, South London and Maudsley NHS Foundation Trust, London SE11 5DL, UK
[3] Department of Brain and Behavioral Sciences, University of Pavia, 27100 Pavia, Italy; umberto.provenzani@unipv.it (U.P.); stefano.damiani@unipv.it (S.D.); natascia.brondino@unipv.it (N.B.)
[4] Department of Biostatistics and Health Informatics, Institute of Psychiatry, Psychology & Neuroscience, King's College London, London SE5 8AB, UK
[5] Department of Psychiatry, University of Oxford, Oxford OX3 7JX, UK; philip.mcguire@psych.ox.ac.uk
[6] NIHR Oxford Health Biomedical Research Centre, Oxford OX3 7JX, UK
[7] OPEN Early Detection Service, Oxford Health NHS Foundation Trust, Oxford OX3 7JX, UK
[8] Department of Psychiatry and Psychotherapy, Ludwig-Maximilian-University Munich, 80336 Munich, Germany
* Correspondence: paolo.fusar-poli@kcl.ac.uk
† These authors contributed equally to this work.

Abstract: Background: The clinical high risk for psychosis (CHR-P) construct represents an opportunity for prevention and early intervention in young adults, but the relationship between risk for psychosis and physical health in these patients remains unclear. Methods: We conducted a RECORD-compliant clinical register-based cohort study, selecting the long-term cumulative risk of developing a persistent psychotic disorder as the primary outcome. We investigated associations between primary outcome and physical health data with Electronic Health Records at the South London and Maudsley (SLaM) NHS Trust, UK (January 2013–October 2020). We performed survival analyses using Kaplan-Meier curves, log-rank tests, and Cox proportional hazard models. Results: The database included 137 CHR-P subjects; 21 CHR-P developed psychosis during follow-up, and the cumulative incidence of psychosis risk was 4.9% at 1 year and 56.3% at 7 years. Log-rank tests suggested that psychosis risk might change between different levels of nicotine and alcohol dependence. Kaplan-Meier curve analyses indicated that non-hazardous drinkers may have a lower psychosis risk than non-drinkers. In the Cox proportional hazard model, nicotine dependence presented a hazard ratio of 1.34 (95% CI: 1.1–1.64) ($p = 0.01$), indicating a 34% increase in psychosis risk for every additional point on the Fagerström Test for Nicotine Dependence. Conclusions: Our findings suggest that a comprehensive assessment of tobacco and alcohol use, diet, and physical activity in CHR-P subjects is key to understanding how physical health contributes to psychosis risk.

Keywords: physical health; psychosis; risk; CHR-P

1. Introduction

The CHR-P—Clinical High Risk for Psychosis—populations [1,2] present a substantially higher risk of transitioning to a first episode of psychosis compared to the general population, recently estimated at around 25% within 3 years [3]. These subjects might develop psychosis up to 10 years after the initial presentation [4], with longer-term longitudinal studies finding a 38% transition rate at 16 years [5].

Most of these patients will develop an ICD/DSM schizophrenia-spectrum disorder [6], but there is more uncertainty around non-transitioned CHR-P subjects as a high percentage do not reach clinical and functional recovery and present at least one mental disorder at long-term follow-ups [7]. Indeed, aside from the classical 3 CHR-P subgroups—Attenuated Psychotic Symptoms (APS), Brief Limited Intermitted Psychotic Symptoms (BLIPS), and Genetic Risk and Deterioration Syndrome (GRD)—that define the construct [8], CHR-P individuals may present comorbidities such as affective or anxiety disorders [9].

Impaired global functioning is a key component of the clinical construct [10] and might represent a predictor of transition to psychosis [11,12]. Amongst the other psychosis risk factors in CHR-P subjects, physical health data are still under-investigated. For example, in one of the most recent meta-analyses on the topic [13], only 3 out of 44 studies investigated physical conditions, whilst more attention was given, for instance, to substance use.

Despite these gaps in the literature and the fact that current CHR-P assessments are entirely based on psychopathological features [8,14], the CHR-P phase represents a window of opportunity for prevention and early intervention in young cohorts (14–35 years), including the opportunity to ameliorate crucial physical ill-health trajectories [15]. This opportunity is particularly relevant in view of the alarming weight of serious mental illnesses on the overall disease burden worldwide, more precisely the 21.2% of total years lived with disabilities [16]. In terms of physical health, subjects affected by schizophrenia have a life expectancy reduced by approximately 10 to 30 years compared to the general population [17–19] and preventable cardiovascular risk factors such as tobacco use, abdominal obesity, a sedentary lifestyle, and a diet with high levels of saturated fats play a main role in this discrepancy [20,21].

Interestingly, some CHR-P subjects also present a higher prevalence of cardiometabolic risk factors compared to age-matched controls (e.g., increased blood pressure, waist circumference, and fasting blood glucose) [22]. This vulnerability has also been associated with modifiable physical health behaviours in CHR-P, such as reduced physical activity and increased rates of smoking and alcohol abuse [23–27].

There are several reasons to promote good physical health and lifestyles during the CHR-P phase. As discussed above, a large proportion of CHR-P subjects develop comorbid disorders (e.g., mood, anxiety) at various stages [9], which are also correlated with physical health deterioration [28]. Second, in CHR-P individuals who will transition to psychosis, adopting a preventative approach in the earliest stage is associated with better long-term outcomes [29], as psychosis is frequently associated with a wide range of comorbid and multiple physical health illnesses [30] and often progresses to chronic, severe conditions [31].

Finally, several physical health outcomes, such as tobacco use [32,33], substance use, including alcohol [34], low levels of physical activity [35], and dietary components such as omega-3 fatty acids [36], have been proposed as risk factors for psychosis, and thus physical health interventions might reduce the risk of transitioning to psychosis for CHR-P subjects. However, only a limited number of studies [37,38] investigated the degree of causality in these relationships.

Even though promoting physical health in these clinical populations is likely to be beneficial [39], physical health outcomes are often not monitored in CHR-P services [40], a problem shared with psychiatric services more broadly [41]. High-profile research focused on physical health is still scarce [40], but recently it was found that well-tolerated exercise in the CHR-P phase might improve fitness, cognitive performance, and the severity of attenuated positive symptoms [42]. Attention to the physical health of patients suffering from mental disorders has been increasing in the last few years. For instance, one of the pillars of the "NHS five year forward view" [43] focused on increasing physical health checks in these clinical populations. However, more robust research evidence is required to help bridge the gap between scientific understanding and clinical need and practice. More comprehensive and precise data would offer a better-informed view of feasible physical health interventions for these patients [44] and an understanding of the significance of these outcomes in CHR-P patients who develop a first episode of psychosis.

Aim of the Study

The primary aim of this study was to illustrate the relationship between the risk of transition to psychosis in a cohort of CHR-P service users and physical health data, routinely collected via Electronic Health Records (EHR) and through validated questionnaires. We hypothesised that CHR-P subjects with poorer physical health and lifestyle (high nicotine or alcohol dependency, low level of physical activity, or unbalanced diet) have an increased risk of transitioning to psychosis, in line with previous findings of studies focusing on physical outcomes in psychosis [33,45]. Potential findings may shed light on the role of physical health outcomes in the genesis of psychosis and call for more preventative interventions tailored to the physical health needs of these patients.

2. Materials and Methods

2.1. Design

A clinical cohort study using Electronic Health Records (EHR) conducted in accordance with the REporting of studies Conducted using Observational Routinely collected health Data (RECORD) Statement [46].

2.2. Data Source

EHR data on routine physical health checks [47] from all individuals from January 2013 until October 2020, managed by the South London and Maudsley (SLaM) National Health Service (NHS) Foundation Trust, UK. The data source EHR employed in the current study provides contemporaneous EHR and 'real-world' data on routine mental healthcare from all patients managed by SLaM. SLaM is a UK NHS mental health trust that provides secondary mental health care to a population of 1.36 million individuals in South London (Lambeth, Southwark, Lewisham, and Croydon boroughs), with around 545,000 subjects aged 16–35. In SLaM, there is one of the highest rates of psychosis in the world [48]. In terms of the quality of SLaM/CRIS records, SLaM was an early pioneer of EHR, and the Trust is effectively digitised and paper-free. SLaM has a near-monopoly in terms of secondary mental healthcare provision in its local catchment area, and it is a legal requirement for SLaM healthcare professionals to keep these records up-to-date [49]. Whereas many national registers capture only those patients who have been hospitalised, the SLaM EHR register contains the full clinical records of all patients, which are continually updated throughout their care, regardless of discharges from and/or referrals to other services.

2.3. Study Population

OASIS (Outreach and Support in South London) was set up in 2001, and it is one of the oldest early detection CHR-P services in the UK [50,51]. The service is focused on the identification, prognostic assessment, treatment (pharmacological, psychological, and psychoeducational), and clinical follow-up of help-seeking CHR-P individuals aged 14–35 years, serving the SLaM catchment area. OASIS is integrated into the Pan-London Network for Psychosis-prevention (PNP) [52]. The study population included a sample of all individuals accessing OASIS in the period from January 2013 to October 2020, assessed with the Comprehensive Assessment of At-Risk Mental State (CAARMS) [8] and meeting CHR-P criteria: Attenuated Psychotic Symptoms (APS), Brief Limited Intermittent Psychotic Symptoms (BLIPS), and Genetic Risk and Deterioration Syndrome (GRD). All OASIS staff undergo extensive psychometric training to ensure high reliability in the designation of at-risk cases [53]. The OASIS population can be considered representative of the general CHR-P sample since the level of risk enrichment observed (pretest risk [54]: 14.6% at more than 3 years [55]) aligns with that observed in CHR-P services worldwide (meta-analytical pretest risk: 15% at more than 3 years [56]).

2.4. Assessment Instruments

Baseline assessment of CHR-P subjects includes a routine and comprehensive medical examination for physical parameters (e.g., BMI, heart rate, systolic pressure; see "Study *measures"*), which is complemented by the following validated questionnaires, in line with NICE (National Institute for Health and Care Excellence) Clinical Guideline 178 [57].

1. The Fagerström Test for Nicotine Dependence (FTND) [58] is a standardised instrument consisting of six questions exploring daily cigarette consumption, compulsive use, and dependence. The score ranges from 0 to 10 (with higher scores indicating a most severe level of dependence on nicotine). More precisely, scores from 0 to 2 indicate a low level of dependence, from 3 to 4 low-moderate dependence, from 5 to 7 moderate dependence, and more than 8 a high level of dependence. For people that use other types of nicotine consumption other than cigarette smoking (e.g., e-cigarette, nicotine gum, or nicotine patches), we have investigated habits and reported information in adapted versions of FTND already used in previous literature (for instance, the equivalence of 10 vape nicotine puffs for a cigarette [59] or a re-worded test for gum users [60]).
2. AUDIT (Alcohol Use Disorder Identification Test) [61] consists of 10 self-administered questions to investigate alcohol use disorder. When the AUDIT-C score, which includes core questions regarding alcohol units consumed and frequency of drinking, is equal to or above 5, it might indicate hazardous drinking. Regarding the AUDIT total score, a low level of risk is identified with an overall score between 0 and 7, and the range from 8 to 15 is the most appropriate for simple advice focused on the reduction of drinking. Higher scores (up to 19) suggest a need for brief counselling and continuous monitoring, while a complete diagnostic evaluation for alcoholic dependence is warranted for scores over 20.
3. DINE (Dietary Instrument for Nutritional Education) [62] is a structured interview investigating dietary fibre and fat (unsaturated and saturated) intake. Scores for fibres and fats are rated into three different categories: low (under 30), medium (between 30 and 40), and high (more than 40). Scores for unsaturated fats are rated as low (less than 6), medium (6–9) and high (more than 9).
4. IPAQ (International Physical Health Questionnaire) [63] rates the level of physical activity. This tool comprises three different categories of physical activity based on intensity (vigorous, moderate, and walking) and quantifies the amount of time spent sitting. Scores can also be expressed as a continuous variable with METs (estimating resting energy expenditure) [64].

2.5. Study Measures

The primary outcome was the long-term (up to 7 years) cumulative incidence (risk) of developing a persistent psychotic disorder, defined as the onset of the first ICD-10 diagnosis of a non-organic psychotic disorder (Table S1) from a CHR-P stage and association of the outcome with the physical health data. The start of the follow-up period was defined as the time of acceptance into the secondary mental health service (OASIS), and the time of an event was defined as the transition to psychosis. The patients' time lost to follow-up was used for censoring and indicated by the last clinical entry to the EHR. Baseline outcome variables included were:

1. Sociodemographic parameters: age, sex, ethnicity.
2. Physical health data:
    o   Tobacco use: tobacco smoker status (yes/no), number of daily cigarettes, FTND score.
    o   Alcohol use: alcohol drinker status (yes/no), AUDIT-C, and AUDIT total score.
    o   Type of diet: DINE fibre score, DINE saturated fat score, DINE unsaturated fat score.
    o   Physical activity: IPAQ vigorous, moderate, and walking activity (minutes per week), IPAQ time spent sitting (minutes per week), MET levels (continuous variable).
    o   Physical parameters: BMI (body mass index), waist circumference in centimetres, heart rate in beats per minute (bpm), respiratory rate in acts per minute (apm), systolic and diastolic pressure in mmHg.

2.6. Statistical Analysis

This clinical register-based cohort study was conducted according to the REporting of studies Conducted using Observational Routinely collected health Data (RECORD) Statement [46] (Table S2). Sociodemographic and physical health data of the sample (including missing data) were described with mean and standard deviation (SD) for continuous variables, and absolute and relative frequencies were used for categorical variables stratified by transition to psychosis.

As previously mentioned, the primary aim of the analysis was to investigate the association between physical health data and the risk of transitioning to psychosis. Firstly, the physical health data were categorised into strata to explore differences between groups through well-established survival analysis methods, by visually examining Kaplan-Maier survival curves [65], and by the formal assessment of between-group differences through the results of log-rank tests [66]. The categorisation of variables was structured as follows: (i) smoking: smokers vs. non-smokers; (ii) nicotine dependence: non-smokers—0 FTND score, low dependence < 4 FTND score, moderate dependence < 7, and high dependence > 7 FTND score; (iii) drinking status: drinkers vs. non-drinkers; (iv) alcohol use: non-drinkers—0 AUDIT score, non-hazardous drinkers < 8 AUDIT score, and hazardous drinkers ≥ 8 AUDIT score; (v) physical activity: vigorous, moderate, and walking activity were transformed into MET scores so that patients with MET scores less than 3000 were assigned to the inactive group and those with MET scores larger than 3000 to the active group; (vi) for DINE questionnaires, we used the categories illustrated in the *"Assessment Instruments"* section for fibre, saturated fat, and unsaturated fat subsets.

The second part of the analysis consisted of quantifying the significance and magnitude of the association between the physical health data and psychosis risk with the Cox proportional hazard model, using recorded time to psychosis and censoring data [67]. Four measures were selected to be investigated by the Cox model. These included the FTND score as a measure of nicotine dependence, the AUDIT score as a measure of alcohol use, the fibre score in the DINE interview, and the MET score as a measure of physical activity. The four measures were selected as they were believed to capture the most information by their continuous nature, indicating the intensity of each physical health data, focusing on some modifiable risk factors, and on measures collected in a more rigorous way. Four Cox proportional hazard models were run with each of the four measures adjusted by the basic confounders of age, gender, and ethnicity. The four Cox models were inspected for influential observations by examining the standardised DFBETA values. Observations exceeding the 0.2 DFBETA threshold were excluded in the sensitivity analysis [68]. To adjust for multiple comparisons, the Benjamini-Hochberg correction was used [69].

All analyses were conducted in R, version 4.2.3 [70], using the 'survival' package.

3. Results

3.1. Sample Characteristics

The final database included 137 CHR-P subjects, 57 (41%) females and 80 (59%) males. The mean age was 23.65 ± 5.38 years (range from 14 to 36). The majority of the sample comprised White (39%) and Black British (21%) subjects. In terms of physical health outcomes, 40% of CHR-P subjects smoked tobacco, 77% drank alcohol, 63% had low fibre intake, and 72% were physically inactive (MET score of less than 3000). The mean follow-up time was 806 ± 634 days (range from 20 to 2785) (Table 1). The clinical characteristics and physical parameters of the full cohort were described elsewhere [24].

We observed 21 (15%) events (transitions to psychotic disorders) during the study period, 9 (16%) among females and 12 among males (15%) CHR-P individuals. The mean time to transition to psychotic disorders was 2098 days (95% CI: 1847–2349). The cumulative incidence (Kaplan-Meier survival function) of risk of developing psychotic disorders was 4.9% at 1 year (95% CI: 1.2–8.6%), 9.6% at 2 years (95% CI: 4.1–15.1%), 19.9% at 3 years (95% CI: 10.1–29.7%), 23.9% at 4 years (95% CI: 11.8–36.1%), 33.3% at 5 and 6 years (95% CI: 17.0–49.6%), and 56.3% at 7 years (95% CI: 27.1–85.5%) (Figure 1).

Table 1. Sample description.

	Patient Characteristics Stratified by Psychosis Transition	
	Non-Transitioned	Transitioned
n	116	21
Gender		
Male	68 (58.6)	12 (57.1)
Female	48 (41.4)	9 (42.9)
Age Group		
<20	34 (29.3)	3 (14.3)
20–25	38 (32.8)	10 (47.6)
26–30	24 (20.7)	4 (19.0)
>30	20 (17.2)	4 (19.0)
Ethnicity		
White	51 (44.0)	2 (9.5)
Asian	2 (1.7)	2 (9.5)
Black African	10 (8.6)	5 (23.8)
Black Caribbean	3 (2.6)	1 (4.8)
Black British	22 (19.0)	7 (33.3)
Other	28 (24.1)	4 (19.0)
Smoker Status		
Yes	47 (40.5)	8 (38.1)
No	69 (59.5)	13 (61.9)
Nicotine Dependence		
Non-Smokers	69 (59.5)	14 (66.7)
Low	40 (34.5)	3 (14.3)
Moderate	3 (2.6)	2 (9.5)
High	4 (3.4)	2 (9.5)
Drinking Status		
Yes	93 (80.2)	12 (57.1)
No	23 (19.8)	9 (42.9)
Alcohol Consumption		
Non-Drinkers	25 (21.6)	9 (42.9)
Non-Hazardous	57 (49.1)	7 (33.3)
Hazardous	34 (29.3)	5 (23.8)
Fibre Consumption		
Low	72 (62.1)	15 (71.4)
Moderate	20 (17.2)	3 (14.3)
High	24 (20.7)	3 (14.3)
Physical Activity		
Active	35 (30.2)	3 (14.3)
Inactive	81 (69.8)	18 (85.7)
BMI Category		
Underweight	7 (6.3)	1 (4.8)
Healthy Range	67 (60.4)	12 (57.1)
Overweight	37 (33.3)	8 (38.1)

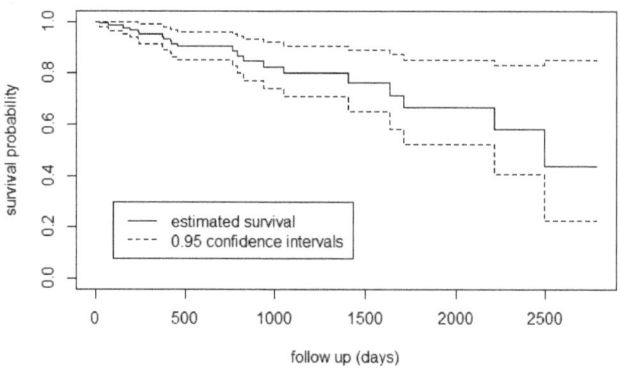

Figure 1. Cumulative incidence of risk of developing psychosis in the OASIS CHR-P sample across the follow-up. The decreasing trajectory is an expression of cumulative transitions to psychosis.

3.2. Physical Health Data and Transition in the CHR-P Sample

3.2.1. Tobacco Use

The comparison between smoker and non-smoker CHR-P subjects (the latter scoring 0 on the FTND) showed that smoking tobacco is associated with a lower risk of transition, especially after 1000 days of follow-up (Figure 2). Considering the different levels of nicotine dependence as per the FTND, relative to non-smokers, it appears that patients with a moderate to high level of tobacco dependence have a higher risk of developing psychosis, and people with a low level of dependence are less prone to developing psychosis (Figure 3).

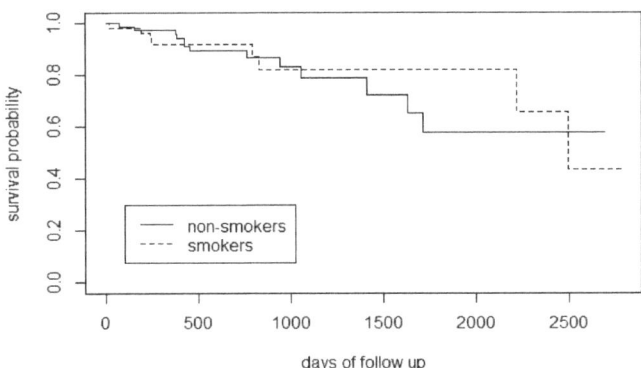

Figure 2. Representation of CHR-P smokers vs. non-smokers (scoring 0 at FTND).

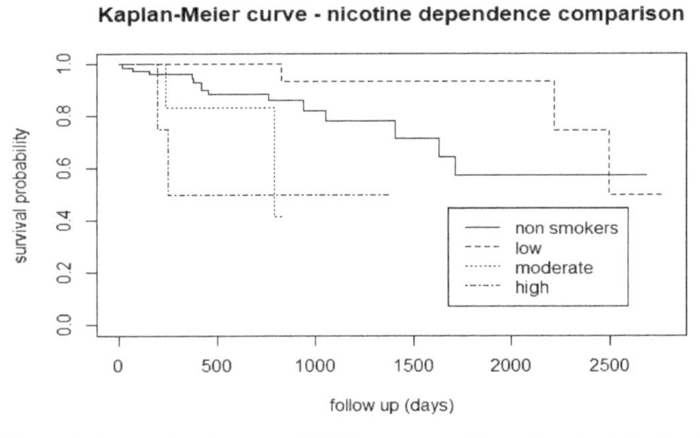

Figure 3. Comparison between CHR-P groups at different levels of nicotine dependence.

3.2.2. Alcohol Use

Figure 4 indicated that for almost the entire follow-up period, CHR-P subjects who drink alcohol were less at risk of developing psychosis than those who do not drink. However, Figure 5 (Kaplan-Maier graph stratified by distinct levels of alcohol dependence) indicated that non-hazardous drinkers may have a lower risk of transition than non-drinkers.

3.2.3. Type of Diet

A visual examination of the Kaplan-Meier curve for fibre intake (Figure 6) showed that CHR-P subjects who self-report high fibre intake present with a lower risk of transitioning to psychosis. Graphs related to saturated and unsaturated fat are appended in Supplementary Materials (Figures S1 and S2).

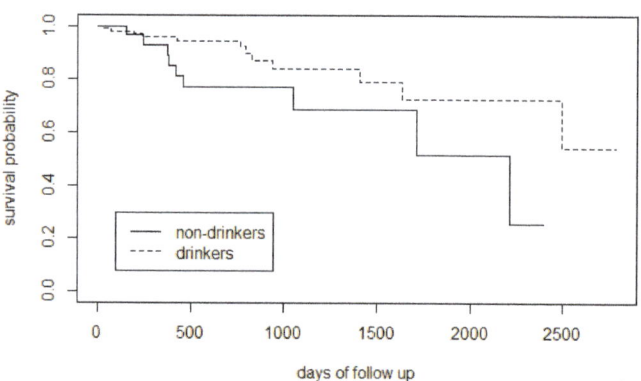

Figure 4. Risk of transition to psychosis between CHR-P individuals that drink alcohol vs. non-drinkers.

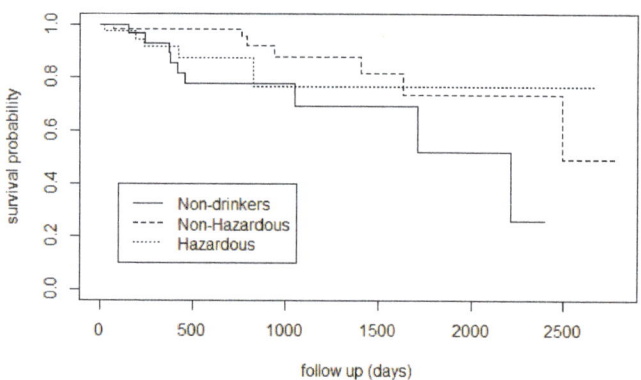

Figure 5. Risk of transition to psychosis in CHR-P subjects, stratified by level of alcohol dependency.

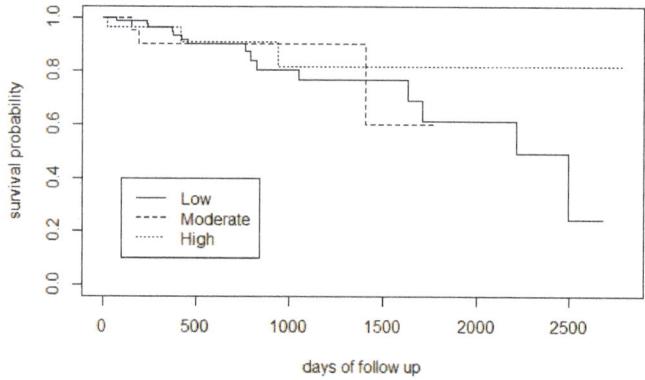

Figure 6. Comparison of the risk of transition to psychosis between CHR-P subjects with a high, moderate, and low fibre intake.

3.2.4. Physical Activity

Visually exploring the Kaplan-Meier graphs suggested that being physically active may be a protective factor against the transition to psychosis (Figure 7).

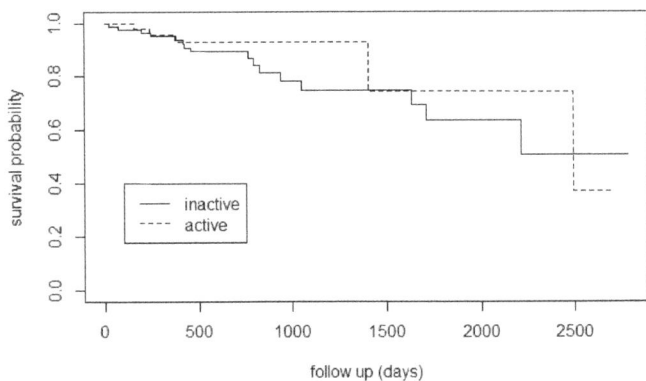

Figure 7. Psychosis risk comparison between physically active CHR-P subjects (>3000 METs) and inactive subjects (<3000 METs).

3.2.5. Physical Parameters

After 1000 days of follow-up, the Kaplan-Meier curve suggested that overweight CHR-P subjects are more at risk of transitioning to psychosis (Figure 8).

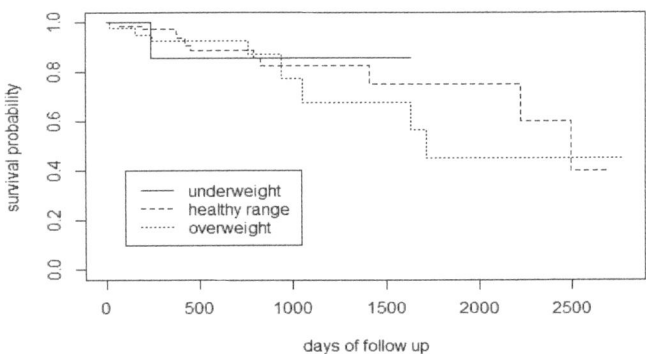

Figure 8. Stratification of psychosis risk in CHR-P subjects with normal, low, and high BMI.

3.3. Log-Rank Tests

The log-rank tests indicated that there may be significant differences between different nicotine dependence groups and psychosis risk. Further exploration of differences between individual nicotine strata revealed that significant differences exist when the low and moderate-high groups are compared, as well as when non-smokers are compared with moderate-high groups (Table 2). The evidence for the difference between various alcohol consumption groups and transition risk is less clear, with a χ^2 of 6 and a corresponding p-value of 0.05. The results of the log-rank tests for fibre intake, physical activity levels, and BMI values did not indicate significant differences between groups.

Table 2. Comparison of differences between groups with a log-rank test.

Feature	χ^2	Degrees of Freedom	p-Value
Log-Rank Test Group Comparison			
Nicotine dependence: low, moderate, high, and non-smokers	12.8	3	0.005
Nicotine dependence: non-smokers and low	3.6	1	0.06
Nicotine dependence: low and moderate or high	14.1	1	0.002
Nicotine dependence: non-smokers and moderate or high	4.7	1	0.03
Alcohol consumption: non-drinkers, non-hazardous, and hazardous	6	2	0.05
Fibre consumption: low, moderate, and high	1.3	2	0.5
Physical activity: active and non-active group	0.8	1	0.4
Body mass index (BMI)	0.3	2	2

3.4. Cox Proportional Hazard Model

The Cox proportional hazard model results are presented in Table 3. Nicotine dependence as measured by the FTND resulted in a Hazard Ratio of 1.34 (95% CI: 1.1–1.64) with an adjusted Benjamini-Hochberg correction p-value of 0.01, which suggests a 34% increase in psychosis risk with every additional point in the FTND score. The confidence intervals of the hazard ratios for the AUDIT score, DINE (fibre score), and the MET physical activity score did not indicate significant associations between these three measures and the transition to psychosis. The DFBETA analysis did not find any influential observations related to the physical health measures at the 0.2 threshold. The only influential observations (DFBETA > 0.2) were found for ethnicity. In sensitivity analysis, after the exclusion of the influential observations, the physical health coefficients changed only marginally, not influencing the interpretation.

Table 3. Hazard ratios obtained from four separate Cox proportional hazard models adjusted by age, gender, and ethnicity.

Feature	Hazard Ratios	Lower 0.95	Upper 0.95	p-Value	Adjusted p-Value
Cox Regression Results					
FTND	1.34	1.1	1.64	0.0034	0.01
AUDIT	1.04	0.95	1.143	0.34	0.45
DINE (fibre score)	0.99	0.96	1.01	0.7	0.7
Physical Act (MET)	0.99	0.96	1.01	0.22	0.44

4. Discussion

We conducted this study on one of the largest CHR-P cohorts (137 subjects) with a long-term follow-up, focusing on physical health data and psychosis risk. This is a subset of a larger dataset we used to describe CHR-P physical health in a cross-sectional design [24]. In the present study, 21 patients transitioned to psychosis across the follow-up period, with a cumulative psychosis risk of 56.3% at 7 years.

From the survival analysis, people who smoke tobacco presented a lower proportion of transition to psychosis (Figure 2), but stratifying the level of nicotine dependence, we noticed that subjects with a moderate to high dependence have a higher risk of psychosis, while people with a low tobacco dependence presented a lower risk than non-smokers (Figure 3). More precisely, we found that smokers with low-dependence are much less at risk than people with moderate-high dependence (Table 2). Kaplan-Meier curves of alcohol status and alcohol dependence showed that patients who are abstinent from alcohol are more prone to developing psychosis (Figure 4). In terms of diet, we found that a low fibre intake might be related to a higher risk of psychosis (Figure 6). In this cohort, higher levels of physical activity seemed to be a protective factor from psychosis (Figure 7), and subjects with a high BMI might have a higher risk after 1000 days of follow-up, but initially underweight is more related to psychosis risk (Figure 8). These results should be interpreted with caution, as log-rank tests showed a significant difference between distinct levels of dependence on nicotine and alcohol and psychosis risk (Table 2), and the

Cox proportional hazard model showed an increment of 34% of psychosis per point only for the FTND (nicotine dependence) score (Table 3).

These latter findings corroborate evidence of the correlation between tobacco use in CHR-P individuals and psychosis. This is in line with the formulation of tobacco smoking as a risk factor [23,32,33], one of the current hypotheses, along with self-medication [71]. Unfortunately, we were not able to control for confounders such as cannabis use, especially high-potency strains, which are also strongly associated with the onset of first-episode psychosis [72,73] and frequently used by subjects that smoke tobacco [74]. Despite the high prevalence of tobacco smoking in CHR-P subjects [23,24], only a few longitudinal studies have investigated the association between tobacco use and transition to psychosis from a CHR-P state [75–78], and our findings require corroboration from future studies that investigate the association in terms of causality. More studies are also needed to investigate the relevant difference in psychosis risk between low and moderate-high nicotine dependence, as it might involve additional confounders, such as potential social factors.

In terms of alcohol use, we replicated the finding of Buchy and colleagues [37,79] who found that low levels of alcohol use were associated with a higher risk of transitioning to psychosis. Again, the result needs to be interpreted with caution, as even though alcohol intake rates are high in CHR-P subjects [24,38], there is a relatively low prevalence of cases of alcohol abuse/high dependence. This may reflect the fact that this subgroup of patients is primarily treated by addiction services, and this might affect the ability to detect the effect of alcohol on psychosis development. We also need to consider the possibility that low alcohol use might be interpreted as a proxy measure for social functioning [80]. Indeed, in the survival analysis, subjects with low alcohol dependence appeared less at risk of transition than abstinent subjects. These findings were also supported by the result of the log-rank test, which found a significant difference in transition risk across different levels of alcohol dependence. Overall, the role of alcohol in the development of psychosis is still not completely clear, as it does not predict the transition to psychosis in different studies [37,79], but it was detected as an important confounder between cannabis use and psychosis conversion in a high-risk sample [81]. These observations underline the importance of developing tailored alcohol intake monitoring and related preventative interventions in the CHR-P phase.

We made one of the first attempts to assess the dietary intake of a CHR-P cohort. Diet has been identified as a modifiable risk factor in depression, and higher dietary intake of energy, sodium [82], refined carbohydrates, and total fats, as well as a lower intake of fibre and omega-3 and omega-6 fatty acids (FA), are related to the psychosis spectrum, but specific dietary guidelines are still not available [83]. This dimension has not been systematically evaluated yet in subjects at risk of developing psychosis. There is evidence [84] that CHR-P subjects report an increased intake of calories and saturated FA and reduced protein consumption compared to healthy controls. Moreover, a prospective study [85] found that CHR-Ps consumed significantly more calories than controls. More recently, a study showed a relatively low red blood cell omega-3 index in CHR-P subjects [86], and cross-sectional data found a positive correlation between intake of omega-3 FA and functional status [86]. In terms of prediction of functional outcomes, results are less clear, but combined concentrations of baseline erythrocyte membrane FA have been found to predict functional enhancement in CHR-P subjects [87]. In one Polish study [36], CHR-P subjects who transitioned to psychosis reported consuming less omega-3 FA than the non-converters. In terms of interventions, a multicentre RCT [88] failed to replicate the result of a single-centre study [89,90], showing that omega-3 polyunsaturated FAs are not effective in preventing transition to psychosis when evidence-based psychological interventions are available. However, a longitudinal analysis of biomarkers showed that an increase in the omega-3 index predicted better symptomatology and functional outcomes [91].

Given the lack of validated dietary assessment tools for patients suffering from serious mental illnesses [92], the DINE questionnaire was challenging to administer, especially in saturated and unsaturated fat sections (e.g., items with a high weight in the total score were particularly difficult to assess). This calls for the implementation of dietary assessment tools tailored for clinical populations suffering from mental disorders [92,93]. The fibre section of the DINE questionnaire was easier to administer, and the results appeared to be more reliable. This is noteworthy, as in our cross-sectional study, 60% of CHR-P subjects presented with a low fibre intake [24], in line with psychosis patients [83]. In our survival analysis, people with a lower fibre intake appeared to transition more than people with a higher proportion of fibre in their diet, but this result was not confirmed by the log-rank test nor the Cox proportional hazard model. In a recent review, Teasdale and colleagues [82] recommended further research into dietary intake in the pre-illness onset phase to understand "whether any dietary factors may indicate the onset of the illness".

People with psychosis present with reduced physical activity levels [94–96] and spend more time in sedentary behaviour [95] than the general population, which may contribute to their increased cardiometabolic risk [97–99]. CHR-P populations also present with reduced levels of physical activity [25], and our cross-sectional study [24] found that in CHR-P subjects, averages of physical activity levels were far below UK national guidelines [100].

A recent meta-analysis found that people with high levels of self-reported physical activity had reduced odds of developing psychosis, but the association was no longer significant when adjusted for covariates [101]. The literature on the topic is still scarce, but one Finnish cohort study identified low levels of physical activity in childhood/early adolescence as an independent predictor of psychosis [35]. Similarly, a birth cohort study found that subjects who later transitioned to psychosis were more inactive during their adolescence [102], and adolescents with parents with psychosis who were more engaged in physical activity were 24% less likely to develop psychosis [103]. This is in line with our survival analysis that showed that physically active CHR-P individuals (IPAQ-MET score) are less likely to develop psychosis, but our result was not confirmed using the log-rank test or the Cox proportional hazard model. The Lancet Psychiatry Commission [104] advocated physical activity as a core component for preventative interventions from the earliest stages of mental illnesses to protect physical health from illness onset and prevent physical health comorbidity from developing. A recent study [105] confirmed that CHR-P individuals are less fit than controls and that their self-report items did not reflect objective indices of fitness, perhaps reflecting elements of grandiosity or avolition. This adds further caution when interpreting results about physical activity that rely exclusively on self-reported measures. Given the effect of physical exercise on brain plasticity [106] and potentially also in CHR-P subjects [42,107], it is plausible that it may help to protect CHR-P against psychosis beyond the improvement of their fitness, global functioning, attenuated symptoms, and cognitive performance [42,107]. There is evidence that service users find interventions on physical activity feasible and acceptable [108].

In terms of physical parameters, our cross-sectional study [24] found that CHR-P physical measures were in line with the matched UK general population, similar to a previous review [25], but in contrast with the NAPLS study, which found high rates of cardiometabolic abnormalities, including obesity [86]. In the current study, CHR-P individuals with high BMI appeared more at risk of developing psychosis after 1000 days of follow-up in the survival analysis, but this result should be interpreted with caution because of the low number of transitions in the later stages of follow-up.

Results from a Finnish birth cohort [109] showed that being underweight but not overweight in adolescence independently predicts the later development of non-affective psychosis. Classically, low birthweight has been interpreted as a risk factor for schizophrenia [110], and several studies have reported associations between non-affective psychosis and low BMI during childhood and adolescence/young adulthood [111]. The literature presents different associations between BMI and different clinical features in the CHR-P phase. For instance, in medicated CHR-P subjects (with antidepressants/antipsychotics) BMI was negatively correlated with positive symptoms [112]. An increase in BMI was associated with baseline molecular circulating lipids [113]. BMI was also positively correlated with leptin levels [114] and was negatively associated with polyunsaturated FA levels [115].

Moreover, in subjects with a familial risk of psychosis, a higher BMI was related to white matter abnormalities [116].

Only a few studies have reported waist circumference values for CHR-P individuals [22,84,114,117].

Overall, BMI and the other anthropometric measures are still not well characterised in CHR-P subjects [105], in line with various other potential risk factors for psychosis. For instance, high systolic blood pressure was found to be weakly correlated to an increased risk of schizophrenia in a recent GWAS study [118]. However, a single study found systolic pressure to be significantly lower in CHR-P individuals than in controls during a stress test [117]. Higher blood pressure and resting heart rate (RHR) values in adolescence predicted schizophrenia in adulthood in male subjects from a large cohort study [119]. Heart rate (HR) is considered an expression of autonomic functioning [120,121], which is altered in many psychiatric syndromes [122,123]. In the CHR-P phase, findings are contradictory: Clamor and colleagues [124] did not find any difference in heart parameters compared to healthy controls, while Counotte et al. [125] reported associations between psychosis liability and increased HR and HR variability (HRV). Furthermore, Kocsis [126] found an increased RHR in CHR-P patients relative to healthy controls, and increased RHR was positively correlated with CAARMS severity and distress scores. Low HRV was instead correlated with antipsychotic/antidepressant use in a longitudinal study [127] in CHR-P individuals.

In the end, only a small proportion of studies systematically report the physical measures of CHR-P cohorts [25], especially in relation to the transition to psychosis. This calls for further high-quality research to facilitate a more comprehensive understanding of the role of physical measures in the context of psychosis onset.

In terms of limitations, we did not assess physical health data at different time points, and so we cannot address potential changes in these habits across the follow-up period. In addition, we mainly used self-report measures, which might be susceptible to recall bias. The use of biomarkers would help to overcome this limitation. As mentioned, due to the lack of validated instruments to assess dietary intake for populations with serious mental illness, the administration of the DINE questionnaire was particularly challenging. We did not control for substance use (cannabis use may be of particular importance), so our findings around tobacco and the transition to psychosis should be interpreted with caution, given the frequent cases of polysubstance abuse. Finally, data on education were not available, and we did not control for religion, spirituality, and family bonds [128], which might also represent potential confounders given their potential influence on alcohol and dietary habits or their reported effects on treatment maintenance, sociality, and health practices [129,130].

5. Conclusions

This study investigated the relationship between different physical health data and the transition to psychosis in a large cohort of CHR-P service users, finding that an increase in nicotine dependence is related to a substantial increase in psychosis risk, as confirmed by the Cox proportional hazard model. We also conducted survival analyses on alcohol use, dietary intake, levels of physical activity, and BMI, finding that non-drinkers were more likely to develop psychosis, as were CHR-P subjects with low fibre intake and low physical activity levels. In terms of anthropometric measures, a higher BMI was associated with greater psychosis risk after the first 1000 days.

These findings call for monitoring data on physical health and lifestyle in CHR-P subjects to increase our understanding of their potential role in psychosis onset and to implement tailored interventions targeting unhealthy daily habits. Indeed, interventions aimed at reducing alcohol and tobacco use, promoting a balanced diet, and promoting physical activity in line with national guidelines would constitute favourable and generalisable treatments for CHR-P, with potential effectiveness in also improving mental health outcomes in this clinical population.

Supplementary Materials: The following supporting information can be downloaded at: https://www.mdpi.com/article/10.3390/biomedicines12030523/s1, Table S1: ICD-10 Diagnoses for non-organic psychotic disorders; Table S2: The RECORD statement—checklist of items, extended from the STROBE statement, that should be reported in observational studies using routinely collected health data; Figure S1: Stratification of psychosis risk in CHR-P subjects with low, medium, and high saturated fat intake; Figure S2: Stratification of psychosis risk in CHR-P subjects with low, medium, and high unsaturated fat intake.

Author Contributions: Conceptualisation, P.F.-P. and A.D.M.; methodology, P.F.-P., U.P. and K.K.; software, U.P., S.D. and K.K.; validation, A.D.M. and P.F.-P.; formal analysis, U.P., S.D. and K.K.; investigation, A.D.M.; writing—original draft preparation, A.D.M., U.P. and K.K.; writing—review and editing, S.D. and D.O.; supervision N.B., P.F.-P. and P.M. All authors have read and agreed to the published version of the manuscript.

Funding: This research received no external funding.

Institutional Review Board Statement: The study was conducted in accordance with the Declaration of Helsinki and approved by Oxfordshire REC C (Ref: 18/SC/0372). The data resource received ethical approval as a deidentified dataset for secondary mental health research analyses from Oxfordshire REC C (Ref: 18/SC/0372).

Informed Consent Statement: Consent is not required to analyse the deidentified dataset for approved research studies. Patients may opt-out of inclusion in the deidentified dataset.

Data Availability Statement: The authors give no permission to share raw data.

Conflicts of Interest: P.F.-P. is supported by #NEXTGENERATIONEU (NGEU), funded by the Ministry of University and Research (MUR), National Recovery and Resilience Plan (NRRP), project MNESYS (PE0000006)—A Multiscale integrated approach to the study of the nervous system in health and disease (DN. 1553 11.10.2022). The other authors declare no conflict of interest.

References

1. Fusar-Poli, P.; Borgwardt, S.; Bechdolf, A.; Addington, J.; Riecher-Rössler, A.; Schultze-Lutter, F.; Keshavan, M.; Wood, S.; Ruhrmann, S.; Seidman, L.J.; et al. The psychosis high-risk state: A comprehensive state-of-the-art review. *JAMA Psychiatry* **2013**, *70*, 107–120. [CrossRef] [PubMed]
2. Yung, A.; McGorry, P. The prodromal phase of first-episode psychosis: Past and current conceptualizations. *Schizophr. Bull.* **1996**, *22*, 353–370. [CrossRef]
3. Salazar de Pablo, G.; Radua, J.; Pereira, J.; Bonoldi, I.; Arienti, V.; Besana, F.; Soardo, L.; Cabras, A.; Fortea, L.; Catalan, A.; et al. Probability of Transition to Psychosis in Individuals at Clinical High Risk: An Updated Meta-analysis. *JAMA Psychiatry* **2021**, *78*, 970–978. [CrossRef]
4. Yung, A.; Nelson, B.; Yuen, H.; Spiliotacopoulos, D.; Lin, A.; Simmons, M.; Bruxner, A.; Broussard, C.; Thompson, A.; McGorry, P. Long term outcome in an ultra high risk ("prodromal") group. *Schizophr. Bull.* **2011**, *37*, 22–23. [CrossRef]
5. Beck, K.; Studerus, E.; Andreou, C.; Egloff, L.; Leanza, L.; Simon, A.; Borgwardt, S.; Riecher-Rössler, A. Clinical and functional ultra-long-term outcome of patients with a clinical high risk (CHR) for psychosis. *Eur. Psychiatry* **2019**, *62*, 30–37. [CrossRef] [PubMed]
6. Fusar-Poli, P.; Bechdolf, A.; Taylor, M.; Bonoldi, I.; Carpenter, W.; Yung, A.; McGuire, P. At risk for schizophrenic or affective psychoses? A meta-analysis of DSM/ICD diagnostic outcomes in individuals at high clinical risk. *Schizophr. Bull.* **2012**, *39*, 923–932. [CrossRef] [PubMed]
7. Beck, K.; Andreou, C.; Studerus, E.; Heitz, U.; Ittig, S.; Leanza, L.; Riecher-Rössler, A. Clinical and functional long-term outcome of patients at clinical high risk (CHR) for psychosis without transition to psychosis: A systematic review. *Schizophr. Res.* **2019**, *210*, 39–47. [CrossRef]
8. Yung, A.; Pan Yuen, H.; McGorry, P.; Phillips, L.; Kelly, D.; Dell'Olio, M.; Francey, S.; Cosgrave, E.; Killackey, E.; Stanford, C.; et al. Mapping the onset of psychosis: The Comprehensive Assessment of At-Risk Mental States. *Aust. N. Z. J. Psychiatry* **2005**, *39*, 964–971. [CrossRef]
9. Rutigliano, G.; Valmaggia, L.; Landi, P.; Frascarelli, M.; Cappucciati, M.; Sear, V.; Rocchetti, M.; De Micheli, A.; Jones, C.; Palombini, E.; et al. Persistence or recurrence of non-psychotic comorbid mental disorders associated with 6-year poor functional outcomes in patients at ultra high risk for psychosis. *J. Affect. Disord.* **2016**, *203*, 101–110. [CrossRef]
10. Haining, K.; Brunner, G.; Gajwani, R.; Gross, J.; Gumley, A.; Lawrie, S.; Schwannauer, M.; Schultze-Lutter, F.; Uhlhaas, P. The relationship between cognitive deficits and impaired short-term functional outcome in clinical high-risk for psychosis participants: A machine learning and modelling approach. *Schizophr. Res.* **2021**, *231*, 24–31. [CrossRef]

11. Fusar-Poli, P.; Byrne, M.; Valmaggia, L.; Day, F.; Tabraham, P.; Johns, L.; McGuire, P. Social dysfunction predicts two years clinical outcome in people at ultra high risk for psychosis. *J. Psychiatr. Res.* **2010**, *44*, 294–301. [CrossRef]
12. Velthorst, E.; Nieman, D.; Linszen, D.; Becker, H.; de Haan, L.; Dingemans, P.; Birchwood, M.; Patterson, P.; Salokangas, R.; Heinimaa, M.; et al. Disability in people clinically at high risk of psychosis. *Br. J. Psychiatry* **2010**, *197*, 278–284. [CrossRef]
13. Fusar-Poli, P.; Tantardini, M.; De Simone, S.; Ramella-Cravaro, V.; Oliver, D.; Kingdon, J.; Kotlicka-Antczak, M.; Valmaggia, L.; Lee, J.; Millan, M.; et al. Deconstructing vulnerability for psychosis: Meta-analysis of environmental risk factors for psychosis in subjects at ultra high-risk. *Eur. Psychiatry* **2017**, *40*, 65–75. [CrossRef]
14. Miller, T.; McGlashan, T.; Rosen, J.; Cadenhead, K.; Cannon, T.; Ventura, J.; McFarlane, W.; Perkins, D.; Pearlson, G.; Woods, S. Prodromal assessment with the structured interview for prodromal syndromes and the scale of prodromal symptoms: Predictive validity, interrater reliability, and training to reliability. *Schizophr. Bull.* **2003**, *29*, 703–715. [CrossRef] [PubMed]
15. Hui, T.; Garvey, L.; Olasoji, M. Improving the physical health of young people with early psychosis with lifestyle interventions: Scoping review. *Int. J. Ment. Health Nurs.* **2021**, *30*, 1498–1524. [CrossRef]
16. GBD 2016 Disease and Injury Incidence and Prevalence Collaborators. Global, regional, and national incidence, prevalence, and years lived with disability for 328 diseased and injuries for 195 countries, 1990-2016 a systematic analysis for the Global Burden of Diseases Study 2016. *Lancet* **2017**, *390*, 1211–1259. [CrossRef]
17. De Hert, M.; Cohen, D.; Bobes, J.; Cetkovich-Bakmas, M.; Leucht, S.; Ndetei, D.; Newcomer, J.; Uwakwe, R.; Asai, I.; Möller, H.; et al. Physical illness in patients with severe mental disorders. II. Barriers to care, monitoring and treatment guidelines, plus recommendations at the system and individual level. *World Psychiatry* **2011**, *10*, 138–151. [CrossRef] [PubMed]
18. Wahlbeck, K.; Westman, J.; Nordentoft, M.; Gissier, M.; Laursen Munk, T. Outcomes of Nordic mental health systems: Life expectancy of patient with mental disorders. *Br. J. Psychiatry* **2011**, *199*, 453–458. [CrossRef] [PubMed]
19. Saha, S.; Chant, D.; McGrath, J. A systematic review of mortality in schizophrenia: Is the differential mortality gap worsening over time? *Arch. Gen. Psychiatry* **2007**, *64*, 1123–1131. [CrossRef]
20. Hjorthøj, C.; Stürup, A.; McGrath, J.; Nordentoft, M. Years of potential life lost and life expectancy in schizophrenia: A systematic review and meta-analysis. *Lancet Psychiatry* **2017**, *4*, 295–301. [CrossRef]
21. Jayatilleke, N.; Hayes, R.; Dutta, R.; Shetty, H.; Hotopf, M.; Chang, C.; Stewart, R. Contributions of specific causes of death to lost life expectancy in severe mental illness. *Eur. Psychiatry* **2017**, *43*, 109–115. [CrossRef] [PubMed]
22. Cordes, J.; Bechdolf, A.; Engelke, C.; Kahl, K.; Balijepalli, C.; Lösch, C.; Klosterkötter, J.; Wagner, M.; Maier, W.; Heinz, A.; et al. Prevalence of metabolic syndrome in female and male patients at risk of psychosis. *Schizophr. Res.* **2017**, *181*, 38–42. [CrossRef] [PubMed]
23. De Micheli, A.; Provenzani, U.; Solmi, M.; Van Pabst, A.; Youssef, E.; McGuire, P.; Fusar-Poli, P. Prevalence of tobacco smoking in people at clinical high-risk for psychosis: Systematic review and meta-analysis. *Schizophr. Res.* **2023**, *254*, 109–115. [CrossRef] [PubMed]
24. Provenzani, U.; De Micheli, A.; Damiani, S.; Oliver, D.; Brondino, N.; Fusar-Poli, P. Physical Health in Clinical High Risk for Psychosis Individuals: A Cross-Sectional Study. *Brain Sci.* **2023**, *13*, 128. [CrossRef] [PubMed]
25. Carney, R.; Cotter, J.; Bradshaw, T.; Firth, J.; Yung, A. Cardiometabolic risk factors in young people at ultra-high risk for psychosis: A systematic review and meta-analysis. *Schizophr. Res.* **2016**, *170*, 290–300. [CrossRef]
26. Newberry, R.; Dean, D.; Sayyah, M.; Mittal, V. What prevents youth at clinical high risk for psychosis from engaging in physical activity? An examination of the barriers to physical activity. *Schizophr. Res.* **2018**, *201*, 400–405. [CrossRef]
27. Mittal, V.; Gupta, T.; Orr, J.; Pelletier-Baldelli, A.; Dean, D.; Lunsford-Avery, J.; Smith, A.; Robustelli, B.; Leopold, D.; Millman, Z.J. Physical activity level and medial temporal health in youth at ultra-high-risk for psychosis. *J. Abnorm. Psychol.* **2013**, *122*, 1101–1110. [CrossRef]
28. Colomer, L.; Anmella, G.; Vieta, E.; Grande, I. Physical health in affective disorders: A narrative review of the literature. *Braz. J. Psychiatry* **2021**, *43*, 621–630. [CrossRef] [PubMed]
29. Tsiachristas, A.; Thomas, T.; Leal, J.; Lennox, B. Economic impact of early intervention in psychosis services: Results from a longitudinal retrospective controlled study in England. *BMJ Open* **2016**, *6*, e012611. [CrossRef] [PubMed]
30. Smith, D.; Langan, J.; McLean, G.; Guthrie, B.; Mercer, S. Schizophrenia is associated with excess multiple physical-health comorbidities but low levels of recorded cardiovascular disease in primary care: Cross-sectional study. *BMJ Open* **2013**, *3*, e002808. [CrossRef]
31. Damiani, S.; Rutigliano, G.; Fazia, T.; Merlino, F.; Berzuini, C.; Bernardinelli, L.; Politi, P.; Fusar-Poli, P. Developing and validating an individualized clinical prediction model to forecast psychotic recurrence in acute and transient psychotic disorders: Electronic health record cohort study. *Schizophr. Bull.* **2021**, *47*, 1695–1705. [CrossRef]
32. Gage, S.; Jones, H.; Taylor, A.; Burgess, S.; Zammit, S.; Munafò, M. Investigating causality in associations between smoking initiation and schizophrenia using Mendelian randomization. *Sci. Rep.* **2017**, *7*, 40653. [CrossRef]
33. Gurillo, P.; Jauhar, S.; Murray, R.; MacCabe, J. Does tobacco use cause psychosis? Systematic review and meta-analysis. *Lancet Psychiatry* **2015**, *2*, 718–725. [CrossRef]
34. Cannon, T.; Cadenhead, K.; Cornblatt, B.; Woods, S.; Addington, J.; Walker, E.; Seidman, L.; Perkins, D.; Tsuang, M.; McGlashan, T.; et al. Prediction of psychosis in youth at high clinical risk: A multisite longitudinal study in North America. *Arch. Gen. Psychiatry* **2008**, *65*, 28–37. [CrossRef]

35. Sormunen, E.; Saarinen, M.; Salokangas, R.; Telama, R.; Hutri-Kähönen, N.; Tammelin, T.; Viikari, J.; Raitakari, O.; Hietala, J. Effects of childhood and adolescence physical activity patterns on psychosis risk-a general population cohort study. *NPJ Schizophr.* **2017**, *3*, 5. [CrossRef]
36. Pawełczyk, T.; Trafalska, E.; Kotlicka-Antczak, M.; Pawełczyk, A. The association between polyunsaturated fatty acid consumption and the transition to psychosis in ultra-high risk individuals. *Prostaglandins Leukot. Essent. Fat. Acids* **2016**, *108*, 30–37. [CrossRef]
37. Buchy, L.; Perkins, D.; Woods, S.; Liu, L.; Addington, J. Impact of substance use on conversion to psychosis in youth at clinical high risk of psychosis. *Schizophr. Res.* **2014**, *156*, 277–280. [CrossRef]
38. Amir, C.; Kapler, S.; Hoftman, G.; Kushan, L.; Zinberg, J.; Cadenhead, K.; Kennedy, L.; Cornblatt, B.; Keshavan, M.; Mathalon, D.; et al. Neurobehavioral risk factors influence prevalence and severity of hazardous substance use in youth at genetic and clinical high risk for psychosis. *Front. Psychiatry* **2023**, *14*, 1143315. [CrossRef]
39. Abarca, M.; Pizarro, H.; Nuñez, R.; Arancibia, M. Physical exercise as an intervention in people at clinical high-risk for psychosis: A narrative review. *Medwave* **2023**, *23*, e2724. [CrossRef]
40. Carney, R.; Bradshaw, T.; Yung, A. Monitoring of physical health in services for young people at ultra-high risk of psychosis. *Early Interv. Psychiatry* **2018**, *12*, 153–159. [CrossRef]
41. Thornicroft, G. Physical health disparities and mental illness: The scandal of premature mortality. *Br. J. Psychiatry* **2011**, *199*, 441–442. [CrossRef]
42. Damme, K.; Gupta, T.; Ristanovic, I.; Kimhy, D.; Bryan, A.; Mittal, V. Exercise intervention in individuals at clinical high risk for psychosis: Benefits to fitness, symptoms, hippocampal volumes, and functional connectivity. *Schizophr. Bull.* **2022**, *48*, 1394–1405. [CrossRef]
43. NHS UK: NHS Five Year Forward View (Page Last Reviewed: 8th March 2019). Available online: https://www.england.nhs.uk/five-year-forward-view/ (accessed on 20 July 2023).
44. Lederman, O.; Rosenbaum, S.; Maloney, C.; Curtis, J.; Ward, P. Modifiable cardiometabolic risk factors in youth with at-risk mental states: A cross-sectional pilot study. *Psychiatry Res.* **2017**, *257*, 424–430. [CrossRef]
45. Bhavsar, V.; Jauhar, S.; Murray, R.; Hotopf, M.; Hatch, S.; McNeill, A.; Boydell, J.; MacCabe, J. Tobacco smoking is associated with psychotic experiences in the general population of South London. *Psychol. Med.* **2018**, *48*, 123–131. [CrossRef]
46. Benchimol, E.; Smeeth, L.; Guttmann, A.; Harron, K.; Moher, D.; Petersen, I.; Sørensen, H.T.; von Elm, E.; Langan, S. The REporting of studies Conducted using Observational Routinely-collected health Data (RECORD) statement. *PLoS Med.* **2015**, *12*, e1001885. [CrossRef]
47. Perera, G.; Broadbent, M.; Callard, F.; Chang, C.; Downs, J.; Dutta, R.; Fernandes, A.; Hayes, R.; Henderson, M.; Jackson, R.; et al. Cohort profile of the South London and Maudsley NHS Foundation Trust Biomedical Research Centre (SLaM BRC) Case Register: Current status and recent enhancement of an Electronic Mental Health Record-derived data resource. *BMJ Open* **2016**, *6*, e008721. [CrossRef]
48. Jongsma, H.; Gayer-Anderson, C.; Lasalvia, A.; Quattrone, D.; Mulè, A.; Szöke, A.; Selten, J.; Turner, C.; Arango, C.; Tarricone, I.; et al. Treated incidence of psychotic disorders in the multinational EU-GEI Study. *JAMA Psychiatry* **2018**, *75*, 36–46. [CrossRef]
49. Stewart, R.; Soremekun, M.; Perera, G.; Broadbent, M.; Callard, F.; Denis, M.; Hotopf, M.; Thornicroft, G.; Lovestone, S. The South London and Maudsley NHS Foundation Trust Biomedical Research Centre (SLAM BRC) case register: Development and descriptive data. *BMC Psychiatry* **2009**, *9*, 51. [CrossRef]
50. Fusar-Poli, P.; Spencer, T.; De Micheli, A.; Curzi, V.; Nandha, S.; McGuire, P. Outreach and support in South-London (OASIS) 2001–2020: Twenty years of early detection, prognosis and preventive care for young people at risk of psychosis. *Eur. Neuropsychopharmacol.* **2020**, *39*, 111–122. [CrossRef]
51. Fusar-Poli, P.; Byrne, M.; Badger, S.; Valmaggia, L.; McGuire, P. Outreach and support in south London (OASIS), 2001–2011: Ten years of early diagnosis and treatment for young individuals at high clinical risk for psychosis. *Eur. Psychiatry* **2013**, *28*, 315–326. [CrossRef]
52. Fusar-Poli, P.; Estradé, A.; Spencer, T.; Gupta, S.; Murguia-Asensio, S.; Eranti, S.; Wilding, K.; Andlauer, O.; Buhagiar, J.; Smith, M.; et al. Pan-London Network for Psychosis-Prevention (PNP). *Front. Psychiatry* **2019**, *10*, 707. [CrossRef] [PubMed]
53. Fusar-Poli, P.; De Micheli, A.; Signorini, L.; Baldwin, H.; Salazar de Pablo, G.; McGuire, P. Real-world long-term outcomes in individuals at clinical risk for psychosis: The case for extending duration of care. *EClinicalMedicine* **2020**, *28*, 100578. [CrossRef]
54. Fusar-Poli, P.; Schultze-Lutter, F. Predicting the onset of psychosis in patients at clinical high risk: Practical guide to probabilistic prognostic reasoning. *Evid. Based Ment. Health* **2016**, *19*, 10–15. [CrossRef]
55. Fusar-Poli, P.; Palombini, E.; Davies, C.; Oliver, D.; Bonoldi, I.; Ramella-Cravaro, V.; McGuire, P. Why transition risk to psychosis is not declining at the OASIS ultra high risk service: The hidden role of stable pretest risk enrichment. *Schizophr. Res.* **2018**, *192*, 385–390. [CrossRef]
56. Fusar-Poli, P.; Schultze-Lutter, F.; Cappucciati, M.; Rutigliano, G.; Bonoldi, I.; Stahl, D.; Borgwardt, S.; Riecher-Rössler, A.; Addington, J.; Perkins, D.; et al. The dark side of the moon: Meta-analytical impact of recruitment strategies on risk enrichment in the clinical high risk state for psychosis. *Schizophr. Bull.* **2016**, *42*, 732–743. [CrossRef]
57. NICE. *Surveillance Report 2017—Psychosis and Schizophrenia in Adults: Prevention and Management (2014) NICE Guideline CG178*; National Institute for Health and Care Excellence (NICE): London, UK, 2017. Available online: https://www.nice.org.uk/guidance/cg178/evidence/full-guideline-490503565/ (accessed on 27 December 2023).

58. Heatherton, T.; Kozlowski, L.; Frecker, R.; Fagerström, K. The Fagerström test for nicotine dependence: A revision of the Fagerström tolerance questionnaire. *Br. J. Addict.* **1991**, *86*, 1119–1127. [CrossRef]
59. Etter, J.; Eissenberg, T. Dependence levels in users of electronic cigarettes, nicotine gums and tobacco cigarettes. *Drug Alcohol Depend.* **2015**, *147*, 68–75. [CrossRef]
60. Etter, J. Dependence on the nicotine gum in former smokers. *Addict. Behav.* **2009**, *34*, 246–251. [CrossRef]
61. Saunders, J.; Aasland, O.; Babor, T.; de la Fuente, J.; Grant, M. Development of the Alcohol Use Disorders Identification Test (AUDIT): WHO Collaborative project on early detection of persons with harmful alcohol consumption—II. *Addiction* **1993**, *88*, 791–804. [CrossRef] [PubMed]
62. Little, P.; Barnett, J.; Margetts, B.; Kinmonth, A.; Gabbay, J.; Thompson, R.; Warm, D.; Warwick, H.; Wooton, S. The validity of dietary assessment in general practice. *J. Epidemiol. Community Health* **1999**, *53*, 165–172. [CrossRef]
63. Hagströmer, M.; Oja, P.; Sjöström, M. The International Physical Activity Questionnaire (IPAQ): A study of concurrent and construct validity. *Public Health Nutr.* **2006**, *9*, 755–762. [CrossRef]
64. Craig, C.; Marshall, A.; Sjöström, M.; Bauman, A.; Booth, M.; Ainsworth, B.; Pratt, M.; Ekelund, U.; Yngve, A.; Sallis, J.; et al. International physical activity questionnaire: 12-country reliability and validity. *Med. Sci. Sports Exerc.* **2003**, *35*, 1381–1395. [CrossRef]
65. Kaplan, E.; Meier, P. Nonparametric Estimation from Incomplete Observations. *J. Am. Stat. Assoc.* **1958**, *53*, 457–481. [CrossRef]
66. Mantel, N. Evaluation of survival data and two new rank order statistics arising in its consideration. *Cancer Chemother. Rep.* **1966**, *50*, 163–170.
67. Cox, D. Regression models and life tables. *J. R. Stat. Soc. Ser. B* **1972**, *34*, 187–220. [CrossRef]
68. Harrell, F. Regression modeling strategies. *Bios* **2017**, *330*, 14. Available online: https://www.google.com/url?sa=t&rct=j&q=&esrc=s&source=web&cd=&ved=2ahUKEwj1_5zsuq6DAxWg8rsIHbexCYYQFnoECBEQAQ&url=https://www.researchgate.net/profile/David-Booth-7/post/What_model_may_i_use_instead_of_multiple_regression_model/attachment/6380dd2a97e2867d5070450f/AS%253A11431281100713611%25401669389609596/download/courseHarrell.pdf&usg=AOvVaw1bAPyF3Kf1cHhxGClsRJX6&opi=89978449/ (accessed on 27 December 2023).
69. Benjamini, Y.; Hochberg, Y. Controlling the False Discovery Rate: A Practical and Powerful Approach to Multiple Testing. *J. R. Stat. Soc. Ser. B* **1995**, *57*, 289–300. [CrossRef]
70. R Core Team. R: A Language and Environment for Statistical Computing. In *R Foundation for Statistical Computing*; R Core Team: Vienna, Austria, 2023; Available online: http://www.R-project.org/ (accessed on 29 August 2023).
71. Parikh, V.; Kutlu, M.; Gould, T. nAChR dysfunction as a common substrate for schizophrenia and comorbid nicotine addiction: Current trends and perspectives. *Schizophr. Res.* **2016**, *171*, 1–15. [CrossRef] [PubMed]
72. Di Forti, M.; Quattrone, D.; Freeman, T.; Tripoli, G.; Gayer-Anderson, C.; Quigley, H.; Rodriguez, V.; Jongsma, H.; Ferraro, L.; La Cascia, C.; et al. The contribution of cannabis use to variation in the incidence of psychotic disorder across Europe (EU-GEI): A multicentre case-control study. *Lancet Psychiatry* **2019**, *6*, 427–436. [CrossRef] [PubMed]
73. Marconi, A.; Di Forti, M.; Lewis, C.; Murray, R.; Vassos, E. Meta-analysis of the Association Between the Level of Cannabis Use and Risk of Psychosis. *Schizophr. Bull.* **2016**, *42*, 1262–1269. [CrossRef]
74. MacCabe, J. It is time to start taking tobacco seriously as a risk factor for psychosis: Self-medication cannot explain the association. *Acta Psychiatr. Scand.* **2018**, *138*, 3–4. [CrossRef] [PubMed]
75. van der Heijden, H.; Schirmbeck, F.; McGuire, P.; Valmaggia, L.; Kempton, M.; van der Gaag, M.; Nelson, B.; Riecher-Rössler, A.; Bressan, R.; Barrantes-Vidal, N.; et al. Association between tobacco use and symptomatology in individuals at ultra-high risk to develop a psychosis: A longitudinal study. *Schizophr. Res.* **2021**, *236*, 48–53. [CrossRef] [PubMed]
76. Ward, H.; Lawson, M.; Addington, J.; Bearden, C.; Cadenhead, K.; Cannon, T.; Cornblatt, B.; Jeffries, C.; Mathalon, D.; McGlashan, T.; et al. Tobacco use and psychosis risk in persons at clinical high risk. *Early Interv. Psychiatry* **2019**, *13*, 1173–1181. [CrossRef]
77. Buchy, L.; Cannon, T.; Anticevic, A.; Lyngberg, K.; Cadenhead, K.; Cornblatt, B.; McGlashan, T.; Perkins, D.; Seidman, L.; Tsuang, M.; et al. Evaluating the impact of cannabis use on thalamic connectivity in youth at clinical high risk of psychosis. *BMC Psychiatry* **2015**, *15*, 276. [CrossRef] [PubMed]
78. Kristensen, K.; Cadenhead, K. Cannabis abuse and risk for psychosis in a prodromal sample. *Psychiatry Res.* **2007**, *151*, 151–154. [CrossRef] [PubMed]
79. Buchy, L.; Cadenhead, K.; Cannon, T.; Cornblatt, B.; McGlashan, T.; Perkins, D.; Seidman, L.; Tsuang, M.; Walker, E.; Woods, S.; et al. Substance use in individuals at clinical high risk of psychosis. *Psychol. Med.* **2015**, *45*, 2275–2284. [CrossRef] [PubMed]
80. Thornton, L.; Baker, A.; Johnson, M.; Kay-Lambkin, F.; Lewin, T. Reasons for substance use among people with psychotic disorders: Method triangulation approach. *Psychol. Addict. Behav.* **2012**, *26*, 279–288. [CrossRef]
81. Auther, A.; Cadenhead, K.; Carrión, R.; Addington, J.; Bearden, C.; Cannon, T.; McGlashan, T.; Perkins, D.; Seidman, L.; Tsuang, M.; et al. Alcohol confounds relationship between cannabis misuse and psychosis conversion in a high-risk sample. *Acta Psychiatr. Scand.* **2015**, *132*, 60–68. [CrossRef]
82. Teasdale, S.; Ward, P.; Samaras, K.; Firth, J.; Stubbs, B.; Tripodi, E.; Burrows, T. Dietary intake of people with severe mental illness: Systematic review and meta-analysis. *Br. J. Psychiatry* **2019**, *214*, 251–259. [CrossRef]

83. Aucoin, M.; LaChance, L.; Cooley, K.; Kidd, S. Diet and Psychosis: A Scoping Review. *Neuropsychobiology* **2020**, *79*, 20–42. [CrossRef]
84. Manzanares, N.; Monseny, R.; Ortega, L.; Montalvo, I.; Franch, J.; Gutiérrez-Zotes, A.; Reynolds, R.; Walker, B.; Vilella, E.; Labad, J. Unhealthy lifestyle in early psychoses: The role of life stress and the hypothalamic-pituitary-adrenal axis. *Psychoneuroendocrinology* **2014**, *39*, 1–10. [CrossRef]
85. Labad, J.; Stojanovic-Pérez, A.; Montalvo, I.; Solé, M.; Cabezas, Á.; Ortega, L.; Moreno, I.; Vilella, E.; Martorell, L.; Reynolds, R.; et al. Stress biomarkers as predictors of transition to psychosis in at-risk mental states: Roles for cortisol, prolactin and albumin. *J. Psychiatr. Res.* **2015**, *60*, 163–169. [CrossRef]
86. Cadenhead, K.; Minichino, A.; Kelsven, S.; Addington, J.; Bearden, C.; Cannon, T.; Cornblatt, B.; Mathalon, D.; McGlashan, T.; Perkins, D.; et al. Metabolic abnormalities and low dietary Omega 3 are associated with symptom severity and worse functioning prior to the onset of psychosis: Findings from the North American Prodrome Longitudinal Studies Consortium. *Schizophr. Res.* **2019**, *204*, 96–103. [CrossRef] [PubMed]
87. Susai, S.; Sabherwal, S.; Mongan, D.; Föcking, M.; Cotter, D. Omega-3 fatty acid in ultra-high-risk psychosis: A systematic review based on functional outcome. *Early Interv. Psychiatry* **2022**, *16*, 3–16. [CrossRef] [PubMed]
88. McGorry, P.; Nelson, B.; Markulev, C.; Yuen, H.; Schäfer, M.; Mossaheb, N.; Schlögelhofer, M.; Smesny, S.; Hickie, I.; Berger, G.; et al. Effect of ω-3 polyunsaturated fatty acids in young people at ultrahigh risk for psychotic disorders: The NEURAPRO randomized clinical trial. *JAMA Psychiatry* **2017**, *74*, 19–27. [CrossRef] [PubMed]
89. Amminger, G.; Mechelli, A.; Rice, S.; Kim, S.; Klier, C.; McNamara, R.; Berk, M.; McGorry, P.; Schäfer, M. Predictors of treatment response in young people at ultra-high risk for psychosis who received long-chain omega-3 fatty acids. *Transl. Psychiatry* **2015**, *5*, e495. [CrossRef]
90. Amminger, G.; Schäfer, M.; Papageorgiou, K.; Klier, C.; Cotton, S.; Harrigan, S.; Mackinnon, A.; McGorry, P.; Berger, G. Long-chain omega-3 fatty acids for indicated prevention of psychotic disorders: A randomized, placebo-controlled trial. *Arch. Gen. Psychiatry* **2010**, *67*, 146–154. [CrossRef]
91. Amminger, G.; Nelson, B.; Markulev, C.; Yuen, H.; Schäfer, M.; Berger, M.; Mossaheb, N.; Schlögelhofer, M.; Smesny, S.; Hickie, I.; et al. The NEURAPRO Biomarker Analysis: Long-Chain Omega-3 Fatty Acids Improve 6-Month and 12-Month Outcomes in Youths at Ultra-High Risk for Psychosis. *Biol. Psychiatry* **2020**, *87*, 243–252. [CrossRef]
92. Teasdale, S.; Moerkl, S.; Moetteli, S.; Mueller-Stierlin, A. The Development of a Nutrition Screening Tool for Mental Health Settings Prone to Obesity and Cardiometabolic Complications: Study Protocol for the NutriMental Screener. *Int. J. Environ. Res. Public Health* **2021**, *18*, 11269. [CrossRef]
93. Hancox, L.; Lee, P.; Armaghanian, N.; Hirani, V.; Wakefield, G. Nutrition risk screening methods for adults living with severe mental illness: A scoping review. *Nutr. Diet.* **2022**, *79*, 349–363. [CrossRef]
94. Firth, J.; Stubbs, B.; Vancampfort, D.; Schuch, F.; Rosenbaum, S.; Ward, P.; Firth, J.A.; Sarris, J.; Yung, A. The validity and value of self-reported physical activity and accelerometry in people with schizophrenia: A population-scale study of the UK Biobank. *Schizophr. Bull.* **2018**, *44*, 1293–1300. [CrossRef]
95. Vancampfort, D.; Firth, J.; Schuch, F.; Rosenbaum, S.; Mugisha, J.; Hallgren, M.; Probst, M.; Ward, P.; Gaughran, F.; De Hert, M.; et al. Sedentary behavior and physical activity levels in people with schizophrenia, bipolar disorder and major depressive disorder: A global systematic review and meta-analysis. *World Psychiatry* **2017**, *16*, 308–315. [CrossRef]
96. Stubbs, B.; Firth, J.; Berry, A.; Schuch, F.; Rosenbaum, S.; Gaughran, F.; Veronesse, N.; Williams, J.; Craig, T.; Yung, A.; et al. How much physical activity do people with schizophrenia engage in? A systematic review, comparative meta-analysis and meta-regression. *Schizophr. Res.* **2016**, *176*, 431–440. [CrossRef]
97. Correll, C.; Solmi, M.; Veronese, N.; Bortolato, B.; Rosson, S.; Santonastaso, P.; Thapa-Chhetri, N.; Fornaro, M.; Gallicchio, D.; Collantoni, E.; et al. Prevalence, incidence and mortality from cardiovascular disease in patients with pooled and specific severe mental illness: A large-scale meta-analysis of 3,211,768 patients and 113,383,368 controls. *World Psychiatry* **2017**, *16*, 163–180. [CrossRef]
98. Vancampfort, D.; Correll, C.; Galling, B.; Probst, M.; De Hert, M.; Ward, P.; Rosenbaum, S.; Gaughran, F.; Lally, J.; Stubbs, B. Diabetes mellitus in people with schizophrenia, bipolar disorder and major depressive disorder: A systematic review and large scale meta-analysis. *World Psychiatry* **2016**, *15*, 166–174. [CrossRef]
99. Vancampfort, D.; Stubbs, B.; Mitchell, A.; De Hert, M.; Wampers, M.; Ward, P.; Rosenbaum, S.; Correll, C. Risk of metabolic syndrome and its components in people with schizophrenia and related psychotic disorders, bipolar disorder and major depressive disorder: A systematic review and meta-analysis. *World Psychiatry* **2015**, *14*, 339–347. [CrossRef]
100. NHS UK: Physical Activity Guidelines for Adults Aged 19 to 64 (Page Last Reviewed: 4th August 2021). Available online: https://www.nhs.uk/live-well/exercise/exercise-guidelines/physical-activity-guidelines-for-adults-aged-19-to-64/ (accessed on 20 July 2023).
101. Brokmeier, L.; Firth, J.; Vancampfort, D.; Smith, L.; Deenik, J.; Rosenbaum, S.; Stubbs, B.; Schuch, F. Does physical activity reduce the risk of psychosis? A systematic review and meta-analysis of prospective studies. *Psychiatry Res.* **2020**, *284*, 112675. [CrossRef] [PubMed]
102. Koivukangas, J.; Tammelin, T.; Kaakinen, M.; Mäki, P.; Moilanen, I.; Taanila, A.; Veijola, J. Physical activity and fitness in adolescents at risk for psychosis within the Northern Finland 1986 Birth Cohort. *Schizophr. Res.* **2010**, *116*, 152–158. [CrossRef] [PubMed]

103. Keskinen, E.; Marttila, R.; Koivumaa-Honkanen, H.; Moilanen, K.; Keinänen-Kiukaanniemi, S.; Timonen, M.; Isohanni, M.; McGrath, J.; Miettunen, J.; Jääskeläinen, E. Search for protective factors for psychosis—A population-based sample with special interest in unaffected individuals with parental psychosis. *Early Interv. Psychiatry* **2018**, *12*, 869–878. [CrossRef]
104. Firth, J.; Siddiqi, N.; Koyanagi, A.; Siskind, D.; Rosenbaum, S.; Galletly, C.; Allan, S.; Caneo, C.; Carney, R.; Carvalho, A.; et al. The Lancet Psychiatry Commission: A blueprint for protecting physical health in people with mental illness. *Lancet Psychiatry* **2019**, *6*, 675–712. [CrossRef] [PubMed]
105. Damme, K.; Sloan, R.; Bartels, M.; Ozsan, A.; Ospina, L.; Kimhy, D.; Mittal, V. Psychosis risk individuals show poor fitness and discrepancies with objective and subjective measures. *Sci. Rep.* **2021**, *11*, 9851. [CrossRef]
106. Firth, J.; Stubbs, B.; Vancampfort, D.; Schuch, F.; Lagopoulos, J.; Rosenbaum, S.; Ward, P. Effect of aerobic exercise on hippocampal volume in humans: A systematic review and meta-analysis. *NeuroImage* **2018**, *166*, 230–238. [CrossRef] [PubMed]
107. Dean, D.; Bryan, A.; Newberry, R.; Gupta, T.; Carol, E.; Mittal, V. A supervised exercise intervention for youth at risk for psychosis: An open-label pilot study. *J. Clin. Psychiatry* **2017**, *78*, e1167–e1173. [CrossRef] [PubMed]
108. Lederman, O.; Ward, P.; Rosenbaum, S.; Maloney, C.; Watkins, A.; Teasdale, S.; Morell, R.; Curtis, J. Stepping up early treatment for help-seeking youth with at-risk mental states: Feasibility and acceptability of a real-world exercise program. *Early Interv. Psychiatry* **2020**, *14*, 450–462. [CrossRef]
109. Sormunen, E.; Saarinen, M.; Salokangas, R.; Hutri-Kähönen, N.; Viikari, J.; Raitakari, O.; Hietala, J. Body mass index trajectories in childhood and adolescence—Risk for non-affective psychosis. *Schizophr. Res.* **2019**, *206*, 313–317. [CrossRef]
110. Abel, K.; Wicks, S.; Susser, E.; Dalman, C.; Pedersen, M.; Mortensen, P.; Webb, R. Birth weight, schizophrenia, and adult mental disorder: Is risk confined to the smallest babies? *Arch. Gen. Psychiatry* **2010**, *67*, 923–930. [CrossRef] [PubMed]
111. Zammit, S.; Rasmussen, F.; Farahmand, B.; Gunnell, D.; Lewis, G.; Tynelius, P.; Brobert, G. Height and body mass index in young adulthood and risk of schizophrenia: A longitudinal study of 1 347 520 Swedish men. *Acta Psychiatr. Scand.* **2007**, *116*, 378–385. [CrossRef] [PubMed]
112. Caravaggio, F.; Brucato, G.; Kegeles, L.; Lehembre-Shiah, E.; Arndt, L.; Colibazzi, T.; Girgis, R. Exploring the relationship between body mass index and positive symptom severity in persons at clinical high risk for psychosis. *J. Nerv. Ment. Dis.* **2017**, *205*, 893–895. [CrossRef]
113. Lamichhane, S.; Dickens, A.; Sen, P.; Laurikainen, H.; Borgan, F.; Suvisaari, J.; Hyötyläinen, T.; Howes, O.; Hietala, J.; Orešič, M. Association between circulating lipids and future weight gain in individuals with an at-risk mental state and in first-episode psychosis. *Schizophr. Bull.* **2021**, *47*, 160–169. [CrossRef]
114. Martorell, L.; Muntané, G.; Porta-López, S.; Moreno, L.; Ortega, L.; Montalvo, I.; Sanchez-Gistau, V.; Monseny, R.; Labad, J.; Vilella, E. Increased levels of serum leptin in the early stages of psychosis. *J. Psychiatr. Res.* **2019**, *111*, 24–29. [CrossRef]
115. Alqarni, A.; Mitchell, T.; McGorry, P.; Nelson, B.; Markulev, C.; Yuen, H.; Schäfer, M.; Berger, M.; Mossaheb, N.; Schlögelhofer, M.; et al. Comparison of erythrocyte omega-3 index, fatty acids and molecular phospholipid species in people at ultra-high risk of developing psychosis and healthy people. *Schizophr. Res.* **2020**, *226*, 44–51. [CrossRef]
116. Koivukangas, J.; Björnholm, L.; Tervonen, O.; Miettunen, J.; Nordström, T.; Kiviniemi, V.; Mäki, P.; Mukkala, S.; Moilanen, I.; Barnett, J.; et al. Body mass index and brain white matter structure in young adults at risk for psychosis—The Oulu Brain and Mind Study. *Psychiatry Res. Neuroimaging* **2016**, *254*, 169–176. [CrossRef]
117. Pruessner, M.; Béchard-Evans, L.; Boekestyn, L.; Iyer, S.; Pruessner, J.; Malla, A. Attenuated cortisol response to acute psychosocial stress in individuals at ultra-high risk for psychosis. *Schizophr. Res.* **2013**, *146*, 79–86. [CrossRef]
118. Veeneman, R.; Vermeulen, J.; Abdellaoui, A.; Sanderson, E.; Wootton, R.; Tadros, R.; Bezzina, C.; Denys, D.; Munafò, M.; Verweij, K.; et al. Exploring the relationship between schizophrenia and cardiovascular disease: A genetic correlation and multivariable Mendelian randomization study. *Schizophr. Bull.* **2022**, *48*, 463–473. [CrossRef]
119. Latvala, A.; Kuja-Halkola, R.; Rück, C.; D'Onofrio, B.; Jernberg, T.; Almqvist, C.; Mataix-Cols, D.; Larsson, H.; Lichtenstein, P. Association of resting heart rate and blood pressure in late adolescence with subsequent mental disorders: A longitudinal population study of more than 1 million men in Sweden. *JAMA Psychiatry* **2016**, *73*, 1268–1275. [CrossRef]
120. Thayer, J.; Hansen, A.; Saus-Rose, E.; Johnsen, B. Heart rate variability, prefrontal neural function, and cognitive performance: The neurovisceral integration perspective on self-regulation, adaptation, and health. *Ann. Behav. Med.* **2009**, *37*, 141–153. [CrossRef]
121. Levy, M. Autonomic interactions in cardiac control. *Ann. N. Y. Acad. Sci.* **1990**, *601*, 209–221. [CrossRef]
122. Montaquila, J.; Trachik, B.; Bedwell, J. Heart rate variability and vagal tone in schizophrenia: A review. *J. Psychiatr. Res.* **2015**, *69*, 57–66. [CrossRef]
123. Chalmers, J.; Quintana, D.; Abbott, M.; Kemp, A. Anxiety disorders are associated with reduced heart rate variability: A meta-analysis. *Front. Psychiatry* **2014**, *5*, 80. [CrossRef]
124. Clamor, A.; Sundag, J.; Lincoln, T. Specificity of resting-state heart rate variability in psychosis: A comparison with clinical high risk, anxiety, and healthy controls. *Schizophr. Res.* **2019**, *206*, 89–95. [CrossRef]
125. Counotte, J.; Pot-Kolder, R.; van Roon, A.; Hoskam, O.; van der Gaag, M.; Veling, W. High psychosis liability is associated with altered autonomic balance during exposure to Virtual Reality social stressors. *Schizophr. Res.* **2017**, *184*, 14–20. [CrossRef]
126. Kocsis, A.; Gajwani, R.; Gross, J.; Gumley, A.; Lawrie, S.; Schwannauer, M.; Schultze-Lutter, F.; Grent-'t-Jong, T.; Uhlhaas, P. Altered autonomic function in individuals at clinical high risk for psychosis. *Front. Psychiatry* **2020**, *11*, 580503. [CrossRef]

127. Nordholm, D.; Jensen, M.; Kristiansen, J.; Glenthøj, L.; Kristensen, T.; Wenneberg, C.; Hjorthøj, C.; Garde, A.; Nordentoft, M. A longitudinal study on physiological stress in individuals at ultra high-risk of psychosis. *Schizophr. Res.* **2023**, *254*, 218–226. [CrossRef] [PubMed]
128. Giannouli, V. Ethnicity, mortality, and severe mental illness. *Lancet Psychiatry* **2017**, *4*, 517. [CrossRef]
129. Glick, I.; Stekoll, A.; Hays, S. The role of the family and improvement in treatment maintenance, adherence, and outcome for schizophrenia. *J. Clin. Psychopharmacol.* **2011**, *31*, 82–85. [CrossRef]
130. McCullough, E.; Hoyt, W.; Larson, D.; Koenig, H.; Thoresen, C. Religious involvement and mortality: A meta-analytic review. *Health Psychol.* **2000**, *19*, 211–222. [CrossRef] [PubMed]

Disclaimer/Publisher's Note: The statements, opinions and data contained in all publications are solely those of the individual author(s) and contributor(s) and not of MDPI and/or the editor(s). MDPI and/or the editor(s) disclaim responsibility for any injury to people or property resulting from any ideas, methods, instructions or products referred to in the content.

MDPI
St. Alban-Anlage 66
4052 Basel
Switzerland
www.mdpi.com

Biomedicines Editorial Office
E-mail: biomedicines@mdpi.com
www.mdpi.com/journal/biomedicines

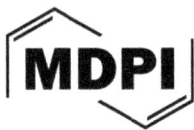

Disclaimer/Publisher's Note: The statements, opinions and data contained in all publications are solely those of the individual author(s) and contributor(s) and not of MDPI and/or the editor(s). MDPI and/or the editor(s) disclaim responsibility for any injury to people or property resulting from any ideas, methods, instructions or products referred to in the content.

www.ingramcontent.com/pod-product-compliance
Lightning Source LLC
LaVergne TN
LVHW070438100526
838202LV00014B/1623